Minimally Invasive Fracture Repair

Guest Editors

BRIAN S. BEALE, DVM
ANTONIO POZZI, DMV, MS

VETERINARY CLINICS
OF NORTH AMERICA:
SMALL ANIMAL PRACTICE

www.vetsmall.theclinics.com

September 2012 • Volume 42 • Number 5

SAUNDERS an imprint of ELSEVIER, Inc.

W.B. SAUNDERS COMPANY
A Division of Elsevier Inc.
1600 John F. Kennedy Blvd. • Suite 1800 • Philadelphia, PA 19103-2899
http://www.vetsmall.theclinics.com

VETERINARY CLINICS OF NORTH AMERICA: SMALL ANIMAL PRACTICE Volume 42, Number 5
September 2012 ISSN 0195-5616, ISBN-13: 978-1-4557-4970-6

Editor: John Vassallo; j.vassallo@elsevier.com
Developmental Editor: John Vassallo; j.vassallo@elsevier.com

Veterinary Clinics of North America: Small Animal Practice (ISSN 0195-5616) is published bimonthly (For Post Office use only: volume 42 issue 1 of 6) by Elsevier Inc., 360 Park Avenue South, New York, NY 10010-1710. Months of issue are January, March, May, July, September, and November. Business and Editorial Offices: 1600 John F. Kennedy Blvd., Ste. 1800, Philadelphia, PA 19103-2899. Customer Service Office: 3251 Riverport Lane, Maryland Heights, MO 63043. Periodicals postage paid at New York, NY and additional mailing offices. Subscription prices are $283.00 per year (domestic individuals), $455.00 per year (domestic institutions), $138.00 per year (domestic students/residents), $375.00 per year (Canadian individuals), $559.00 per year (Canadian institutions), $416.00 per year (international individuals), $559.00 per year (international institutions), and $201.00 per year (international and Canadian students/residents). To receive student/resident rate, orders must be accompanied by name of affiliated institution, date of term, and the *signature* of program/residency coordinator on institution letterhead. Orders will be billed at individual rate until proof of status is received. Foreign air speed delivery is included in all *Clinics* subscription prices. All prices are subject to change without notice. **POSTMASTER:** Send address changes to *Veterinary Clinics of North America: Small Animal Practice*, Elsevier Health Sciences Division, Subscription Customer Service, 3251 Riverport Lane, Maryland Heights, MO 63043. Customer Service (orders, claims, online, change of address): Elsevier Periodicals Customer Service, Elsevier Health Sciences Division Subscription Customer Service 3251 Riverport Lane Maryland Heights, MO 63043. Tel: 1-800-654-2452 (U.S. and Canada); 314-447-8871 (outside U.S. and Canada). Fax: 314-447-8029. E-mail: journalscustomerservice-usa@elsevier.com (for print support); journalsonlinesupport-usa@elsevier.com (for online support).

Reprints. For copies of 100 or more of articles in this publication, please contact the Commercial Reprints Department, Elsevier Inc., 360 Park Avenue South, New York, NY 10010-1710. Tel.: 212-633-3812; Fax: 212-462-1935; E-mail: reprints@elsevier.com.

Veterinary Clinics of North America: Small Animal Practice is also published in Japanese by Inter Zoo Publishing Co., Ltd., Aoyama Crystal-Bldg 5F, 3-5-12 Kitaaoyama, Minato-ku, Tokyo 107-0061, Japan.

Veterinary Clinics of North America: Small Animal Practice is covered in *Current Contents/Agriculture, Biology and Environmental Sciences, Science Citation Index, ASCA, MEDLINE/PubMed (Index Medicus), Excerpta Medica,* and *BIOSIS.*

Printed and bound by CPI Group (UK) Ltd, Croydon, CR0 4YY
Transferred to digital print 2012

Contributors

GUEST EDITORS

BRIAN S. BEALE, DVM
Diplomate, American College of Veterinary Surgeons, Gulf Coast Veterinary Specialists, Houston, Texas

ANTONIO POZZI, DMV, MS
Diplomate, American College of Veterinary Surgeons, Assistant Professor Small Animal Surgery, Department of Small Animal Clinical Sciences, College of Veterinary Medicine, University of Florida, Gainesville, Florida

AUTHORS

ALESSANDRO BOERO BARONCELLI, DVM, PhD
Department of Animal Pathology - School of Veterinary Medicine, University of Turin, Grugliasco, Turin, Italy

BRIAN S. BEALE, DVM
Diplomate, American College of Veterinary Surgeons, Gulf Coast Veterinary Specialists, Houston, Texas

PEINI CHAO, DVM, MS
College of Veterinary Medicine, University of Florida, Gainesville, Florida

GRAYSON COLE, DVM
Gulf Coast Veterinary Specialists, Houston, Texas

LOÏC M. DÉJARDIN, DVM, MS
Diplomate, American College of Veterinary Surgeons and European College of Veterinary Surgeons, Associate Professor, Head of Orthopaedic Surgery, Department of Small Animal Clinical Sciences, Director, Collaborative Orthopaedic Investigations Laboratory, College of Veterinary Medicine, Michigan State University, East Lansing, Michigan

TOMÁS G. GUERRERO, Dr med vet
Diplomate, European College of Veterinary Surgeons, Professor of Small Animal Surgery, St. George's University, Grenada, West Indies

LAURENT P. GUIOT, DVM
Diplomate, American College of Veterinary Surgeons and European College of Veterinary Surgeons, Assistant Professor, Department of Small Animal Clinical Sciences, College of Veterinary Medicine, Michigan State University, East Lansing, Michigan

CALEB C. HUDSON, DVM, MS
Clinical Lecturer Small Animal Surgery, Department of Small Animal Clinical Sciences, College of Veterinary Medicine, University of Florida, Gainesville, Florida

DON HULSE, DVM
Professor of Surgery, Department of Small Animal Surgery, College Veterinary Medicine, Texas A&M University, College Station, Texas

STANLEY E. KIM, BVSc, MS
Department of Small Animal Clinical Sciences, College of Veterinary Medicine, University of Florida, Gainesville, Florida

MICHAEL P. KOWALESKI, DVM
Diplomate, American College of Veterinary Surgeons and European College of Veterinary Surgeons, Associate Professor of Orthopedic Surgery, Department of Clinical Sciences, Cummings School of Veterinary Medicine, Tufts University, North Grafton, Massachusetts

DANIEL D. LEWIS, DVM
Diplomate, American College of Veterinary Surgeons, Professor Small Animal Surgery, Jerry and Lola Collins Eminent Scholar in Canine Sports Medicine and Comparative Orthopedics, Department of Small Animal Clinical Sciences, College of Veterinary Medicine, University of Florida, Gainesville, Florida

RYAN MCCALLY, DVM
Gulf Coast Veterinary Specialists, Houston, Texas

ROSS H. PALMER, DVM, MS
Diplomate, American College of Veterinary Surgeons, Associate Professor, Orthopedic Surgery, Department of Clinical Sciences, College of Veterinary Medicine & Biomedical Sciences, Colorado State University, Fort Collins, Colorado

BRUNO PEIRONE, DVM, PhD
Department of Animal Pathology, School of Veterinary Medicine, University of Turin, Grugliasco, Turin, Italy

ALESSANDRO PIRAS, DVM, MRCVS
Italian Specialist in Veterinary Surgery, Adjunct Professor, University College Dublin, Dublin, Ireland

LISA PIRAS, DVM, PhD
Department of Animal Pathology - School of Veterinary Medicine, University of Turin, Grugliasco, Turin, Italy

ANTONIO POZZI, DMV, MS
Diplomate, American College of Veterinary Surgeons, Assistant Professor Small Animal Surgery, Department of Small Animal Clinical Sciences, College of Veterinary Medicine, University of Florida, Gainesville, Florida

GIAN LUCA ROVESTI, DVM
Diplomate, European College of Veterinary Surgeons, Clinica Veterinaria Miller - Via della Costituzione, Cavriago, Reggio Emilia, Italy

JAMES TOMLINSON, DVM, MVSc
Diplomate, American College of Veterinary Surgeons, Professor of Small Animal Orthopedic Surgery, Department of Veterinary Medicine and Surgery, College of Veterinary Medicine, University of Missouri, Columbia, Missouri

DIRSKO J.F. VON PFEIL, DVM
Diplomate, American College of Veterinary Surgeons and European College of Veterinary Surgeons, Veterinary Specialists of Alaska, PC, Anchorage, Alaska

Contents

Preface: Minimally Invasive Fracture Repair   xi

Brian S. Beale and Antonio Pozzi

Biomechanical Concepts in Small Animal Fracture Fixation   853

Peini Chao, Daniel D. Lewis, Michael P. Kowaleski, and Antonio Pozzi

> Understanding the basic biomechanical principles of surgical stabilization of fractures is essential for developing an appropriate preoperative plan as well as making prudent intraoperative decisions. This article aims to provide basic biomechanical knowledge essential to the understanding of the complex interaction between the mechanics and biology of fracture healing. The type of healing and the outcome can be influenced by several mechanical factors, which depend on the interaction between bone and implant. The surgeon should understand the mechanical principles of fracture fixation and be able to choose the best type of fixation for each specific fracture.

Minimally Invasive Plate Osteosynthesis Fracture Reduction Techniques in Small Animals   873

Bruno Peirone, Gian Luca Rovesti, Alessandro Boero Baroncelli, and Lisa Piras

> Indirect fracture reduction is used to align diaphyseal fractures in small animals when using minimally-invasive fracture repair. Indirect reduction achieves functional fracture reduction without opening the fracture site. The limb is restored to length and spatial alignment is achieved to ensure proper angular and rotational alignment. Fracture reduction can be accomplished using a variety of techniques and devices, including hanging the limb, manual traction, distraction table, external fixators, and a fracture distractor.

Perioperative Imaging in Minimally Invasive Osteosynthesis in Small Animals   897

Laurent P. Guiot and Loïc M. Déjardin

> Perioperative imaging using various appropriate modalities is critical to the successful planning and performance of any orthopedic surgery. Although not an absolute prerequisite, the use of intraoperative imaging considerably facilitates the smooth and effective execution of minimally invasive osteosynthesis (MIO). However, the risk of overexposure to radiation is real, particularly when considering its insidious effect over time. Therefore, the primary concern of the surgeon must be safety of the surgical team. This article outlines basic, simple steps that will be effective in reducing radiation exposure, which in turn will make MIO a safe alternative to open reduction and internal fixation.

External Fixators and Minimally Invasive Osteosynthesis in Small Animal Veterinary Medicine   913

Ross H. Palmer

> Modern external skeletal fixation (ESF) is a very versatile system that is well suited to the ideals of minimally invasive osteosynthesis (MIO). It offers

variable-angle, locked fixation that can be applied with minimal to no disruption of the fracture zone. Technological advances in ESF have fostered the ability to use more simple frame applications than in previous generations. Even when rigid bilateral or multiplanar frames are required, timely staged-disassembly is easy to perform and allows for a gradual shift of loading from the frame to the healing bony column. Hybrid ESF is ideally suited for the MIO treatment of many juxta-articular fractures and osteotomies. Adherence to the principles of ESF and postoperative care is essential to overcome the various disadvantages that are inherent to ESF.

Interlocking Nails and Minimally Invasive Osteosynthesis   935

Loïc M. Déjardin, Laurent P. Guiot, and Dirsko J.F. von Pfeil

Interlocking nailing of long bone fractures has long been considered the gold standard osteosynthesis technique in people. Thanks to improvements in the locking mechanism design and nail profile, a recently developed veterinary angle stable nail has become the first true intramedullary fixator providing accurate and consistent repair stability while allowing semirigid fixation. As a result, indications for interlocking nailing have expanded to include treatment of periarticular fractures, corrections of angular deformities and revisions of failed plate osteosyntheses. Perfectly suited for minimally invasive osteosynthesis, interlocking nailing is an attractive and effective alternative to bone plating and plate-rod fixation technique.

Percutaneous Pinning for Fracture Repair in Dogs and Cats   963

Stanley E. Kim, Caleb C. Hudson, and Antonio Pozzi

This article describes the technique of percutaneous pinning in dogs and cats. Only acute fractures evaluated within the first 48 hours after trauma are selected for percutaneous pinning. Reduction is performed with careful manipulation of the fracture to minimize the trauma to the growth plate. After ensuring the fracture is reduced anatomically, smooth pins of appropriate size are inserted through stab incisions. Depending on the anatomic location, the pins are cut flush with bone or bent. The main advantages of this technique are the minimal surgical trauma and lower perioperative morbidity.

MIPO Techniques for the Humerus in Small Animals   975

Don Hulse

Knowledge of regional and topographic anatomy is paramount for success when using minimally invasive plate osteosynthesis (MIPO) for fracture management. Preoperative planning is essential for an optimal outcome and reducing stress among the surgical team; factors to consider include biologic assessment, mechanical assessment, clinical assessment, portal placement, and implant selection. MIPO is a useful technique for the direct or indirect reduction of humeral diaphyseal fractures. Implants should span the length of the bone for ease of implant application and to optimize the mechanical advantage of the implant. After surgery, incision care and controlled activity are 2 primary considerations.

Minimally Invasive Plate Osteosynthesis in Small Animals:
Radius and Ulna Fractures   983

Caleb C. Hudson, Daniel D. Lewis, and Antonio Pozzi

Minimally invasive plate osteosynthesis (MIPO) is a biologically friendly approach to fracture reduction and stabilization that is applicable to many radius and ulna fractures in small animals. An appropriate knowledge of the anatomy of the antebrachium and careful preoperative planning is essential. This article describes the MIPO technique, which entails stabilization of the fractured radius with a bone plate and screws that are applied without performing an extensive open surgical approach. This technique results in good outcomes, including a rapid time to union and return of function.

Minimally Invasive Osteosynthesis Techniques of the Femur   997

Michael P. Kowaleski

Indirect reduction techniques and carefully planned and executed direct reduction techniques result in maximal preservation of the biology of the fracture site and bone fragments. These techniques, coupled with the use of small soft tissue windows for the insertion of instruments and implants, result in minimal additional trauma to the soft tissues and fracture fragments. Without direct visualization, minimally invasive osteosynthesis (MIO) techniques are more demanding than open reduction and internal fixation; however, the biologic advantages are vast. As such, MIO techniques represent a fascinating new armamentarium in fracture fixation.

Minimally Invasive Plate Osteosynthesis: Tibia and Fibula   1023

Brian S. Beale and Ryan McCally

Fractures of the tibia and fibula are common in dogs and cats and occur most commonly as a result of substantial trauma. Tibial fractures are often amenable to repair using the minimally invasive plate osteosynthesis (MIPO) technique because of the minimal soft tissue covering of the tibia and relative ease of indirect reduction and application of the implant system on the tibia. Treatment of tibial fractures by MIPO has been found to reduce surgical time, reduce the time for fracture healing, and decrease patient morbidity, while at the same time reducing complications compared with traditional open reduction and internal fixation.

Minimally Invasive Repair of Meta-bones   1045

Alessandro Piras and Tomás G. Guerrero

Metacarpal and metatarsal fractures are common injuries in small animals and, in most of the cases, can be treated by minimally invasive techniques. Bone plates applied through epi-periosteal tunnels can stabilize meta-bones. Meta-bones III and IV are stabilized by dorsally applied plates. Meta-bones II and V are stabilized using plates applied medially and laterally. The scarcity of soft tissue coverage and the simple anatomy of meta-bones make these fractures amenable to fixation by using minimally invasive techniques. This practice should reduce morbidity and enhance healing time.

Minimally Invasive Osteosynthesis Technique for Articular Fractures   1051

Brian S. Beale and Grayson Cole

Articular fractures require accurate reduction and rigid stabilization to decrease the chance of osteoarthritis and joint dysfunction. Articular fractures have been traditionally repaired by arthrotomy and internal fixation. Recently, minimally invasive techniques have been introduced to treat articular fractures, reducing patient morbidity and improving the accuracy of reduction. A variety of techniques, including distraction, radiographic imaging, and arthroscopy, are used with the minimally invasive osteosynthesis technique of articular fractures to achieve a successful repair and outcome.

Minimally Invasive Repair of Sacroiliac Luxation in Small Animals   1069

James Tomlinson

Sacroiliac fracture-luxation is a common injury that is associated with ilial and acetabular fractures of the opposite hemipelvis. Sacroiliac fracture-luxation results in an unstable pelvis and potentially collapse of the pelvic canal. A minimally invasive technique for repair of sacroiliac-fracture luxation is a viable option for repair of this injury and has considerable benefits. Reduction and fixation using a minimally invasive technique provides results comparable to an open technique without the associated morbidity of an open technique. Exact screw placement is facilitated by fluoroscopy to make sure that the disk space or vertebral canal is not penetrated yet allows an adequate length of screw purchase in the sacrum.

Percutaneous Plate Arthrodesis in Small Animals   1079

Antonio Pozzi, Daniel D. Lewis, Caleb C. Hudson, and Stanley E. Kim

Arthrodesis is an elective surgical procedure designed to eliminate articular pain and dysfunction by deliberate osseous fusion. A percutaneous approach can be used to perform tarsal and carpal arthrodeses in dogs and cats. Intraoperative imaging facilitates cartilage debridement performed with a burr inserted through stab incisions. The plate is introduced through an epiperiosteal tunnel and secured with screws inserted through the skin insertion incisions. Additional screws can be placed through separate stab incisions. The primary advantage of this technique is a decreased risk of soft tissue complications such as plantar necrosis or wound dehiscence. Preliminary clinical results are promising.

Index   1097

VETERINARY CLINICS OF NORTH AMERICA: SMALL ANIMAL PRACTICE

FORTHCOMING ISSUES

November 2012
Otology and Otic Disease
Bradley Njaa, BSc, DVM, MVSc, and
Lynette Cole, DVM, PhD, *Guest Editors*

January 2013
Clinical Dermatology
Daniel O. Morris, DVM, MPH, and Robert
A. Kennis, DVM, MS, *Guest Editors*

March 2013
Feline Diabetes
Jacquie Rand, BVSc, DVSc, *Guest Editor*

RECENT ISSUES

July 2012
Geriatrics
William D. Forgone, DVM, *Guest Editor*

May 2012
Small Animal Theriogenology
Catherine G. Lamm, DVM, MRCVS, and
Chelsea L. Makloski, DVM, MS,
Guest Editors

March 2012
Common Toxicologic Issues in Small Animals
Safdar A. Khan, DVM, MS, PhD, and
Stephen B. Hooser, DVM, PhD, *Guest
Editors*

RELATED INTEREST

Veterinary Clinics of North America: Exotic Animal Practice
May 2010 (Vol. 13, No. 2)
Endoscopy and Endosurgery
Stephen J. Divers, BvetMed, DzooMed, FRCVS
Guest Editor

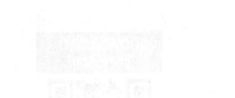

Preface

Minimally Invasive Fracture Repair

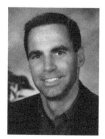 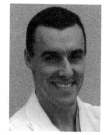

Brian S. Beale, DVM   Antonio Pozzi, DMV, MS
Guest Editors

Fracture stabilization techniques continue to evolve and to provide approaches that minimize iatrogenic trauma associated with surgery. This issue includes a comprehensive look at the current status of treatment of fractures using minimally invasive plate osteosynthesis (MIPO) and minimally invasive surgery. Principles of minimally invasive fracture repair are included as well as case examples of different fracture types of all the major long bones. The editors sincerely appreciate the efforts of the individual article authors as much time and effort were put forth to bring together an issue that provides a clear view of the principles and clinical recommendations needed to help surgeons develop the skills to successfully manage simple and comminuted fractures in dogs and cats using minimally invasive fracture repair.

The concept of biological internal fixation has been predicated for years with the goal of maximizing preservation of the blood supply to the fractured bone. This trend resulted in new implants and new techniques that allowed surgeons to approach fracture fixation with smaller, less invasive approaches. The principal concept is to gain access to the bone via small incisions away from the fracture zone, thus preserving blood supply to the fracture fragments. The small incisions provide a means of inserting a bone plate and placing screws to achieve stabilization and osteosynthesis. In this issue we included a description of the techniques of indirect reduction as well as fracture fixation using minimally invasive techniques.

The logical evolution of biologic fracture fixation has been minimally invasive fracture fixation. Although young surgeons consider minimally invasive fracture fixation a novel approach, history would prove them wrong, as percutaneous nailing was already performed by Kuntscher in the 1940s. However, the technique was not readily used until the 1990s. So, what is really new about minimally invasive fracture fixation? The answer is probably technology. Improvements in fixation implants and imaging techniques allow the surgeon to achieve more consistent results with fewer complications. Advanced imaging techniques such as fluoroscopy and arthroscopy allow a method of guiding the reduction of the fracture and the application of the implants. New implants such as locking plates facilitate reduction and fixation of fractures, while

Vet Clin Small Anim 42 (2012) xi–xii
http://dx.doi.org/10.1016/j.cvsm.2012.08.007
0195-5616/12/$ – see front matter © 2012 Elsevier Inc. All rights reserved.

keeping a balance between biomechanics and biology. While bone plates are used most commonly for minimally invasive fracture repair, other implant systems such as the interlocking nail and external fixator can be used with success too.

An obvious question arises: is minimally invasive fracture fixation better than open reduction and fracture fixation? A reasonable answer would be that it depends on the fracture type. The benefits of a minimally invasive approach may be more evident for specific types of fractures. However, this question can only be answered with well-designed future prospective studies. Early studies suggest fracture repair using the MIPO technique benefits the patient by providing less morbidity and accelerated fracture healing. With this issue our intention is to present an up-to-date description of the techniques of minimally invasive fracture fixation used in small animals. We hope that this issue will trigger interest and motivate more surgeons to use these new techniques and help spawn future techniques that will continue to improve our outcome with minimally invasive fracture repair.

Brian S. Beale, DVM
Gulf Coast Veterinary Specialists
1111 West Loop South #160
Houston, TX 77027, USA

Antonio Pozzi, DMV, MS
College of Veterinary Medicine
University of Florida
2015 SW 16th Avenue
PO Box 100126
Gainesville, FL 32610-0126, USA

E-mail addresses:
brianbeale@me.com (B.S. Beale)
pozzia@ufl.edu (A. Pozzi)

Biomechanical Concepts Applicable to Minimally Invasive Fracture Repair in Small Animals

Peini Chao, DVM, MS[a], Daniel D. Lewis, DVM[a],
Michael P. Kowaleski, DVM[b], Antonio Pozzi, DMV, MS[a],*

KEYWORDS

- Small animals • Fracture fixation • Biomechanics • Fracture implants

KEY POINTS

- The strength of an implant depends on its ability to resist deformation or breakage from an applied stress. An implant's stiffness defines its ability to resist deformation resulting from an applied force, but does not directly correlate with the implant's strength.
- The mechanical performance of an implant is dictated by its material composition, conformation, and dimensions. The area moment of inertia describes the resistance of an implant to bending and is related to the implant's shape and cross-sectional area relative to an applied bending load.
- In fractures with adequate vascularity, fracture healing is influenced by mechanical stimuli at the fracture gap.

INTRODUCTION

Over the past 2 decades, there has been a paradigm shift regarding the approach to internal fixation of long-bone fractures with bone plates. The prerequisite for open anatomic reduction and rigid stabilization has given way to less invasive application of more flexible constructs with bridging plates.[1–3] The use of locking technology allows the plate to function as an internal fixator.[4–9] Surgeons can choose among a variety of implant systems to employ a more or less flexible bone-plate construct.[8,10–29] Furthermore, the design and type of plate utilized can play a primary role in fracture reduction.[12,26,29–32] Whereas plates with a compression or neutralization function require precise reconstruction and provide rigid stabilization, plates applied in a bridging fashion circumvent the need for anatomic reduction of the fracture to obtain functional alignment and length of the fractured limb segment.[33] Bridging plates are often applied

[a] College of Veterinary Medicine-University of Florida, PO Box 100126, 2015 Southwest 16th Avenue, Gainesville, FL 32610-0126, USA; [b] Department of Clinical Sciences, Cumming School of Veterinary Medicine, Foster Hospital for Small Animals, Tufts University, 200 Westboro Road, North Grafton, MA 01536, USA
* Corresponding author.
E-mail address: pozzia@ufl.edu

Vet Clin Small Anim 42 (2012) 853–872
http://dx.doi.org/10.1016/j.cvsm.2012.07.007
0195-5616/12/$ – see front matter © 2012 Elsevier Inc. All rights reserved.
vetsmall.theclinics.com

using indirect reduction techniques, which mitigates the degree of iatrogenic trauma while preserving fracture vascularity.[1,3,4,32,34–38] Understanding the basic biomechanical principles of surgical stabilization of fractures is essential for developing an appropriate preoperative plan as well as making prudent intraoperative decisions.

The objective of this article is to provide basic biomechanical knowledge essential to the understanding of the complex interaction between the mechanics and biology of fracture healing. It is clearly understood that limited soft-tissue manipulation is very important in preserving the blood supply to the injured bone. However, the type of healing and the outcome can be influenced by several mechanical factors, which depend on the interaction between the bone and the implant.[31,39–42] The main objective for using less invasive fracture stabilization techniques is to optimize the healing potential by achieving a symbiotic balance between the biological and the mechanical factors of fracture fixation. Thus the surgeon should understand the mechanical principles of fracture fixation and be able to choose the best type of fixation for each specific fracture.

BASIC MECHANICS OF MATERIALS
Force, Deformation, Stress, and Strain

The strength of a material depends on its ability to resist failure from an applied stress. Stress is the force acting on an area, and can be compressive, tensile, or shear. The unit for stress is force divided by area, such as Newtons per square millimeter (N/mm^2).[43] When stress is applied to an object, deformation may occur. Thus, the term deformation is used to describe the change in shape or size of an object caused by an applied load.[43] Depending on the size, shape, material composition of the object, and the force applied, various types of deformation may occur. Elastic deformation is reversible: an object may deform when subjected to an applied load, but the object returns to its original shape once the load is released. Plastic deformation, in contrast, is irreversible and the object does not return to its original shape once the applied load is released. Another type of deformation, unique to ductile metals, is metal fatigue. This phenomenon describes the progressive formation of cracks, which develop in a material subjected to numerous cycles of elastic deformation.[44] The behaviour of a material is illustrated with a stress-strain curve (**Fig. 1**), which shows the relationship between stress (force applied)

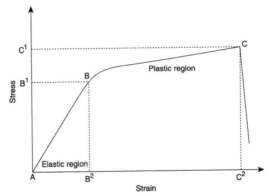

Fig. 1. Stress-strain curve. Yield point (B): permanent deformation occurs beyond the yield point. Yield strain (B^1): amount of deformation sustained before plastic deformation occurred. Yield stress (B^2): load per unit area sustained by this material before plastic deformation. Ultimate failure point (C): failure of this material occurs at this point. Ultimate strain (C^1): amount of deformation sustained by the sample before failure. Ultimate stress (C^2): load per unit area sustained by the sample before failure.

and strain (deformation) of the material.[43] The elastic range of the curve ends when the object reaches its yield strength and begins to undergo permanent plastic deformation. If continued load is applied, material failure may occur in the form of a fracture, or the object may just continue to undergo further plastic deformation depending on the brittleness or ductibility of the material. When applying these concepts to fracture fixation, a bone plate should function within the elastic region, and should not be subjected to loads that exceed the plate's yield strength. Therefore, yield strength is a very useful parameter for comparing the mechanical properties of different plates; however, this information is most meaningful when the applied load in vivo is known.

The term strain is used to give a more standardized and quantified description of material deformation resulting from an applied stress. Strain is defined as the ratio between the measured change in length during loading and the original length. Strain refers to a change in shape of a specified segment that undergoes either elongation or shortening depending on the nature of the applied stress. Strain is a unitless ratio (length over length), but is commonly reported in units of microstrain, so that a strain of 0.01 (1%) would be 10,000 microstrain. Interfragmentary strain is a term used to describe the mechanical environment within a fracture gap subjected to axial loading.[45,46] Interfragmentary strain is defined as the relative change in the fracture gap divided by the original width of the fracture gap.[1,42,45,46]

Stiffness

A structure's stiffness defines its ability to resist deformation resulting from an applied force.[43] For so-called linear elastic materials (such as most metals), the elastic region of the load-displacement curve is linear, because deformation is directly proportional to the applied load (**Fig. 2**). The slope of the linear portion of the load-displacement

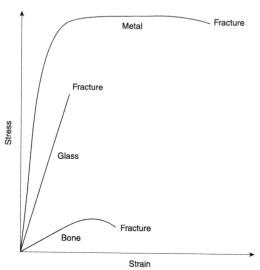

Fig. 2. Stress-strain curves of 3 materials. Metal has the steepest slope in the elastic region; therefore it is the stiffest material. The elastic portion of the curve for the metal is straight, indicating linearly elastic behavior. The long plastic region of the metal indicates that this material deforms extensively before failure. By contrast, glass fails abruptly with minimal deformation, as shown by the lack of a plastic region on the stress-strain curve. Bone, like most biological tissues, typically is nonlinear throughout its physiologic range owing to the nonlinear characteristics of its component.

curve is the structural stiffness. Elasticity is a characteristic of a material or object to return to its original shape after an applied load is released. Plasticity, in contrast to elasticity, describes residual deformation of a material or object as a result of loading, and is an unrecoverable status. More elastic materials can usually sustain considerable plastic deformation, whereas more brittle materials will fracture soon after reaching yield load, rather than deform. As an example, the stress-strain curves of the same object with 3 different materials such as bone, glass, and metal would differ substantially (see **Fig. 2**). A more brittle rigid body such as glass undergoes minimal plastic deformation before reaching its failure point, whereas metal has an elongated linear elastic portion of the curve, indicating linearly elastic behavior. The long plastic region of the metal indicates that this material deforms extensively before failure. Bone differs from glass and metal because bone, like other heterogenous biologic tissues, exhibits non-linear mechanical properties in the elastic portion of the curve.

Another concept that helps elucidate the biomechanical characteristics of orthopedic implants such as plates, screws, intramedullary pins, and interlocking nails is the area moment of inertia.[47] The bending stiffness of an object (such as an orthopedic implant) is the product of the elastic modulus of the material composition of the object and the area moment of inertia which is determined by the cross section of the object (**Fig. 3**). The area moment of inertia describes the capacity of the cross-sectional profile of an object to resist bending in response to an applied bending load. The greater the area moment of inertia, the less a structure will deflect (higher bending stiffness) when subjected to a bending load. The area moment of inertia is dependent on an object's cross-sectional geometry and dimensions and the direction of applied load (see **Fig. 3**; **Table 1**). The further the object's mass is distributed from the neutral axis, the larger the moment of inertia. For this reason, area moment of inertia is always considered with respect to a reference axis, in the x, y, or z direction, which is usually located at the center of an object's cross section. The area moment of inertia of an object having

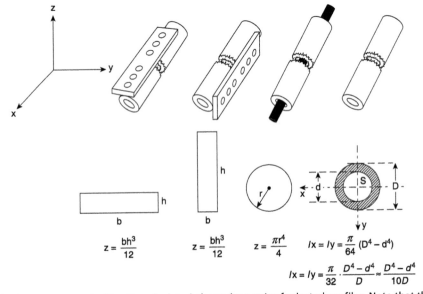

$$z = \frac{bh^3}{12} \qquad z = \frac{bh^3}{12} \qquad z = \frac{\pi r^4}{4} \qquad Ix = Iy = \frac{\pi}{64}(D^4 - d^4)$$

$$Ix = Iy = \frac{\pi}{32} \cdot \frac{D^4 - d^4}{D} \approx \frac{D^4 - d^4}{10D}$$

Fig. 3. Area moment of inertia calculated about the z-axis of selected profiles. Note that the orientation of the plate to applied bending loads has a profound effect on the implant's area of moment of inertia.

Table 1
Plate profile and area of moment of inertia of commonly used locking compression plates (LCP) of different sizes

Plate	Thickness (mm)	Width (mm)	Area of Moment of Inertia (mm^4)
2.0-mm/1.5-mm LCP	1.2	5.5	0.513
2.0-mm/1.5-mm LCP	1.5	5.5	0.894
2.4-mm LCP	1.7	6.5	1.900
2.4-mm LCP	2.0	6.5	2.613
2.7-mm LCP	2.6	7.5	4.078
3.5-mm LCP	3.3	11	13.445
3.5-mm broad LCP	4.2	13.5	40.580

The area of moment of inertia was calculated based on an axis perpendicular to the plate's thickness. Note how the area of moment of inertia increases as the thickness of the plate increases.

a rectangular cross-sectional profile, such as a plate, can be derived by the equation $bh^3/12$, where b is the base and h is the height. The base dimension is oriented parallel to the axis of the moment of inertia, and height is defined as the dimension parallel to the direction of the applied load. Thus the position of a plate on a bone and the plate's orientation to applied bending load can have a profound effect on a construct's bending stiffness (see **Fig. 3**). This effect becomes even more important when fractures are not anatomically reconstructed and plates are applied in bridging fashion. Understanding the area moment of inertia is important when comparing the mechanical properties of implants with different shapes and dimensions, such as when comparing an interlocking nail, a bone plate, and a plate-rod construct (**Fig. 4**). As shown in the calculation, the interlocking nail has the largest area of moment of inertia because of its large radius. It should also be noted that the area of moment of inertia of an intramedullary pin occupying 40% of the medullary canal has a significant contribution to the total area of moment of inertia of a plate-rod construct (see **Fig. 4**), justifying the recommendation to use this combination construct as bridging implants for comminuted fractures.[17,48] Another approach to stabilize a fracture with a gap is to increase the size of the plate. As shown in the calculation (see **Fig. 4**), a 3.5-mm broad locking compression plate has an area of moment of inertia 3 times larger than a 3.5-mm locking compression plate and almost twice as much as a 3.5-mm locking compression plate construct–intramedullary rod.

Although the stiffness of a plate is an important predictor of the implant's behavior under applied load, the mechanical properties of the combined plate-bone construct are more relevant to predict the type of fracture healing.[14] For this reason, it is important to distinguish between implant stiffness, structural stiffness of the construct, and stiffness across the fracture gap.[8,49–51] The construct stiffness is determined by numerous variables, including the plate's composition and geometry, the distance between plate and bone surface, plate length, type of screws, and the plate working length.[4,8,10,16,27,28,52–59] The plate working length is defined as the distance between the proximal and distal screws positioned closest to the fracture.[34] The gap stiffness is derived from the load-displacement curve describing the mechanical behavior of the fracture gap. Interfragmentary strain is defined as the relative displacement of the fracture-gap ends divided by the initial fracture-gap width.[45,60] For this reason the size of the initial fracture gap is an important factor in determining the interfragmentary strain. The relationship between gap strain and fracture healing has been extensively studied and is discussed in the next section.

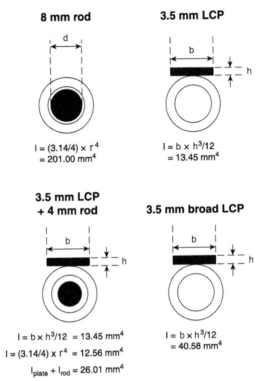

Fig. 4. The area of moment of inertia of an 8-mm diameter intramedullary rod, a 3.5-mm locking compression plate (LCP), a plate-rod construct composed of a 3.5-mm LCP and a 4-mm diameter intramedullary rod, and a 3.5-mm broad LCP. Note the 2-fold increase in area of moment of inertia from the isolated 3.5-mm LCP to the plate-rod combination. The area of moment of inertia of the 3.5-mm broad LCP alone is greater than both the 3.5-mm LCP alone and the plate-rod construct.

Fatigue Failure

Mechanical failure of plates can be broadly divided into 3 categories: plastic, brittle, and fatigue failure. Plastic failure is the failure of an implant to maintain its original shape, resulting in altered reduction and alignment and potentially clinical failure. Brittle failure, an unusual course of implant failure, results from a defect in design or metallurgy. Fatigue failure occurs as a result of repetitive loading at an intensity considerably below the normal yield strength of the implant.[43,44] Cyclic loading can lead to the formation of microscopic cracks that can propagate until these cracks reach a critical size, which then cause sudden failure of the implant. Although the propagation of the microcracks can take a considerable amount of time, there is typically very little, if any, warning preceding ultimate failure. Crack formation is commonly initiated at a "stress concentrator" or a "stress riser" such as a scratch on the plate or at a location where there is a change in the plate's cross-sectional geometry, such as a screw hole. The stress that is focused in these areas can be relatively higher than the average stress of the whole construct. Therefore, local material failure can occur at one of these stress concentrators and eventually propagate through the implant.[44] The number of cycles required to cause fatigue failure decreases as the magnitude of the stress increases. Fatigue failure is a genuine concern following fracture stabilization because of the high number of repetitive loads that implants are subjected to during the postoperative convalescent period. Therefore, surgeons must be cognizant when repairing any fracture that they have entered the proverbial race between fatigue failure of the implant and healing of the fracture.

Cyclic testing is useful for detecting the performance of an implant in resisting fatigue failure. In general, a predetermined load is applied during each cycle of the test, until plastic, brittle, or fatigue failure occurs, or the sample survives the planned number of cycles, termed run out. The principle of this type of testing is to determine the total number of loading cycles that a particular construct can withstand before failing. A construct's fatigue behavior can be described in an S-N curve; in which the stress to failure, S, is plotted against the number of cycles to failure, N (**Fig. 5**).[43] A construct's failure point is termed allowable stress. Typically a construct subjected to a small applied stress can withstand a large numbers of cycles and vice versa. However, the number of cycles to failure at a constant stress level can be affected by many factors such as the material composition and the geometry of the construct, the size of the gap or the stiffness of the developing fracture callus.

APPLIED BIOMECHANICS
Biomechanics of Fracture Healing

Numerous studies have shown that the mechanical conditions affecting the fracture site, principally the stability afforded by the fixation and the width of the fracture gap, influence callus formation during the healing process.[28,45,61-71] The process of bone healing depends on numerous interactions between biological and mechanical factors. The type of injury, the location and configuration of the fracture, the magnitude of load acting on the fracture, and systemic factors all play a role in the type and efficiency of bone healing.[42,61,72] Two principal concerns are whether there is adequate

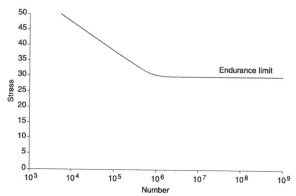

Fig. 5. The stress–number of cycles (S-N) curve of a specific material represents that material's resistance to fatigue failure. When performing a fatigue test of an implant such as a bone plate, the resulting data are presented as a plot of stress against the number of cycles to failure. During the mechanical test the implants are cycled at different stresses and their failure values are plotted in the graph. The S-N curve can be obtained with a minimum of 4 test specimens, but a larger number is preferable. In this case, testing began at a stress value of 50, thus the curve begins there. Fatigue life is the number of cycles that will cause failure at a defined stress level. Fatigue or endurance limit describes the resistance of the material and its geometry to failure. If an implant is loaded below the fatigue limit, the implant will not fail, regardless of the number of cycles. Fatigue strength is the stress at which failure occurs for a given number of cycles.

blood supply and the requisite stability necessary to obtain fracture union. If the local circulation is adequate to support fracture healing, the pattern of bone healing is then dependent on the surrounding biomechanical environment.[42,45,61,66,69–72] Several mechanoregulation theories of skeletal tissue differentiation have been developed that predict many aspects of bone healing under various mechanical conditions.[60,67–71,73] The theory proposed by Perren[45,60] is based on the interfragmentary strain present in the fracture gap. This theory suggests that the type of tissue formed in a healing fracture gap is dependent on the strain environment within the gap. The tissues that are stressed beyond their ultimate strain could not form in the gap. If interfragmentary strain exceeds 100%, nonunion may occur, because this degree of strain exceeds the allowable strain of biological tissues. Gap strains between 10% and 100% allow for formation of granulation and fibrous tissue. Strains between 2% and 10% allow for cartilage formation and subsequent endochondral ossification. Strains of less than 2% allow for bone formation and strains of 0% allow for primary fracture healing. Perren proposed that as tissue is formed, it would progressively stiffen the fracture gap. In turn, the tissue formed in the gap would lead to lower strains, which would allow formation of the sequentially stiffer tissue, and the cycle would repeat until bone formed within the gap. An alternative theory relating mechanical stimulus to fracture healing was proposed by Carter and Blenman,[69,71,74] purposed that tissue differentiation within the fracture gap depends on the magnitude and the type of local stress, including hydrostatic pressure and octahedral shear stress. This theory purports that the vascular supply to the tissues at the fracture site is the primary factor in determining tissue differentiation. With adequate circulation, Carter and Blenman proposed that fibrocartilage will form if high hydrostatic compressive stresses are present. In an analysis of fracture healing, Carter and Blenman[69–71] correlated compressive hydrostatic stress with cartilage formation (chondrogenesis), whereas low hydrostatic stress corresponded to bone formation (osteogenesis). However, the relationship between the ossification pattern and the loading history was described only qualitatively and not quantitatively. More recently, Claes and Heigele[67] have proposed and tested the quantitative tissue differentiation theory which relates interfragmentary tissue formation to the local stress and strain in a fracture gap. The results regarding the global strain and hydrostatic pressure fields correlate with the principal results of Carter and Blenman. In contrast to Carter and Blenman's work,[69,71,74] the quantitative tissue differentiation theory is based on the assumption that new bone formation only occurs on existing osseous surfaces and under defined ranges of strain and hydrostatic pressure. The tissue differentiation hypothesis predicts intramembranous bone formation will proceed once interfragmentary strain decrease to less than 5% while endochondral ossification can occur at interfragmentary strains approximating 15% in a diaphyseal fracture, which obtain union by secondary bone healing.[46,67] Another recent theory on mechanobiology of fracture healing proposed a model dependent on 2 biophysical stimuli: tissue shear strain and interstitial fluid flow.[68] The rationale for this approach is that fluid flow increases the biomechanical stress and deformation on the cells above what the strain of the collagenous material generated.[68]

Although Perren's theory on interfragmentary strain is important in understanding the concept of tissue mechanobiology at the fracture gap, several studies have demonstrated that gap strain higher than 2% is tolerated and that the strain patterns within a fracture gap are heterogenous.[75,76] It is well accepted that interfragmentary movement is the most important biomechanical factor in fracture healing, but the optimal range for callus formation and bone healing is still unknown.

Bone Healing Under Conditions of Absolute and Relative Stability

The term stability is defined as the load-dependent displacement of the fracture surfaces. Stability in osteosynthesis covers a spectrum from minimal to absolute. Absolute stability is present only when there is no displacement of the stabilized fracture segments under loading (**Fig. 6**). Absolute stability is achieved by (1) applying a compressive preload that exceeds the traction force acting at the segments, and (2) counteracting the shear forces acting on the fracture surfaces with friction. The elimination of relative motion between the bone segments results from the application of interfragmentary compression, and requires anatomic reduction.[9] Placement of a lag screw is an excellent example of a fixation that can provide absolute stability (see **Fig. 6**). In vivo experiments have shown that a lag screw can produce high compressive forces (>2500 N) across a fracture.[9] Although absolute stability was originally thought to be necessary for successful management of most fractures, current thinking suggests that absolute stability is only obligatory when stabilizing articular fractures and only when interfragmentary compression can be achieved without inducing excessive iatrogenic damage to blood supply and surrounding soft tissues.[9] Limiting soft-tissue trauma is an essential tenet of any fracture repair. Even when performing a direct open reduction, efforts should be made to minimize iatrogenic trauma to the regional soft tissues and the periosteum.

Fractures stabilized under conditions of absolute stability will heal by primary or direct fracture healing, if anatomically reduced.[77–79] Because there is no motion at the fracture site, there will be negligible callus formation. The fracture heals through

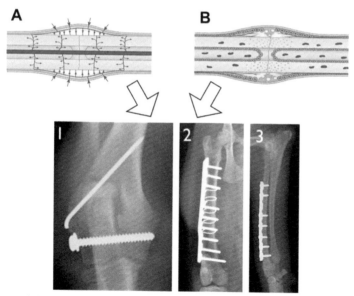

Fig. 6. Successful fracture healing under conditions of absolute stability depends on the mechanical conditions at the fracture gap and the presence of an adequate vascular supply. As depicted with the arrows directed towards the fracture, the blood supply originates from the peripheral soft tissue. Fixation providing absolute stability aims to produce a mechanical environment that eliminates motion at the fracture site, as demonstrated in these fractures stabilized with lag screw and Kirschner wire (*1*), cerclage wires and neutralization plate (*2*), and compression plate (*3*). Limited callus formation is expected under these mechanical conditions (*B*).

the formation of osteonal cutting cones and Haversian remodeling of the compressed cortical bone.[78,79] Direct bone healing can be further subdivided into 2 types based on the width of the fracture gap. Contact healing occurs when the ends of the bone segments are in direct contact, the gap between the 2 bone segments is less than 0.01 mm, and when interfragmentary strain is less than 2%.[78] If the fracture gap is larger but does not exceed 1 mm, and an interfragmentary strain again is less than 2%, gap healing will occur, whereby intramembranous bone will be formed directly in the fracture gap.[45] In both types, a process called Haversian remodeling begins with osteoclastic resorption, which results in resorption cavities formed by groups of osteoclasts, also called a cutting cone.[79] Bone resorption is followed by osteoblast activity. The osteoblasts line the resorption cavities and produce layers of new bone. The resorption cavity is filled in with new bone to form a new osteon. Gap healing results from the development of lamellar bone forming from granulation tissue in small gaps.[78,79] Intramembranous bone formation occurs during direct bone healing; the surrounding environment can impose up to 5% strain as long as it allows the differentiation of mesenchymal cells into osteoblasts.

Relative stability is a condition whereby an acceptable amount of interfragmentary displacement compatible with fracture healing is present (**Fig. 7**).[80] Relative stability

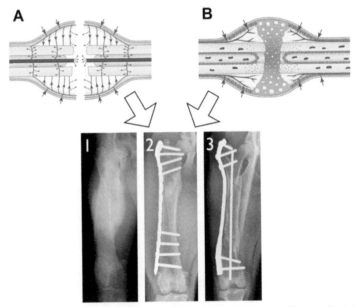

Fig. 7. Successful fracture healing under conditions of relative stability, as depicted in this diagram of a fracture that healed by the process of secondary bone healing, depends on maintaining adequate circulation to the fracture and appropriate gap motion. Immediately after the fracture is sustained (A), there is hematoma formation caused by disruption of blood vessels. The fracture hematoma is gradually replaced by granulation tissue. Under conditions of controlled gap motion, soft callus is progressively replaced with hard callus (B). As depicted with the arrows directed towards the callus in both A and B, the major source of blood vessels supporting the callus formation is the surrounding soft tissues. Secondary bone healing noted in 3 diaphyseal femoral fractures healed under conditions of relative stability: (1) femoral functional malunion healed without surgical fixation; (2) femoral fracture stabilized with bridging plate (3.5-mm broad locking compression plate); (3) femoral fracture stabilized with plate-rod combination (4.5-mm narrow dynamic compression plate and 5-mm intramedullary pin).

involves placement of implants that provide somewhat flexible fixation, which allow an acceptable degree of fracture-segment displacement. Fixation modalities that can be used to provide relative stability include plates, plate-rod constructs, interlocking nails, and external fixators applied in bridging fashion to span a bone defect.[72,81]

Relative stability provides a mechanical environment that promotes indirect or secondary bone healing.[66,80] Indirect bone healing is very similar to embryologic bone development, and occurs via both endochondral and intramembranous ossification.[66,80,82] The healing process by formation of callus can be divided into 4 stages: inflammation, soft callus, hard callus, and remodeling.[82,83] Mineralized cartilaginous callus develops at the ends of the fracture segments (gap callus), along the medullary canal (medullary callus), and on the outer cortex (periosteal callus).[82,83] The majority of the vascular circulation to the callus is derived from the surrounding soft tissues.[84] Therefore, surgical techniques that preserve the soft-tissue envelope adjacent to the fracture are advantageous and promote fracture healing.

The indications for using techniques that achieve absolute or relative stability differ according to fracture location, fracture configuration, soft tissue conditions, and vascularity of the bone. Simple transverse, spiral, or oblique fractures that can be readily anatomically reconstructed are good candidates for anatomic reconstruction and compression or neutralization plating. More complex comminuted fractures that cannot be reconstructed should be treated with bridging fixation. Articular fractures should be anatomically reduced and stabilized with fixation that generates interfragmentary compression, such as lag screws.[72] It is always important to consider whether it is possible to implement anatomic reconstruction when choosing the type of fixation. For example, fractures that may initially appear as simple, reconstructable fractures may instead have fragments that are too small for anatomic reconstruction. In these cases, an open or closed indirect reduction technique and a bridging stabilization technique may be indicated. Because the success of the technique depends on the precision of the reduction, critical preoperative planning should always be performed.

Factors Affecting Stiffness of the Plate-Bone Construct

The stiffness of the bone-plate construct is a major determinant of the mechanism and progression of bone healing.[1,28,51,69,70] There are several parameters in addition to the material properties of the implants that need to be considered when applying a bone plate. Understanding the effect of plate type, size, length, position, screw type, and screw placement is important because successful fracture healing depends on appropriate fixation stability.[54,56,58,59,85–88] Furthermore, a multitude of plate types and concepts have been described and proposed in the last decade, in an attempt to decrease complications and improve the reliability of bone plating. The development of new implants and techniques have followed a shift in emphasis of the Arbeitsgemeinschaft für Osteosynthesefragen/Association for the Study of Internal Fixation philosophy, from obtaining anatomic reconstruction and absolute stability to obtaining anatomic alignment and appropriate stability using more atraumatic application techniques.[9,72] Concurrent with this change in emphasis in internal fixation, newer implant systems such as internal fixators, locking plates, or angle stable devices have been developed to improve bone plating technique.[9] Understanding the mechanical properties of locking plates and conventional plates is important for choosing an appropriate implant system.

Choosing the Type of Plate: Locking Versus Nonlocking Plates

Gautier and Sommer[31] recently presented prudent guidelines that may improve the individual learning curve of surgeons who are less familiar with locking plates.

However, it is important to understand the concepts behind these recommendations for successful use of the vast choice of plates available.[10,27] There are distinct principal biomechanical differences between bridging plates and locked internal fixators with regard to load transfer through a fractured bone. In conventional compression plate constructs or nonlocking bridging plate constructs, fixation stability is limited by the frictional force generated between the plate and the bone. This force is created by axial screw forces and the coefficient of friction between the plate and the bone.[8,89] If the force exerted on the bone while the patient is ambulating exceeds the frictional limit, relative shear displacement will occur between the plate and the bone, causing a loss of reduction between the bone segments (known as secondary loss of reduction), or loosening of the screws, or both. Conventional plates, including dynamic compression plates[90] and limited-contact dynamic compression plates,[91] allow for compression of bone segments using dynamic compression holes. In a transverse fracture that has been anatomically reduced, stability can be further increased by using the plate to generate interfragmentary compression between the ends of the fracture segments. When the screws are inserted eccentrically at the end of the oval hole located remote to the fracture, the lower hemispherical part of the screw head will contact the dynamic compression incline of the compression hole. This interaction between the screw head and the compression incline results in translation of the screw centrally with the hole in the plate, producing compression of the ends of the fracture segments during screw tightening.[90,91]

Locking plates differ from nonlocking plates because stability is not dependent on the frictional forces generated at the bone-plate interface. The first plate that functioned as an internal fixator (Zespol system) was developed in 1970 in Poland.[92] Since then, several locking plates have been developed that use the concept of angular stability. These implants consist of a plate and locking head screws, which together act as an internal fixator. Locking the head screw into the plate hole confers axial and angular stability of the screw, relative to the plate. Because the stability of the construct does not depend on frictional forces generated between plate and bone, the bone-screw threads are unlikely to strip during insertion. The fixed-angle connection between the screw and the plate clearly affords improved long-term stability. Plate failure by "pullout" is unlikely because the screws cannot be sequentially loaded or pulled out.[9,25,93]

Locking plates have both mechanical and biological advantages. The periosteal blood supply beneath the plate is not compromised because compression between plate and bone does not occur. Preservation of the periosteal vasculature may improve healing and decrease the risk of cortical bone necrosis and infection.[81] Another advantage is that the plate does not need to be perfectly contoured, because the bone is not "pulled towards" the plate while tightening the screw. For this reason, locking plates are often used for minimally invasive plate osteosynthesis (MIPO), which involves closed reduction and percutaneous fixation of the fracture.[34–36,94,95] Several locking plate systems are available. Some plates may have combination holes that allow placement of a locking screw or a conventional nonlocking screw in either a compressive or neutral fashion.[9,96,97]

Several biomechanical studies have compared locking and nonlocking plates in dogs. These studies have conflicting results. Whereas some studies demonstrated that locking plate constructs were stiffer than nonlocking plate constructs when tested in axial compression, torsion, and bending,[16,22,52,89,96,98–104] others did not find any significant differences between the two.[12,20,26,29,55,86,98,105–108] The most consistent finding has been that locking plates perform better than nonlocking plates in osteoporotic bone.[4,89,99,109] The biomechanical advantages of locking plates may be less evident in normal bone, particularly when tested in gap models under single cycle (acute) loading, because these models predominantly test the plate stiffness rather than the interaction between the plate, screws, and the bone.

Choosing the Length of the Plate

The selection of an appropriate length of plate is a very important step in the preoperative plan. Appropriate plate length is dependent on the location and configuration of the fracture as well as the intended functional application of the plate. In bridge plating, longer plates lower the pullout force acting in screws because of an improvement of the working leverage for the screws and better distribution of the bending forces along the plate.[31] The theoretical advantage of using a longer plate without placing screws in the center portion of the plate is supported by several biomechanical studies. Sander and colleagues[88] compared 3 different plate lengths, 6-, 8-, or 10-hole 3.5-mm dynamic compression plates fixed on ulnae harvested from dogs, tested in 4-point bending to failure. The results revealed that 10-hole plates with 4 screws (widely spread on the fracture segment) failed at higher peak loads than 6-hole plates with 6 screws, supporting the recommendation that longer plates with fewer screws provide superior bending strength than shorter plates with a greater number of screws. In another study, Weiss and colleagues evaluated 8- and 10-hole 3.5-mm locking compression plates used to stabilize human cadaveric ulnas. This study found that 10-hole plates secured with 2 nonlocking screws placed in a near-far configuration on either side of the fracture demonstrated an increased yield strength compared with 8-hole plates with the same number of screws and configuration in 4-point bending to failure.[86] Iatrogenic trauma associated with the open application of a long plate can be substantially mitigated by using less invasive application techniques such as MIPO.

Two values have been used to determine the length of the plate to be used. The plate span ratio is a quotient derived by dividing plate length by the segmental length of the fracture gap or zone of comminution. Based on guidelines developed for fracture fixation in human patients, the plate span should be more than 2 to 3 in comminuted fractures and more than 8 to10 in simple fractures.[9] Plate-screw density is the quotient derived by dividing the number of screws inserted by the number of holes in the plate. Empirically, values below 0.4 to 0.3 when applied in simple fractures and a value below 0.5 to 0.4 when applied in comminuted fractures have been recommended.[9,31] These guidelines were formulated for the application of plates in human patients, and need to be evaluated in dogs.

Effect of the Position of Screws in the Plate

In comminuted fractures that have not been reconstructed, stress is distributed over the fracture gap and depends on the number and location of screws placed,[9,54] in addition to other factors. The lowest stress in the plate occurs when the screws are positioned as close as practical to the fracture.[54] However, this leads to the highest axial stiffness as well as very small interfragmentary movements and strains beneath the plate. It has been recommended to increase the plate working length to reduce axial stiffness of a plate-bone construct[9,31,110]; however, previous mechanical studies have yielded conflicting results.[54,87,111] Based on mechanical tests performed in their laboratory, the authors suspect that the variability in the results among reported studies might be attributable to how the plate is applied to the bone. In constructs that use nonlocking plates, the contact between the plate and the bone segments appears to cause the bending moment to concentrate within the plate between the ends of the bone segments, regardless of the positioning of the screws. Therefore, the functional plate working length does not correspond to the distance between the screws placed closest to the fracture gap, but rather to the length of the fracture gap. By contrast, the physical offset of a locking plate that is applied without the bone and plate in intimate contact enables a locking plate to bend along the entire segment of the plate between the 2 most centrally positioned screws.

More recent strategies to decrease the stiffness of locking plate–bone constructs include new designs of locking screws that allow increased fracture-gap micromotion with axial loading.[112–114] The goal of this novel approach is to promote more reliable healing and prevent late failures observed in several clinical studies in people.[115–117] The far cortex locking screw has a smooth shaft with threads at its tip which only engage the far cortex.[51,112,113,118] The smooth shaft of this screw decreases the stiffness of the plating construct and allows greater callus compared with standard locked implants.[113] Another screw design attempting to combine the advantages of locking screws and controlled axial micromotion is the dynamic locking screw.[114] This dynamic locking screw is composed of an outer sleeve with threads that engage the bone and an inner pin with threads that lock to the plate. By allowing motion between inner pin and the outer sleeve, dynamic compression screws reduced the axial stiffness by 16%.[114]

SUMMARY

Fracture stabilization involves establishing the proper balance between reducing the potential for implant failure while providing optimal interfragmentary motion to stimulation of callus formation. Overcoming the conflict between stiffness, strength, and interfragmentary strain is challenging because numerous factors affect the biomechanical properties of a fracture-fixation construct. Minimally invasive bridging osteosynthesis techniques take advantage of the concept of flexible fixation. Locking plates are theoretically ideally suited for techniques such as MIPO because these techniques do not require precise anatomic reconstruction of the fracture, and the plates do not need to be precisely contoured and in direct contact with the surface of the stabilized bone. Recent studies, however, suggest that locking plate constructs can be too stiff to promote callus formation and rapid secondary fracture healing.[51,113] Future studies should critically evaluate the advantages and indications for locking implants in animals, and define optimal constructs to achieve appropriate stability, thus to facilitate early, uneventful fracture healing.

REFERENCES

1. Perren SM. Evolution of the internal fixation of long bone fractures. J Bone Joint Surg Am 2002;84:1093–110.
2. Miclau T, Martin RE. The evolution of modern plate osteosynthesis. Injury 1997; 1(Suppl):A3–6.
3. Rozbruch RS, Muller U, Gautier E, et al. The evolution of femoral shaft plating technique. Clin Orthop Relat Res 1998;354:195–208.
4. Egol KA, Kubiak EN, Fulkerson E, et al. Biomechanics of locked plates and screws. J Orthop Trauma 2004;18:488–93.
5. Smith WR, Ziran BH, Anglen JO, et al. Locking plates: tips and tricks. Instr Course Lect 2008;57:25–36.
6. Smith WR, Ziran BH, Anglen JO, et al. Locking plates: tips and tricks. J Bone Joint Surg Am 2007;89:2298–307.
7. Frigg R. Development of the locking compression plate. Injury 2003;34(Suppl 2): B6–10.

8. Miller DL, Goswami T. A review of locking compression plate biomechanics and their advantages as internal fixators in fracture healing. Clin Biomech 2007;22: 1049–62.

9. Wagner M, Frigg R. Background and methodological principles. In: Buckley R, Gautier B, Schutz M, et al, editors. AO manual of fracture management, internal fixators: concepts and cases using LCP and LISS. Stuttgart (Germany): Thieme; 2006. p. 1–57.

10. Blake CA, Boudrieau RJ, Torrance BS, et al. Single cycle to failure in bending of three standard and five locking plates and plate constructs. Vet Comp Orthop Traumatol 2011;24:408–17.

11. Zahn K, Frei R, Wunderle D, et al. Mechanical properties of 18 different AO bone plates and the clamp-rod internal fixation system tested on a gap model construct. Vet Comp Orthop Traumatol 2008;21:185–94.

12. Aguila AZ, Manos JM, Orlansky AS, et al. In vitro biomechanical comparison of limited contact dynamic compression plate and locking compression plate. Vet Comp Orthop Traumatol 2005;18:220–6.

13. Filipowicz D, Lanz O, McLaughlin R, et al. A biomechanical comparison of 3.5 locking compression plate fixation to 3.5 limited contact dynamic compression plate fixation in a canine cadaveric distal humeral metaphyseal gap model. Vet Comp Orthop Traumatol 2009;22:270–7.

14. Gauthier CM, Conrad BP, Lewis DD, et al. In vitro comparison of stiffness of plate fixation of radii from large- and small-breed dogs. Am J Vet Res 2011;72: 1112–7.

15. Goh CS, Santoni BG, Puttlitz CM, et al. Comparison of the mechanical behaviors of semicontoured, locking plate-rod fixation and anatomically contoured, conventional plate-rod fixation applied to experimentally induced gap fractures in canine femora. Am J Vet Res 2009;70:23–9.

16. Gordon S, Moens NM, Runciman RJ, et al. The effect of the combination of locking screws and non-locking screws on the torsional properties of a locking-plate construct. Vet Comp Orthop Traumatol 2010;23:7–13.

17. Hulse D, Hyman W, Nori M, et al. Reduction in plate strain by addition of an intramedullary pin. Vet Surg 1997;26:451–9.

18. Hammel SP, Elizabeth Pluhar G, Novo RE, et al. Fatigue analysis of plates used for fracture stabilization in small dogs and cats. Vet Surg 2006;35:573–8.

19. Johnston SA, Lancaster RL, Hubbard RP, et al. A biomechanical comparison of 7-hole 3.5 mm broad and 5-hole 4.5 mm narrow dynamic compression plates. Vet Surg 1991;20:235–9.

20. Leitner M, Pearce SG, Windolf M, et al. Comparison of locking and conventional screws for maintenance of tibial plateau positioning and biomechanical stability after locking tibial plateau leveling osteotomy plate fixation. Vet Surg 2008;37:357–65.

21. Silbernagel JT, Johnson AL, Pijanowski GJ, et al. A mechanical comparison of 4.5 mm narrow and 3.5 mm broad plating systems for stabilization of gapped fracture models. Vet Surg 2004;33:173–9.

22. Sod GA, Mitchell CF, Hubert JD, et al. In vitro biomechanical comparison of locking compression plate fixation and limited-contact dynamic compression plate fixation of osteotomized equine third metacarpal bones. Vet Surg 2008;37: 283–8.

23. Sod GA, Riggs LM, Mitchell CF, et al. An in vitro biomechanical comparison of a 5.5 mm locking compression plate fixation with a 4.5 mm locking compression plate fixation of osteotomized equine third metacarpal bones. Vet Surg 2010;39: 581–7.

24. Strom AM, Garcia TC, Jandrey K, et al. In vitro mechanical comparison of 2.0 and 2.4 limited-contact dynamic compression plates and 2.0 dynamic compression plates of different thicknesses. Vet Surg 2009;39:824–8.

25. Uhl JM, Seguin B, Kapatkin AS, et al. Mechanical comparison of 3.5 mm broad dynamic compression plate, broad limited-contact dynamic compression plate, and narrow locking compression plate systems using interfragmentary gap models. Vet Surg 2008;37:663–73.

26. DeTora M, Kraus K. Mechanical testing of 3.5 mm locking and non-locking bone plates. Vet Comp Orthop Traumatol 2008;21:318–22.

27. Cabassu JB, Kowaleski MP, Shorinko JK, et al. Single cycle to failure in torsion of three standard and five locking plate constructs. Vet Comp Orthop Traumatol 2011;24:418–25.

28. Terjesen T, Apalset K. The influence of different degrees of stiffness of fixation plates on experimental bone healing. J Orthop Res 1988;6:293–9.

29. Miclau T, Remiger A, Tepic S, et al. A mechanical comparison of the dynamic compression plate, limited contact-dynamic compression plate, and point contact fixator. J Orthop Trauma 1995;9:17–22.

30. Tan SL, Balogh ZJ. Indications and limitations of locked plating. Injury 2009;40: 683–91.

31. Gautier E, Sommer C. Guidelines for the clinical application of the LCP. Injury 2003;34:63–76.

32. Johnson AL, Smith CW, Schaeffer DJ. Fragment reconstruction and bone plate fixation versus bridging plate fixation for treating highly comminuted femoral fractures in dogs: 35 cases (1987-1997). J Am Vet Med Assoc 1998;213:1157–61.

33. Johnson AL. Current concepts in fracture reduction. Vet Comp Orthop Traumatol 2003;16:59–66.

34. Pozzi A, Hudson C, Gauthier C, et al. A retrospective comparison of minimally invasive plate osteosynthesis and open reduction and internal fixation for radius-ulna fractures in dogs. Vet Surg, in press.

35. Pozzi A, Risselada M, Winter M. Ultrasonographic and radiographic assessment of fracture healing after minimally invasive plate osteosynthesis and open reduction and internal fixation of radius-ulna fractures in dogs. J Am Vet Med Assoc, in press.

36. Guiot LP, Dejardin LM. Prospective evaluation of minimally invasive plate osteosynthesis in 36 nonarticular tibial fractures in dogs and cats. Vet Surg 2011;40:171–82.

37. Boero A, Peirone B, MD W, et al. Comparison between minimally invasive plate osteosynthesis and open plating for tibial fractures in dogs. Vet Comp Orthop Traumatol 2012 Jul 25;25(5) [Epub ahead of print].

38. Palmer RH. Biological osteosynthesis. Vet Clin North Am Small Anim Pract 1999; 29:1171–85, vii.

39. Claes L, Heitemeyer U, Krischak G, et al. Fixation technique influences osteogenesis of comminuted fractures. Clin Orthop Relat Res 1999;365:221–9.

40. Stoffel K, Klaue K, Perren SM. Functional load of plates in fracture fixation in vivo and its correlate in bone healing. Injury 2000;31(Suppl 2):37–86.

41. Claes LE, Heigele CA, Neidlinger-Wilke C, et al. Effects of mechanical factors on the fracture healing process. Clin Orthop Relat Res 1998;355:S132–47.

42. Claes L. Biomechanical principles and mechanobiologic aspects of flexible and locked plating. J Orthop Trauma 2011;25:S4–7.

43. Tencer A, Johnson K. Biomechanics in orthopedic trauma—bone fracture and fixation. In: Tencer A, Johnson K, editors. London: Martin Dunitz; 1994. p. 13–6.

44. Taylor D. Fracture mechanics: how does bone break? Nat Mater 2003;2:133–4.

45. Perren SM. Physical and biological aspects of fracture healing with special reference to internal fixation. Clin Orthop Relat Res 1975;138:175–94.
46. Cheal EJ, Mansmann KA, Digioia AM, et al. Role of interfragmentary strain in fracture healing: ovine model of a healing osteotomy. J Orthop Res 1991;9: 131–42.
47. Muir P, Johnson KA, Markel MD. Area moment of inertia for compression of implant cross-sectional geometry and bending stiffness. Vet Comp Orthop Traumatol 1995;8:146–52.
48. Reems MR, Beale BS, Hulse DA. Use of a plate-rod construct and principles of biological osteosynthesis for repair of diaphyseal fractures in dogs and cats: 47 cases (1994-2001). J Am Vet Med Assoc 2003;223:330–5.
49. Lill H, Hepp P, Korner J, et al. Proximal humeral fractures: how stiff should an implant be? Arch Orthop Trauma Surg 2003;123:74–81.
50. Oh JK, Sahu D, Ahn YH, et al. Effect of fracture gap on stability of compression plate fixation: a finite element study. J Orthop Res 2010;28:462–7.
51. Bottlang M, Doornink J, Lujan TJ, et al. Effects of construct stiffness on healing of fractures stabilized with locking plates. J Bone Joint Surg Am 2010;92: 12–22.
52. Snow M, Thompson G, Turner PG. A mechanical comparison of the locking compression plate (LCP) and the low contact-dynamic compression plate (DCP) in an osteoporotic bone model. J Orthop Trauma 2008;22:121–5.
53. Woo SL, Lothringer KS, Akeson WH, et al. Less rigid internal fixation plates: historical perspectives and new concepts. J Orthop Res 1983;1:431–49.
54. Stoffel K, Dieter U, Stachowiak G, et al. Biomechanical testing of the LCP—how can stability in locked internal fixators be controlled? Injury 2003;34:11–9.
55. Stoffel K, Lorenz KU, Kuster MS. Biomechanical considerations in plate osteosynthesis: the effect of plate-to-bone compression with and without angular screw stability. J Orthop Trauma 2007;21:362–8.
56. Tornkvist H, Hearn TC, Schatzker J. The strength of plate fixation in relation to the number and spacing of bone screws. J Orthop Trauma 1996;10:204–8.
57. ElMaraghy AW, ElMaraghy MW, Nousiainen M, et al. Influence of the number of cortices on the stiffness of plate fixation of diaphyseal fractures. J Orthop Trauma 2001;15:186–91.
58. Ellis T, Bourgeault CA, Kyle RF. Screw position affects dynamic compression plate strain in an in vitro fracture model. J Orthop Trauma 2001;15:333–7.
59. Field JR, Tornkvist H, Hearn TC, et al. The influence of screw omission on construction stiffness and bone surface strain in the application of bone plates to cadaveric bone. Injury 1999;30:591–8.
60. Perren M. The concept of interfragmentary strain. In: Perren M, Cordey J, editors. Current concepts of internal fixation of fractures. Berlin: Springer; 1980. p. 63–77.
61. Jagodzinski M, Krettek C. Effect of mechanical stability on fracture healing–an update. Injury 2007;38(Suppl 1):3–10.
62. Augat P, Merk J, Wolf S, et al. Mechanical stimulation by external application of cyclic tensile strains does not effectively enhance bone healing. J Orthop Trauma 2001;15:54–60.
63. Claes L, Wolf S, Augat P. Mechanical modification of callus healing. Chirurg 2000;71:989–94 [in German].
64. Wolf S, Augat P, Eckert-Hubner K, et al. Effects of high-frequency, low-magnitude mechanical stimulus on bone healing. Clin Orthop Relat Res 2001;385: 192–8.

65. Hente R, Fuchtmeier B, Schlegel U, et al. The influence of cyclic compression and distraction on the healing of experimental tibial fractures. J Orthop Res 2004;22:709–15.

66. Goodship AE, Kenwright J. The influence of induced micromovement upon the healing of experimental tibial fractures. J Bone Joint Surg Br 1985;67:650–5.

67. Claes LE, Heigele CA. Magnitudes of local stress and strain along bony surfaces predict the course and type of fracture healing. J Biomech 1999;32:255–66.

68. Prendergast PJ, Huiskes R, Soballe K. ESB Research Award 1996. Biophysical stimuli on cells during tissue differentiation at implant interfaces. J Biomech 1997;30:539–48.

69. Blenman PR, Carter DR, Beaupre GS. Role of mechanical loading in the progressive ossification of a fracture callus. J Orthop Res 1989;7:398–407.

70. Carter DR, Beaupre GS, Giori NJ, et al. Mechanobiology of skeletal regeneration. Clin Orthop Relat Res 1998;355:S41–55.

71. Carter DR, Blenman PR, Beaupré GS. Correlations between mechanical stress history and tissue differentiation in initial fracture healing. J Orthop Res 1988; 6(5):736–48.

72. Griffon D. Fracture healing. In: Johnson AL, Houlton JE, Vannini R, et al, editors. AO principles of fracture management in the dog and cat. Stuttgart (Germany): Thieme; 2005. p. 72–97.

73. Isaksson H, Wilson W, van Donkelaar CC, et al. Comparison of biophysical stimuli for mechano-regulation of tissue differentiation during fracture healing. J Biomech 2006;39:1507–16.

74. Carter DR. Mechanical loading history and skeletal biology. J Biomech 1987;20: 1095–109.

75. Kenwright J, Goodship AE. Controlled mechanical stimulation in the treatment of tibial fractures. Clin Orthop Relat Res 1989;241:36–47.

76. Claes L, Grass R, Schmickal T. Monitoring and healing analysis of 100 tibial shaft fractures. Langenbecks Arch Surg 2002;387:146–52.

77. Olerud S, Danckwardt-Lilliestrom G. Fracture healing in compression osteosynthesis. An experimental study in dogs with an avascular, diaphyseal, intermediate fragment. Acta Orthop Scand Suppl 1971;137:1–44.

78. Rahn BA, Gallinaro P, Baltensperger A, et al. Primary bone healing. An experimental study in the rabbit. J Bone Joint Surg Am 1971;53:783–6.

79. Schenk R, Willenegger H. On the histological picture of so-called primary bone healing of compression osteosynthesis in experimental osteotomies in the dog. Experientia 1963;19:593–5.

80. Goodship AE, Cunningham JL, Kenwright J. Strain rate and timing of stimulation in mechanical modulation of fracture healing. Clin Orthop Relat Res 1998; 355(Suppl):S105–15.

81. Baumgaertel F, Buhl M, Rahn BA. Fracture healing in biological plate osteosynthesis. Injury 1998;29:3–6.

82. Remedios A. Bone and bone healing. Vet Clin North Am Small Anim Pract 1999; 29:1029–44.

83. Klaushofer K, Peterlik M. Pathophysiology of fracture healing. Radiologe 1994; 34:709–14 [in German].

84. Rhinelander F. Tibial blood supply in relation to fracture healing. Clin Orthop Relat Res 1974;105:34–81.

85. Hoffmeier KL, Hofmann GO, Muckley T. Choosing a proper working length can improve the lifespan of locked plates: a biomechanical study. Clin Biomech 2011 May;26(4):405–9.

86. Weiss DB, Kaar SG, Frankenburg EP, et al. Locked versus unlocked plating with respect to plate length in an ulna fracture model. Bull NYU Hosp Jt Dis 2008;66:5–8.

87. Kanchanomai C, Muanjan P, Phiphobmongkol V. Stiffness and endurance of a locking compression plate fixed on fractured femur. J Appl Biomech 2010; 26:10–6.

88. Sanders R, Haidukewych GJ, Milne T, et al. Minimal versus maximal plate fixation techniques of the ulna: the biomechanical effect of number of screws and plate length. J Orthop Trauma 2002;16:166–71.

89. Fulkerson E, Egol KA, Kubiak EN, et al. Fixation of diaphyseal fractures with a segmental defect: a biomechanical comparison of locked and conventional plating techniques. J Trauma 2006;60:830–5.

90. Perren S, Russenberger M, Steinemann S, et al. A dynamic compression plate. Acta Orthop Scand Suppl 1969;125:31–41.

91. Perren SM, Klaue K, Pohler O. The limited contact dynamic compression plate (LC-DCP). Arch Orthop Trauma Surg 1990;109:304–10.

92. Hopf T, Osthege S. Interfragmental compression of the ZESPOL osteosynthesis system—an exploratory biomechanic experiment. Z Orthop Ihre Grenzgeb 1987;125:546–52 [in German].

93. Greiwe RM, Archdeacon MT. Locking plate technology: current concepts. J Knee Surg 2007;20:50–5.

94. Hasenboehler E, Rikli D, Babst R. Locking compression plate with minimally invasive plate osteosynthesis in diaphyseal and distal tibial fracture: a retrospective study of 32 patients. Injury 2007;38:365–70.

95. Khong K, Kotlanka R, Ghista DN. Mechanobiology. In: Tong GO, Bavonratanavech S, Stuttgart DE, editors. AO manual of fracture management. Minimally invasive plate osteosynthesis (MIPO). Stuttgart (Germany): Thieme; 2007. p. 9–21.

96. Gardner MJ, Griffith MH, Demetrakopoulos D, et al. Hybrid locked plating of osteoporotic fractures of the humerus. J Bone Joint Surg 2006;88:1962–7.

97. Doornink J, Fitzpatrick DC, Boldhaus S, et al. Effects of hybrid plating with locked and nonlocked screws on the strength of locked plating constructs in the osteoporotic diaphysis. J Trauma 2010;69:411–7.

98. Stoffel K, Booth G, Rohrl SM, et al. A comparison of conventional versus locking plates in intraarticular calcaneus fractures: a biomechanical study in human cadavers. Clin Biomech (Bristol, Avon) 2007;22:100–5.

99. Kim T, Ayturk UM, Haskell A, et al. Fixation of osteoporotic distal fibula fractures: a biomechanical comparison of locking versus conventional plates. J Foot Ankle Surg 2007;46:2–6.

100. Florin M, Arzdorf M, Linke B, et al. Assessment of stiffness and strength of 4 different implants available for equine fracture treatment: a study on a 20° oblique long-bone fracture model using a bone substitute. Vet Surg 2005;34: 231–8.

101. Burkhart KJ, Mueller LP, Krezdorn D, et al. Stability of radial head and neck fractures: a biomechanical study of six fixation constructs with consideration of three locking plates. J Hand Surg 2007;32:1569–75.

102. Siffri PC, Peindl RD, Coley ER, et al. Biomechanical analysis of blade plate versus locking plate fixation for a proximal humerus fracture: comparison using cadaveric and synthetic humeri. J Orthop Trauma 2006;20:547–54.

103. Boswell S, McIff TE, Trease CA, et al. Mechanical characteristics of locking and compression plate constructs applied dorsally to distal radius fractures. J Hand Surg 2007;32:623–9.

104. Weinstein DM, Bratton DR, Ciccone Ii WJ, et al. Locking plates improve torsional resistance in the stabilization of three-part proximal humeral fractures. J Shoulder Elbow Surg 2006;15:239–43.

105. Korner J, Diederichs G, Arzdorf M, et al. A biomechanical evaluation of methods of distal humerus fracture fixation using locking compression plates versus conventional reconstruction plates. J Orthop Trauma 2004;18:286–93.

106. O'Toole RV, Andersen RC, Vesnovsky O, et al. Are locking screws advantageous with plate fixation of humeral shaft fractures? A biomechanical analysis of synthetic and cadaveric bone. J Orthop Trauma 2008;22:709–15.

107. Chiodo TA, Ziccardi VB, Janal M, et al. Failure strength of 2.0 locking versus 2.0 conventional Synthes mandibular plates: a laboratory model. J Oral Maxillofac Surg 2006;64:1475–9.

108. Amato NS, Richards A, Knight TA, et al. Ex vivo biomechanical comparison of the 2.4 mm UniLOCK® reconstruction plate using 2.4 mm locking versus standard screws for fixation of acetabular osteotomy in dogs. Vet Surg 2008;37:741–8.

109. Sommer C, Babst R, Muller M, et al. Locking compression plate loosening and plate breakage: a report of four cases. J Orthop Trauma 2004;18:571–7.

110. Kubiak EN, Fulkerson E, Strauss E, et al. The evolution of locked plates. J Bone Joint Surg Am 2006;88:189–200.

111. Maxwell M, Horstman CL, Crawford RL, et al. The effects of screw placement on plate strain in 3.5 mm dynamic compression plates and limited-contact dynamic compression plates. Vet Comp Orthop Traumatol 2009;22:125–31.

112. Bottlang M, Lesser M, Koerber J, et al. Far cortical locking can improve healing of fractures stabilized with locking plates. J Bone Joint Surg Am 2010;92:1652–60.

113. Bottlang M, Doornink J, Fitzpatrick DC, et al. Far cortical locking can reduce stiffness of locked plating constructs while retaining construct strength. J Bone Joint Surg Am 2009;91:1985–94.

114. Döbele S, Horn C, Eichhorn S, et al. The dynamic locking screw (DLS) can increase interfragmentary motion on the near cortex of locked plating constructs by reducing the axial stiffness. Langenbecks Arch Surg 2010;395:421–8.

115. Vallier H, Hennessey T, Sontich J. Failure of LCP condylar plate fixation in the distal part of the femur. A report of six cases. J Bone Joint Surg Am 2006;88:846–53.

116. Lujan T, Henderson C, Madey S. Locked plating of distal femur fractures leads to inconsistent and asymmetric callus formation. J Orthop Trauma 2010;24:156–62.

117. Kregor P, Stannard J, Zlowodzki M. Treatment of distal femur fractures using the less invasive stabilization system: surgical experience and early clinical results in 103 fractures. J Orthop Trauma 2004;18:509–20.

118. Bottlang M, Doornink J, Byrd GD, et al. A nonlocking end screw can decrease fracture risk caused by locked plating in the osteoporotic diaphysis. J Bone Joint Surg Am 2009;91:620–7.

Minimally Invasive Plate Osteosynthesis Fracture Reduction Techniques in Small Animals

Bruno Peirone, DVM, PhD[a],*, Gian Luca Rovesti, DVM, ECVS[b],
Alessandro Boero Baroncelli, DVM, PhD[a], Lisa Piras, DVM, PhD[a]

KEYWORDS

- MIPO • Fracture • Reduction • Alignment • Traction • Distractor

KEY POINTS

- Anatomic fracture reduction is not typically achieved with minimally-invasive fracture repair in small animals.
- Indirect fracture reduction is used with minimally invasive plate osteosynthesis to restore limb's length and alignment.
- Indirect fracture reduction preserves soft tissue attachment to fracture fragments, speeding healing and reducing complications.
- Many techniques are available to facilitate fracture reduction, including hanging the limb, manual traction, distraction table, external fixators, and a fracture distractor.

INTRODUCTION

Minimally invasive plate osteosynthesis (MIPO) in small animals involves the application of a bone plate, typically in a bridging fashion, without performing a surgical approach to expose the fracture site.[1]

Treatment of a diaphyseal fracture with MIPO does not usually require the anatomic reduction of the fracture. Functional reduction is the goal; it restores bone length and correct alignment in the frontal, sagittal, and axial planes. Indirect reduction is used to obtain functional fracture reduction without opening the fracture site. This method allows the fracture fragments to remain connected to the adjacent soft tissues. This is the key to improve bone healing because viable bone rapidly unites by callus formation.[2]

[a] Dipartimento di Patologia Animale, Facoltà di Medicina Veterinaria, via Leonardo da Vinci 44, Grugliasco, Turin 10095, Italy; [b] Clinica Veterinaria Miller - Via della Costituzione 10, 42025 Cavriago, Reggio Emilia, Italy
* Corresponding author.
E-mail address: bruno.peirone@unito.it

Vet Clin Small Anim 42 (2012) 873–895
http://dx.doi.org/10.1016/j.cvsm.2012.06.002
0195-5616/12/$ – see front matter © 2012 Elsevier Inc. All rights reserved.

Indirect reduction is the "blind" repositioning of bone fragments using some form of distraction and translation. This method relies on aligning fragments and restoring bone length by distracting the bone ends instead of manipulating the fracture site. It is achieved using a remote instrument so that there is no disturbance of the soft tissues around the fracture site. Indirect reduction may require exposure to apply the reduction devices, but not for visualization of the fracture site.

The general principle involved in indirect reduction is the use of the soft-tissue envelope to help stabilize and reduce the fracture fragments indirectly. This can be achieved through forces applied either on the adjacent bone segments or on the epiphyseal or metaphyseal regions of the fractured bone. The former is commonly referred to as ligamentotaxis.[3] Traction table and limb hanging techniques are prime examples. In the latter, the tension on the soft tissues surrounding the fracture site guides the fragments into alignment as the bone ends are distracted. Intramedullary (IM) pinning, temporary application of a linear or circular external skeletal fixator, bone-holding forceps, bone distractor, or the plate itself are examples of this. These techniques can be used as a sole method of reduction or in any combination.

Fracture reduction can be accomplished completely closed or with the help of small incisions (portals). Proximal and distal incisions are needed to insert the plate and screws when using MIPO technique. A small third portal (observation portal) can be used to view the fracture zone to facilitate placement of an IM pin (see later discussion). It should be emphasized that manipulation of the fracture fragments should be avoided when using an observation portal. If fracture reduction is unsuccessful using the following techniques, the surgeon should consider using a technique described by Hulse as "open but don't touch."[4] A long incision is made over the length on the bone, but the fracture fragments are not manipulated. This more generous approach allows an improved view of the fracture, facilitating indirect reduction of the fracture.

SKELETAL TRACTION TABLE

Traction tables are commonly used in human trauma patients and standardized reproducible techniques are routinely used for fracture reduction. These techniques include proper patient positioning, specific instrumentation, and application of intraoperative skeletal traction (IST).[5,6] The rationale behind fracture reduction by IST is counteracting the muscle contraction and regaining the original limb length. In this way, the bone segments are not overlapped and easily fit each other. When fragmentation is present, the fragments are pulled back in the area they came from by their muscular attachments, which exert a centripetal force. This philosophy of reduction, called ligamentotaxis, has the main objective of achieving fracture reduction by a minimally invasive or close approach.

Recently, a skeletal traction table (Ergomed 99, Ad Maiora, Cavriago, Italy) was specifically designed for veterinary traumatology.[7] This table allows IST to be consistently applied in small animals with safe application of opposition and anchorage points.[8]

The opposition points are defined as the points on the body where stabilization can be applied to counteract the traction forces and avoid translation, without injuring the patient. Anchorage points are defined as the points where traction can be applied distal to the fractured skeletal segment, without damaging the bone or the soft tissues (**Fig. 1**).

Indications

The veterinary traction table has been used to apply IST and reduce different fracture patterns of the appendicular skeleton.[7] It is mandatory to thoroughly follow the

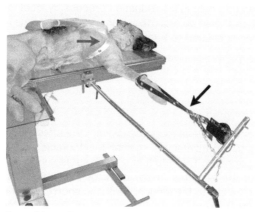

Fig. 1. Skeletal traction table and patient positioning for the craniomedial approach to the antebrachium in a cadaver. Traction is applied via coupled bands connected to the elongating stand (*black arrow*). The animal's body is held in position by two nylon bands crossed over the sternum (*red arrow*).

suggested steps in applying the technique. It is a powerful technique that can be potentially dangerous if applied in the wrong way.

Application of IST with Traction Table

The anchorage devices used for application of traction are represented by anchorage belts for the antebrachium and tibia and a traction stirrup attached to a transcondylar Kirschner wire (K-wire) in the humerus and femur.

The belts are coupled, to evenly distribute the traction forces to both sides of the limb, and then applied in the metacarpal or metatarsal area.

The traction stirrup is used in conjunction with a transosseous K-wire through the condylar region of the humerus or the femur, in a position that is compatible with the site of fracture and the proposed osteosynthesis technique. The wire ends are connected to the stirrup arms by means of bolts. Once secured, the wire is tensioned by the stirrup lever mechanism. This tensioning avoids wire bending and prevents soft tissues from being cut by the bent wire.

The traction is exerted by means of a micrometric traction stand that can be lengthened by up to 20 cm.

The traction stand has an L shape: the long component has a micrometric movement that allows stand elongation. One end of the stand is attached to the table rails with a clamp. The short component has three pins that allow the connection to either of the belts or the stirrup.

Traction is applied progressively and incrementally increased at a rate of about 50 N every 2 minutes and more traction is applied as needed to maintain the scheduled force. The amount of load applied is related to the patient body weight, muscular strength, and time between trauma and surgery, but especially to the quality of fracture alignment obtained. The fracture distraction and alignment achieved can be judged by palpation of the fractured site and or with intraoperative imaging.

During the application of traction, the maximal traction load is measured using a dynamometer. For safety reasons, the maximum load applied to each limb is never allowed to exceed 250 N. If the reduction is not achieved with this amount of load, some kind of interference should be suspected. A reduced approach to the fracture area can be considered to help in the reduction process by local direct manipulation. The duration of traction should be recorded. A shorter traction time reduces the potential damage to tissues subjected to traction.

The positioning for the traction of each bone segment is as follows.

Patient Positioning

Antebrachium
The animal is positioned in lateral recumbency with the affected limb lowermost and the contralateral forelimb maintained against the thoracic wall with the shoulder flexed. The neck is extended. The limb that is to be subjected to traction is positioned with the midshaft of the humerus at the edge of the table. The traction stand is attached to the table caudal to the forelimb, with the short component oriented cranially so that traction can be exerted with the craniomedial region of the radius remaining completely unobstructed.

Opposition points Two bands are crossed over the sternum. A dorsal stabilizer is used on the dorsal area of the neck. The band crossing the upper side surface of the neck region is passed over the stabilizer so that excessive pressure on the base of the neck by this band is avoided.

Anchorage points For this traction technique, traction belts applied to the carpometacarpal region of the forelimb are usually used. A transosseous K-wire can also be inserted through the distal epiphyseal region of the radius or through the metacarpal bones for anchorage in the case of older, displaced, or overriding fractures.

Humerus
Lateral plate application The animal is positioned in lateral recumbency with the affected limb uppermost. The contralateral forelimb is flexed at the elbow and secured with the carpus under the animal's muzzle. The traction stand is placed caudal to the forelimb with the short component oriented caudally to exert axial traction on the humerus.

Opposition points A single band is passed circumferentially around the thorax in the region caudal to the axilla. Sometimes the application of a second K-wire and traction stirrup to the proximal metaphysis of the humerus is required. This approach is adopted because humeral traction applied with a single distal stirrup causes significant distal translation of the scapula without obtaining satisfactory alignment of the fracture segments.

Anchorage points For this technique, the traction stirrup is used. A K-wire is inserted with lateromedial direction across the condylar region or, instead, across the proximal ulna just following the humeral axis. Traction exerted with the bands applied to the carpometacarpal region can damage the distal structures before exerting a useful traction on the humerus because the musculature surrounding the humerus is usually very strong.

Medial and caudomedial plate application The patient is positioned similar to that used for the antebrachium. The body of the patient is slightly tilted by interposition of sand bags between the thorax and the table. In all other respects, traction stand position and opposition points are the same as for the antebrachium (**Fig. 2**).

Anchorage points These are the SAME as described for the humeral lateral approach.

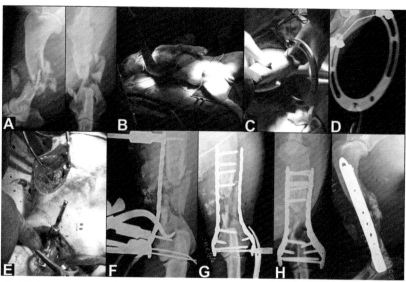

Fig. 2. (*A*) Preoperative radiographs of a comminuted humeral fracture. (*B*) Patient positioning. (*C*) Anchorage point: K-wire inserted in the proximal ulna and connected to an arch. (*D*) Intraoperative radiograph. (*E*) Temporary plate stabilization with push-pull devices on the medial side. (*F*) Intraoperative radiograph. (*G*) Intraoperative radiograph of temporary plate stabilization on the lateral side. (*H*) Immediate postoperative radiographs.

Tibia

Medial plate application: lateral recumbency The animal is positioned in lateral recumbency with the affected limb lowermost and the contralateral hindlimb secured caudally with the stifle flexed and the hip extended. The limb that is to be subjected to traction is positioned with the midpoint of the femoral diaphysis overlying the border of the table. The traction stand is positioned caudal to the limb, with the shorter component of the stand oriented cranially, to keep the craniomedial aspect of the tibia completely unobstructed.

Medial plate application: dorsal recumbency This positioning is very useful because allows a better assessment of the limb alignment on the frontal plane. The animal is positioned in dorsal recumbency. The limb being subjected to traction is extended caudally, with a support placed in the popliteal region. The contralateral hindlimb is positioned in abduction with the joints flexed and secured such that the calcaneus is as close as possible to the ischiatic tuberosity. The traction stand is connected to the end of the table. Usually, a dorsal positioner is put underneath the thoracic region to maintain this position during traction.

Opposition points For the craniomedial approach to the tibia, two nylon bands are applied. One band is passed over the uppermost ilium, across the inguinal region, and under the scrotum of male animals, and then secured to the table caudodorsally. It is useful to add a protective polyurethane cushion to this band, to prevent any harm to the patient. The second band is passed circumferentially around the caudal region of the abdomen and both ends are secured to the table dorsally.

For the craniomedial approach with dorsal recumbency, the oppositional forces are applied to the caudal part of the thigh by means of a limb rest placed in the popliteal region.

Anchorage points Coupled nylon bands are applied to the tarsometatarsal region of the limb for traction to evenly distribute the forces along the longitudinal axis of the tibia. The traction stirrup can be anchored to a transosseous K-wire inserted in the distal epiphysis of the tibia (**Fig. 3**) or to the metatarsal bones in cases of distal, over-riding fractures.

Femur

The animal is positioned in lateral recumbency with the limb being subjected to traction uppermost. The contralateral limb is secured to the table caudally with the stifle flexed and the calcaneus positioned close to the ischiatic tuberosity. The traction stand is attached to the table cranial to the limb, with the shorter component oriented caudally to exert the traction along the longitudinal axis of the femur. A limb rest is used to support the tarsus to maintain the limb in a horizontal plane.

Opposition points A band is passed across the abdomen caudally, just under the iliac wing, then across the inguinal region and under the scrotum of male animals. It is useful to add a protective polyurethane cushion to this band, to prevent any harm to the patient. The band is secured caudodorsally to the table. A second band is passed around the caudal region of the abdomen and both ends of this band are secured to the table dorsally.

Anchorage points For this traction technique, the traction stirrup anchored to a trans-condylar K-wire placed at distal end of the femur is used, because of the strength of the thigh muscles.

Procedure Technique

Traction modalities vary in each case, mostly based on fracture location.

Usually, the animals affected by radius-ulna and tibia closed fractures are positioned on the traction table and traction is applied before the limb is scrubbed. Once the fracture segments are realigned, the fracture reduction is confirmed by digital palpation, radiology, fluoroscopy, or a combination of them. In this setting, the reduction procedure is performed without scrubbing of the limb. Once the fracture is satisfactorily realigned, the limb is maintained in traction, scrubbed, and prepared for surgery as usual. With this traction modality, the traction devices are nonsterile and are not included in the surgical field.

For open fractures stabilization, the limb is prepared for surgery, as usual, and traction is applied in a sterile surgical field.

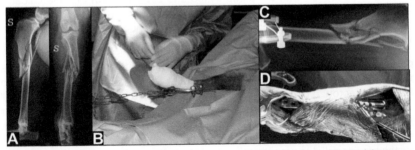

Fig. 3. (*A*) Preoperative radiographs of a comminuted tibial fracture. (*B*) IST. (*C*) Intraoperative medio-lateral radiograph showing the fracture indirect reduction. (*D*) Plate insertion in MIPO fashion. S, Sinistra (Left, in Italian).

For fractures of the humerus and femur, the limb is first scrubbed and prepared for surgery as usual. After performing the surgical approaches, the transcondylar K-wire is inserted and the sterile traction stirrup is applied and then connected to the micrometric traction stand with a small sterile chain. The end of this chain connected to the stirrup is kept sterile, while the end connected to the dynamometer and distraction stand becomes contaminated. An unscrubbed operating room assistant, who sets the load on the surgeon's request, applies the load required to distract the fracture segments. Contamination of the surgical field is avoided, because the assistant can set the traction stand from its top, far from the surgical field, while the portion of the traction stand close to the surgical field remains covered by sterile towels.

Correction of malalignment

Correction of intraoperative angular malalignment of fractures is performed entirely by the unscrubbed assistant who moves the traction stand under the direction of the surgeon, as described above.[6] Correction of varus or valgus malalignment is achieved by rotating the short portion of the traction stand in a clockwise or counterclockwise direction, after temporarily loosening the lock of the clamp holding this bar. In this way, the tip of the bar is moved higher or lower than the starting point. For example, elevation of the tip of the bar results in correction of a valgus malalignment of the tibia with the animal in lateral recumbency and the operated limb in lowermost position. However, the direction of the correction in relation to the animal's position should be evaluated. For example, when the animal is in dorsal recumbency, the correction of valgus or varus deformity is performed by loosening the clamp and sliding the entire traction stand, along the lateral rail of the table, either in a medial or lateral direction.

To correct procurvatum or recurvatum malalignment, for all the positions but for the tibia with the animal in dorsal recumbency, the clamp is loosened and the entire traction stand is pushed horizontally along the lateral rail of the table. The clamp and the connected traction stand are pushed toward the cranial part of the animal for the correction of procurvatum and toward the caudal part for the correction of recurvatum. For the approach to the tibia with the animal in dorsal recumbency, the upward or downward rotation of the shorter part of the traction stand is used for the correction of procurvatum and recurvatum malalignment, respectively.

Potential Complications

This system of skeletal traction for fracture reduction has some elasticity that is inherent to the animal's tissues and the anchoring and opposition bands, which renders the process nonlinear during the initial stages. Although the application of opposition and anchorage belts is relatively simple, slippage of these belts may also contribute to this problem[7] or result in local tissue injury. On the other hand, the traction applied with a traction stirrup results in negligible elastic drop and does not cause any compressive soft tissue injury. It is important to use the opposition points that were developed from the cadaver study[7] and to monitor duration and magnitude of the loading force to avoid any tissue damage.

Excessive traction also potentially results in compromise of the nervous and vascular systems. In circumstances in which an elevated load must be applied, it may be prudent to minimize its duration to reduce the likelihood of complications. When the procedure cannot be completed in a sufficiently brief period, it is preferable to consider temporary stabilization of the fracture (ie, long oblique fracture) with either a point-reduction forceps or a K-wire applied percutaneously, releasing the traction to allow tissues to be better perfused, and then resuming traction after a short period.

Proper patient positioning and the use of skeletal traction are easily learned techniques that can rapidly become standard procedure. Although the time required for setting up of the table, positioning of the patient, and performing traction is somewhat lengthy, this time is regained during the osteosynthesis phase. In fact, plate application in an MIPO fashion is greatly simplified once the desired reduction is achieved because the osseous segments are steadily maintained in correct alignment for the necessary amount of time.

However, the technique may be potentially dangerous and, therefore, should be applied cautiously to avoid iatrogenic trauma. It is imperative that the application of opposition and anchorage points is correct, and prolonged and unnecessary loading is avoided.

LIMB HANGING

Suspending the limb from an infrastructure or from the ceiling orients the limb in a vertical position. By lowering the surgical table the animal's own weight distracts the fracture and helps aligning the joint surfaces.[9,10] Intraoperative imaging is greatly facilitated because both frontal and sagittal planes are unobstructed and the C-arm or portable radiograph machine can be freely moved around the patient.

Indications

This technique is mostly indicated for comminuted fractures of the antebrachium and tibia when used alone.

The subsequent application of a temporary circular or linear external fixator can greatly improve the stability of the fracture reduction.

Procedure Technique

The animal is positioned for surgery in dorsal recumbency, with the affected limb suspended and draped. The anchorage point should be exactly over the limb, to exert a linear traction along the long axis of the fractured bone (**Fig. 4**). The use of a sterile snap-hook system allows the surgeon to disconnect the limb from the anchorage point to evaluate joints' flexion and plane of motion after temporary plate application.[9]

Potential Complications

The weight of the animal restricts the achievement of the fracture reduction.

This technique does not provide control over the horizontal plane. It is, therefore, important to verify rotational alignment after temporary fixation by disconnecting the

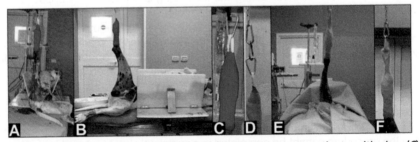

Fig. 4. (A, B) Hanging limb technique for tibial fracture treatment: patient positioning. (C) A nonsterile pulley system is used to suspend the limb. (D) A sterile snap-hook system is secured to the paw. (E) The paw and the pulley system are wrapped with sterile self-adherent tape, (F) allowing the surgeon to disconnect the leg during the procedure.

limb from the suspending hook and flexing and extending the adjacent joints. In tibial fractures, traction applied to the pes frequently results in a caudal translation of the distal fragment. This phenomenon must be taken into account before plate positioning.

IM PINNING

An IM pin used as a distraction device is an effective method to overcome muscle resistance and gradually restoring length and axial alignment of a fractured bone.[9]

The IM pin placed near the neutral axis of the bone is very resistant to bending forces and, therefore, capable of maintaining axial alignment.[11]

Advantages in using an IM pin for indirect reduction in MIPO include:

1. An additional surgical approach is usually not required for normograde pin insertion
2. Pin progression in the distal fragment allows fracture distraction by overcoming the muscles contraction
3. The bone surface is free for further plate application
4. Plate application is easier owing to partial stabilization and alignment of the fracture
5. Proper limb alignment can be confirmed by observing joint orientation during flexion and extension of the proximal and distal joints.

Indication

All long-bone fractures can be treated with indirect reduction achieved by means of an IM pin but, in the case of a radius fracture, the IM pin would be inserted in the ulna.

Long oblique and comminuted fractures with a large fracture gap are suitable for IM pin reduction. Pin progression in the distal bone segment is especially simple in the case of comminuted fractures, because usually there is no overriding of the main segments.

If the fracture pattern is characterized by a small proximal or distal segment it will be more challenging to obtain and temporarily maintain a correct axial alignment. This is due to the small bone stock and consequent inadequate pin-bone purchase.

Short oblique or transverse fractures are more demanding. Muscle contraction produces large fracture dislocation and segment overriding is always present. Gradual and progressive traction has to be applied over a period of time to overcome muscle contraction and achieve fracture alignment. Elevating and distracting the fractured bone ends using bone-holding forceps through the surgical approaches reduces segment overriding and allows pin progression in the distal fragment.[9]

Smooth pins with tips at one or both ends are used, and their size normally ranges from 1.2 to 4 mm in diameter. Correct pin selection is related to bone diameter and determined from preoperative radiographs during surgical planning. The diameter of the pins used should be approximately 30% to 50% of the diameter of the bone's medullary cavity.[4]

Procedure Technique

Surgical proximal and distal approaches, as described for MIPO application in animals, have to be performed before IM pin insertion.[1,12]

The proximal intact bone segment is secured with a bone-holding forceps and the pin is advanced distally. If the pin is properly aligned, it progresses easily in the medullary cavity. In case of difficult progression, the pin is penetrating the cortex and should be redirected.

The pin tip is cut and the pin passed carefully through the fragmented area of the bone.

To cut the distal tip of the pin two options are available:

1. Withdraw the inserted pin, cut the tip, and reinsert it with the same direction
2. Proceed with pin insertion until the tip emerges from the distal approach, then cut the tip.

The pin can be advanced by drill, pushed through using the drill with the motor stopped,[10] or by hand using a mallet.

Without the pointed tip, the distal part of the IM pin leans against the metaphyseal bone of the distal segment, distracting the fracture gap while restoring bone length and aligning the main bone segments.[4,13]

Long pins left out from the entrance point help in the intraoperative evaluation of pin direction.

A second pin with the same length can be used to evaluate IM pin depth in the distal segment's medullary canal.

Holding the distal segment with point-reduction forceps percutaneously, or with bone-holding forceps applied through the distal approach, helps in maintaining the correct axial alignment during pin progression. To achieve adequate stability, the pin must be seated in the cancellous bone of the distal metaphyseal region.

Once in place, the IM pin assists in maintaining the axial alignment of the bone in both frontal and sagittal planes. However, because it does not effectively counteract torsional forces, it is important to check torsional alignment before plate application, especially in comminuted fractures.

Proper pin positioning and bone alignment can be assessed clinically, but thorough intraoperative diagnostic imaging is recommended, especially in proximal bone segments. Once correct pin placement is confirmed, the IM pin can be left in place to function as a plate-rod construct or removed when the plate has been sufficiently secured to the major bone segments.[4,12] If the pin is left in place, the proximal portion could be cut close to its exit from the bone. More commonly, if the diameter of the pin allows it, the pin is bent at its exit from the proximal segment and cut to allow its removal following fracture healing.

Humerus

Lateral approach The lateral approach is mainly used in proximal and middle-third fractures.

The patient is positioned in lateral recumbency with the affected limb uppermost. The proximal approach is performed on the medial aspect of the greater tubercle. The curvature of the bone and the level of the shaft fracture determine the point for insertion of the pin on the cranial crest of the greater tubercle. A point-reduction forceps can be used to hold the proximal segment during pin insertion.

The IM pin is driven from the proximal segment by entering the bone on the lateral slope of the ridge of the greater tubercle near its base.[10,11] Initial drilling is done with the pin held perpendicular to the bone surface. After tip penetration of the outer cortex, the pin is redirected distally into the medullary canal to shift parallel to the caudomedial cortex. The pin must be seated just proximal to the supratrochlear foramen.[10]

Medial approach This approach is mainly used in distal-third fractures.

The patient is positioned in lateral recumbency with the affected limb lowermost and the contralateral retracted caudally. The distal approach is performed along the caudal cortex of the medial epicondyle and soft tissue dissection is performed, being mindful of the ulnar nerve, which should be identified and retracted cranially. Bone-holding forceps can be used to secure the distal fragment during pin insertion. The IM pin enters the bone just distally to the square corner of the medial portion of the condyle, directed parallel to its caudal cortex. Proper pin size must be determined on preoperative radiographs so that it can pass along the medullary canal of the medial epicondyle. The pin progresses through the fracture site and advances proximally along the cranial cortex of the proximal segment.[14]

Femur

The patient is positioned in lateral recumbency with the affected limb uppermost.

Once the proximal approach has been performed, the pin is inserted through the subcutaneous fat and the gluteal muscles until the top of the great trochanter is felt with the tip of the pin. During pin insertion, the proximal femur is held with a bone-holding forceps at the angle and rotation of the normal standing position.[10] Maintaining the same axis as the femur, the pin is gently moved medially off the trochanter into the trochanteric fossa, where it will center itself with some pressure. To avoid slippage, the tip of the pin is first seated into the metaphyseal bone of the trochanteric fossa in a cranial direction. Once penetration begins, the pin is aligned with the long axis of the proximal femoral segment.

Tibia

The patient is positioned in dorsal recumbency with the stifle flexed at a right angle.

The proximal approach is performed on the medial aspect of the proximal tibia over the medial collateral ligament and slightly extended proximally to the medial aspect of the stifle joint (**Fig. 5**).

The pin is then inserted along the medial border of the patellar ligament, entering the proximal end of the tibia between the cranial surface of the tibial tubercle and the medial condyle of the tibia.[10]

Radius and ulna

Fractures affecting the antebrachium can be reduced both with retrograde and normograde IM pinning of the ulna.

The size of the pin should be as large as it can fit in the distal medullary canal of the ulna. The patient is positioned in dorsal recumbency, allowing an easy approach to the radius by extending the elbow and to the ulna by flexing the elbow joint. With minimal soft tissue dissection, the deep flexor muscles on the caudal aspect of the ulna are

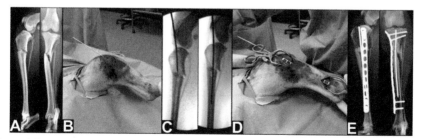

Fig. 5. (*A*) Preoperative radiographs of a mildly comminuted proximal tibia and fibula fracture. (*B*) Normograde IM pinning of the tibia. (*C*) Intraoperative fluoroscopy images showing the indirect reduction of the fracture. (*D*) Plate insertion through medial proximal and distal incisions using an MIPO technique. (*E*) Immediate postoperative radiographs. (*Courtesy of* A. Pozzi, Gainesville, FL.)

elevated to expose the fractured ends of the ulna. The pin is retrograde inserted in the proximal segment to exit at the olecranon. The ulnar fracture is reduced and the pin normograde driven across the fracture site and ideally seated in the distal metaphysis of the ulna.[15] Normograde pin insertion is also possible, but more challenging (**Fig. 6**).

Potential Complications

If a plate and rod technique is selected to treat the fracture, the IM pin can interfere with bicortical screw insertion, especially in the diaphyseal region.

Joint penetration could be possible during pin progression in the distal segment, but is unlikely to occur once the tip has been severed.

When a plate and rod construct is applied, pin migration can occur during the postoperative period and pin removal is, therefore, recommended.[4]

LINEAR EXTERNAL FIXATION

Full pin frames allow correction of angular deformity and maintenance of bone length.

This technique requires shorter setup times, provides complete access to the bone, and allows complete manipulation of the limb, thereby facilitating plate application while avoiding the use of excessive traction because the reduction force is applied solely to the bone and not across the proximal and distal joints.

Indication

Linear external fixation is indicated in fractures of the antebrachium and tibia because of the relative paucity of soft tissues surrounding them. Humerus and femur are not recommended because of the large muscle bellies.

Procedure Technique

During the surgical positioning of the patient, the affected limb is securely suspended from a ceiling hook and draped. Using a sterile hook system allows the surgeon to disconnect the leg during the procedure.[9] Transfixating full-threaded pins are placed in the proximal and distal metaphyses of each bone segment. Their diameter must not exceed 20% to 30% of the width of the medullary canal.[16] The pins are centered in the bone on the sagittal plane and parallel to their respective joint surface. The proximal pin should be placed sufficiently posterior so as not to interfere with plate positioning.[17] It is mandatory to place fixation elements only in safe soft tissues

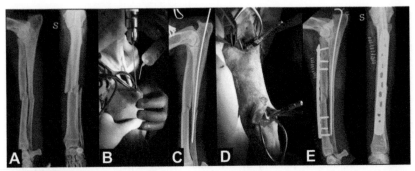

Fig. 6. (*A*) Preoperative radiographs of a comminuted radius and ulna fracture. (*B*) Normograde IM pinning of the ulna. (*C*) Intraoperative radiograph. (*D*) Temporary plate stabilization with push-pull devices. (*E*) Immediate postoperative radiographs. S, Sinistra (Left, in Italian).

corridors.[18] Care must be taken before pin insertion to avoid multiple attempts that would increase the risk of iatrogenic fracture or bone necrosis. Intraoperative radiographic control or fluoroscopy is used to assess correct pin placement.

The table is then lowered or a pulley system used to raise the limb, suspending the patient by the fractured limb. The weight of the patient distracts the fracture and helps aligning the joint surfaces. If necessary, manual distraction on the threaded pin can improve alignment. The connecting bars are placed and limb alignment clinically evaluated. Intraoperative fluoroscopy or radiology is valuable in the assessment of correct alignment.[9]

Only after good reduction and alignment have been achieved the plate can be inserted and secured to the bone.

Potential Complications

Special care is needed to avoid intraarticular pin placement and to ensure that the pins are effectively parallel to the proximal and distal joint surfaces to prevent malalignment.

It is important to avoid pin placement into fissures or superficial cortical areas, possibly resulting in fractures.

Attention must be paid to avoid nerve or vessel injury during pin insertion, respecting safe corridors.

Leaving empty holes is not ideal because this can lead to subsequent bone fracture, probably because of the stress riser effect caused by creating a defect in the cortical bone. Placing a hole too close to one cortex, eccentrically, rather than penetrating the bone in its middle area could also create a stress riser.

CIRCULAR EXTERNAL FIXATION

Tensioned small diameter wires and circular rings can be used with a simple, efficient technique, described by Jackson and colleagues,[17] which allows for precise reduction, length restoration, excellent control of rotation, and easy access for imaging. Once held at the correct length, the frame construct will resist shortening and, perhaps, distraction forces during plate positioning. The application of the frame is straightforward and may be rapidly accomplished and the insertion of fine wires is minimally invasive, causing little tissue trauma.

Indication

Circular external fixation indirect reduction technique is indicated in tibia, radius and ulna fractures. Humerus and femur fractures are less commonly reduced by this technique because of the large muscle bellies and the impingement given by the thorax and the abdomen. When used for those segments, half-rings are used.

This method is particularly useful in fragmented or segmental fractures where the reduction is difficult to maintain. It is challenging in proximal and distal-third fractures, where the frame can interfere with proper plate positioning and fixation. When this is the case, the reduction can be maintained by a transarticular frame.

Procedure Technique

The frame is preassembled with two rings or arches (partial rings) arranged in a single block configuration for the proximal and distal fragment. When arches are used, the proximal one is oriented with the open portion cranially for the radius and caudally for the tibia to avoid interference with elbow or stifle flexion. The distal arch is oriented with the open portion caudally for the radius and cranially for the tibia to avoid interference with the carpus and hock flexion. This frame construct allows for a better limb alignment evaluation during the surgical procedure.

The surgeon must choose a ring or arch size that can be placed around the animal's limb while still having enough space between the skin and the inner margin of the ring to position the plate.

The rings or arches are connected using two threaded rods, positioned to avoid interference with safe corridors and subsequent plate application.

The transosseous wire size is selected according to established guidelines.[19]

A standard hanging limb preparation is performed with the animal in dorsal recumbency in a way that to retains the possibility of attaching and detaching the limb from the hanging support.

The first transosseous wire is placed in the proximal radius or tibia, parallel to the mediolateral axis of the elbow or stifle joint and perpendicular to the longitudinal axis of the proximal segment. The proximal wire should be placed sufficiently posterior so as not to interfere with plate positioning.[17]

The preassembled frame is passed over the limb and connected to the proximal wire. The distal transosseous wire is inserted in a direction that is parallel to the antebrachiocarpal, or hock joint, and perpendicular to the longitudinal axis of the distal segment.

It is recommended that fixation elements be placed only in safe soft tissue corridors. Care must be taken before wire insertion to avoid multiple attempts that would increase the risk of iatrogenic fracture or bone necrosis.

Proper placement of the wires is confirmed through intraoperative radiographs or fluoroscopy. The distal wire is then connected to the frame. The wires are tensioned to a maximum of 30 kg to avoid arch deformation.[19]

Fracture reduction is achieved by gentle and progressive distraction of the rings or arches. Distraction is applied by turning the nuts on the threaded rods. By ensuring that the two wires are inserted perpendicular to the longitudinal axis and parallel to each other in both frontal and sagittal planes, correction of alignment and rotation will be achieved because bone length is restored (**Fig. 7**).

Reduction and axial alignment can be improved by modifying the frame's spatial alignment, using the following methods[20]:

- The angled bar technique. This is used with systems that do no have hemispheric nuts and washers available and consists of changing the angle of a threaded bar between the rings or arches. This bar is connected to the rings or arches, offset by the amount of the deformity to be corrected but in the opposite direction. When the nuts on the previous straight connecting bars are loosened and the nuts on this angled bar are tightened, the angled bar becomes perpendicular to the rings, rotating the bone segment in the direction opposite to that of the deformity.
- Hemispheric nuts and washer technique. This method can be used with systems in which hemispheric nuts and washers are available. The nuts are loosened, the distal ring or arch is rotated in the direction opposite to the deformity, and the nuts are tightened again after deformity correction, leaving the threaded bars at an angle to the rings. Hemispheric nuts and washers can also be used to correct angular deformities. For example, if a valgus deformity is present, the length of the lateral threaded bar connecting the rings may be increased, while the nuts of the threaded bar on the medial side may be released to avoid them holding the rings in the previous position, preventing the frame construct from moving.
- Shifting of the bone along the wire. If a dislocatio ad latum is present, it can be corrected by shifting the bone along the wire, thus changing its position on the horizontal plane.

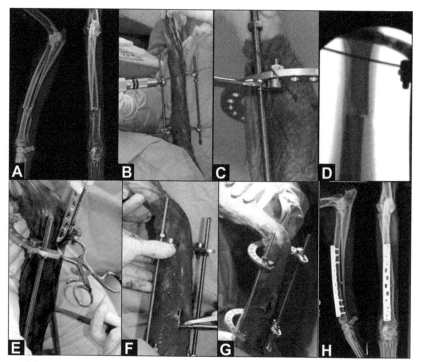

Fig. 7. (A) Preoperative radiographs of a comminuted radius and ulna fracture. (B) Application of the circular fixator (Imex Veterinary Inc, Longview, TX, USA). (C) Fracture distraction applied by turning the nut. (D) Intraoperative fluoroscopy showing fracture reduction. (E) Plate insertion in an MIPO fashion. (F) Screw insertion. (G) Limb alignment evaluation. (H) Immediate postoperative radiographs. (*Courtesy of* A. Pozzi, Gainesville, FL.)

- Rotation of the bone along the fulcrum of the wire. Once distraction of the fracture segments has been achieved, a residual angular deformity may still be present. The bone segment may be aligned using the wire as a fulcrum, thus changing its axis. For this procedure to be performed, it is mandatory that just one wire is inserted in each segment. If more than one wire is inserted in the bone segment, it will be locked.

Potential Complications

Special care has to be put to avoid intraarticular wire placement[18] and to ensure that the wires are effectively parallel to the proximal or distal joint surfaces respectively to prevent malalignment. It is important to avoid the placing of the transfixation pin into fissures or superficial cortical areas, possibly resulting in fractures. Care must be put to avoid nerve or vessel injury during wire insertion.

The use of small-size wires leaves a very small empty hole, diminishing the risk of stress riser effect and secondary fractures.

BONE-HOLDING FORCEPS

Small bone-holding forceps inserted far from the fracture site through the proximal and distal surgical approaches can be used to align the fracture.[21] The most distal and proximal parts of the bone segments are secured with the bone-holding forceps and the segments are distracted and manipulated to reduce the fracture.

This method is most successful in radius-ulna and tibia fractures in which the reduced muscle mass allows more accurate palpation and easier reduction.[1,10]

Nevertheless, a forceps is a space-occupying device and should be applied to the bone in a position that allows subsequent plate application. For example, in a tibial fracture the bone-holding forceps grip the cranial and caudal bone aspects to allow medial plate placement.

It should also be noted that bone-holding forceps are passive devices, requiring an assistant to maintain reduction until plate fixation is completed.

In humerus and femur fractures it is often more challenging to achieve and maintain proper fracture reduction with this method because of the large surrounding muscle. Therefore, in such cases, bone-holding forceps are mostly used in combination with other reduction techniques, such as IM pinning.

For example, in a femoral fracture the bone-holding forceps could be applied through the proximal surgical approach at the level of the subtrochanteric region to hold and maintain the proximal segment in a levered position during pin insertion (**Fig. 8**). A second bone-holding forceps, applied through the distal surgical approach at the level of the supratrochlear region, can be used to distract and manipulate the distal segment allowing pin insertion and progression.

Bone-holding forceps can also be used as an aid to further improve segment alignment when other indirect reduction techniques are used.

Occasionally, a point-reduction forceps can be used percutaneously (**Fig. 9**) to approximate a severely displaced fragment or long oblique fractures.[21]

FRACTURE DISTRACTOR

The fracture distractor is a mechanical device that applies the forces directly to the bone segments. It is composed of a threaded spindle that is fixed on one end while the other end features a sliding carriage that can be moved proximally or distally by tightening the two nuts placed above and below the carriage.

Adjacent parts of the body remain unobstructed. The fracture distractor allows easy distraction of the bone segments, even when severe muscle contraction is present.

Dynamizable linear fixators (Ad Maiora, Cavriago, Italy) that can exert distraction and compression are now available. They work like a temporary fracture distractor if plating is the scheduled procedure, or like a definitive stabilization device if more pins are added once the fracture reduction is achieved. The special clamps allow bone segment movement in all the planes, thus facilitating reduction maneuvers (**Fig. 10**).

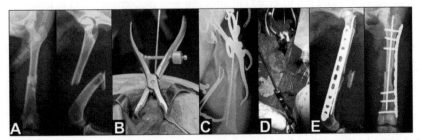

Fig. 8. (*A*) Preoperative radiographs of a butterfly femoral fracture. (*B*) The forceps holds the proximal segment during normograde IM pinning. (*C*) Intraoperative radiograph. (*D*) Temporary plate stabilization with push-pull devices. (*E*) Immediate postoperative radiographs.

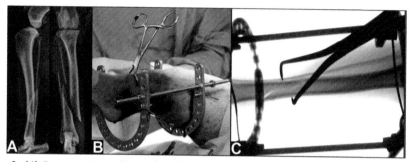

Fig. 9. (*A*) Preoperative radiographs of a long oblique tibia and fibula fracture. (*B*) The point-reduction forceps is used percutaneously to approximate the fracture. (*C*) Intraoperative fluoroscopy. (*Courtesy of* A. Pozzi, Gainesville, FL.)

In very unstable fractures, or when the plate could be potentially weak because of the features of the fracture or the patient's temperament, it can be used like a temporary ancillary stabilization device, to be removed after the early bony callus developed.

Indication

The fracture distractor is generally reserved for use in femur fractures in very large animals, with significant muscle contraction and fragment overriding, or in old fractures in which callus and muscle contracture must be overcome.

The extensible linear fixator can be used in almost all sizes of patients.

Procedure Technique

Two threaded pins are inserted in the metaphyseal area of both the proximal and distal segments.

The fracture distractor is then attached to the pins and the sliding carriage can then be moved distally, distracting the fracture. The offset position of the distractor allows the surgeon to access the fracture site for implant application. Varus, valgus, or rotational malalignment are corrected before pin placement and fracture distraction, using fluoroscopy to confirm proper alignment.

The technique is similar for the dynamizable linear fixator, but it does not require that the angular and torsional deformities be corrected before pin placement because the clamps allow the bone segments connected to the pins to be moved in every plane to achieve fracture reduction. When used like an ancillary temporary device, the distance from the bone and the clamp should be reduced to increase its stiffness, until the plate is secured to the bone.

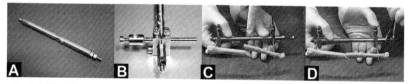

Fig. 10. (*A*) The dynamizable linear fixator. (*B*) Fixator clamp that allows multiplanar fracture segment adjustment. (*C*) Application of the dynamizable fixator to a plastic model simulating an overlapped fracture. Note the central part of the fixator body that is almost closed. (*D*) After fracture reduction, the central part of the fixator body is larger than before distraction. The clamps can now be set to better adjust the fracture reduction.

Potential Complications

Although the fracture distractor can be used to indirectly reduce comminuted fractures, it can be difficult to apply bridging plates in an MIPO fashion with the distractor in place.[8]

The dynamizable linear fixator should be used with long pins, to avoid interference with plate positioning. It should also be placed so that it does not interfere with plate positioning. For example, if a craniomedial plate is scheduled, it should be placed laterally.

REDUCTION THROUGH PLATE APPLICATION

The use of anatomically precontoured standard or locking plates in MIPO treatment of diaphyseal fractures helps to ensure proper reduction and correct limb alignment.[22]

Indication

This technique should be combined with one of the previously described methods of indirect reduction, to restore the correct bone length before plate application.

Only small displacements and angulations on both the frontal and the sagittal planes can be corrected while maintaining stability as the reduction occurs.[1]

Procedure Technique

Plate precontouring

The orthogonal radiographic views of the contralateral intact limb are used to select the adequate plate whole length and to contour the plate preoperatively.[21]

Plate length is evaluated on the mediolateral view and should be close to the length of the whole bone. Schmokel recommends the use of a long plate in MIPO applications to dissipate the stress on the construct.[23] Furthermore, longer plates with a limited number of screws positioned at the plate ends have shown to sustain greater loads before failing than shorter plates with a screw placed in each plate hole.[24]

Accurate plate precontouring is usually performed on the craniocaudal view to ensure proper axial alignment of the main fragments and correct bone length.[23]

Plate bending and twisting are performed to adapt plate ends to the shape of both the proximal and the distal metaphyseal regions of the fractured bone.

Standard plates

With standard bone plates, screw tightening produces frictional forces between the plate and the bone and, during weight bearing, the shearing load is transferred directly from the bone to the plate.[25] Therefore, accurate anatomic plate contouring is mandatory to maintain primary fracture reduction during screw tightening.[26]

After plate insertion, the proximal plate end is positioned on the center of the bone and fixed with a cortical screw inserted perpendicular to the cortex. This screw is not fully tightened to allow movement of the distal plate end. Bone-holding forceps can be used to center the plate over the bone or to achieve plate-bone contact. The bone cortex of the distal segment is then exposed and the plate end centered over the bone and fixed with a second cortical screw. Plate position is then checked by means of intraoperative imaging, after which both screws are tightened and fracture reduction is controlled before the final fixation.

If the axial alignment is not satisfactory, another cortical screw should be inserted closer to the fracture site through a separate stab incision, to act as a reduction screw. This allows the displaced segment to be pulled against the plate and reduced in a more anatomically correct position.[27]

Locking plates

With locking plates, a rigid connection between the plate hole and the screw is achieved; therefore, no frictional forces are produced between the plate and the bone.[25]

The advantage of locking plates is the minimal contouring required for their application in comparison to standard plates. The locking plate acts as an internal fixator and, therefore, does not displace the fracture segments during locking-screw tightening, regardless of the precision of contouring.[26]

To provide stable fixation, proper locking of the screw is essential. Temporary stable plate fixation to the bone is recommended before the insertion of the first locking screws.

The push-pull device (Synthes, Solothurn, Switzerland) is a temporary reduction device applied through a plate hole to hold the locking compression plate against the bone (**Fig. 11**). This device is self-drilling and connects with the quick coupling for power insertion. After monocortical insertion, the flange is turned clockwise until it pulls the plate securely against the bone. Once the plate is secured by the other screws, the push-pull device is removed and a screw can be inserted in the same hole.[28]

Another temporary reduction device is the pin-stopper, part of the Fixin system (Traumavet, Rivoli, Italy). The pin-stopper is a perforated stainless steel cylinder that can be inserted over a smooth pin and locked with a small screw nut (**Fig. 12**). The pin is inserted in the plate hole through a dedicated conical drill guide. Bicortical pin insertion is recommended to improve torsional stability. Pin insertion progresses until the stainless steel cylinder reaches the top of the conical drill guide and consequently pushes the plate against the bone. The use of a threaded pin can improve this action once the threaded tip enters the bone cortex.[29]

With a properly contoured implant, positioning temporary reduction devices in a hole that is further away from the ends of the plate allows better plate-bone contact and consequently more accurate fracture reduction (See **Fig. 12**).

Potential Complications

Inadequate plate contouring may result in loss of primary reduction and axial malalignment during cortical screw tightening or temporary plate fixation.

Axial malalignment can also occur, if bone length is not completely restored and segment overlapping is still present before plate application.

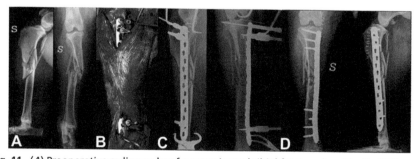

Fig. 11. (*A*) Preoperative radiographs of a comminuted tibial fracture (see **Fig. 3**). (*B*) Temporary plate stabilization with two push and pull devices. (*C*) Intraoperative radiographs showing the indirect reduction of the fracture. (*D*) Immediate post-operative radiographs. S, Sinistra (Left, in Italian).

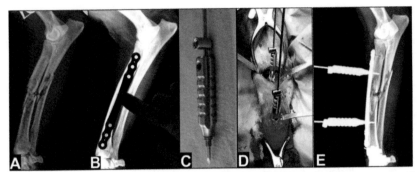

Fig. 12. (A) Preoperative mediolateral radiograph of a comminuted radius and ulna fracture. (B) Plate length assessment on the contralateral limb. (C) Pin-stopper with dedicated guide. (D) Two pin stoppers are inserted through the plate. (E) Intraoperative mediolateral radiograph showing indirect fracture reduction and temporary plate fixation.

If the proximal and distal screws are not inserted into the center of the bone, because of the plate being offset, or if their direction is not perpendicular to the cortical surface, segment rotation and translation may occur at the fracture site.[27]

Care must be taken during tightening of the first screws. The insertion torque applied could still result in dislocation of the bone segments. Therefore, palpation and assessment through visual or intraoperative imaging is recommended to avoid poor fracture reduction.

ASSESSMENT OF ALIGNMENT

After fracture indirect reduction has been achieved, care must be taken to carefully assess limb alignment. Malalignment is the most common complication associated with MIPO, because the fracture site is not exposed and the surgeon cannot rely on direct visualization of correct reduction to restore alignment.

It must be underlined that a loss of length or a moderate malalignment on the sagittal plane (procurvatum or recurvatum) does not affect the patient's functional outcome, whereas malalignment on the frontal (varus or valgus) or axial plane can severely compromise limb function.

Limb alignment can be assessed both by clinical evaluation and intraoperative fluoroscopy or radiology.

Proper patient positioning and surgical draping are mandatory to allow correct alignment evaluation. The limb should still be completely visible in both sagittal and frontal planes after draping, and the distalmost and proximalmost joints should be evaluated in their range of motion. This setting will allow the identification of anatomic landmarks, which is fundamental for clinical evaluation. Familiarity with the normal relationship between external anatomic landmarks is as essential as in depth knowledge of bone anatomy in preventing malalignment.[30]

The availability of a sterile bone model in the operating room can also help the surgeon to recognize these landmarks on the fractured limb.

Clinical evaluation can easily be performed on the antebrachium and crus, but it can be challenging for the arm and thigh, due to the presence of large muscle bellies.

Therefore, for the proximal bone segments, reliance on intraoperative diagnostic imaging is strongly recommended.

Access to a C-arm should be ensured to provide complete visualization of the proximal and distal joints in both frontal and sagittal planes. If fluoroscopy is not available, intraoperative radiographs can be obtained with a portable radiograph machine. Intraoperative radiographs are satisfactory for distal limb segments but suboptimal for proximal ones. Furthermore, the issue of radioprotection for the personnel is raised by the latter technique.

Clinical Evaluation

Tibia

The rotational and frontal alignment are subjectively evaluated with the stifle and hock joints flexed at 90°, by aligning the patella, the tibial crest, and the long axis of the III and IV metatarsal bones, and by reestablishing the sagittal plane of the hind limb. Furthermore, the position of the calcaneus can be assessed during flexion and extension of the stifle. If internal tibial torsion is present, the calcaneus appears to be displaced laterally, whereas, with external tibial torsion, it appears to be displaced medially. Moreover, observing the orientation of the pes with respect to the sagittal plane of the crus while palpating the malleoli is very helpful.[30]

Antebrachium

The same clinical assessment described for the tibia is used to evaluate the alignment of the forearm. The humeral condyle, the radius, and the long axis of the III and IV metacarpal bones are used to reestablish the sagittal plane of the forearm. The position of the flexed manus is useful to assess axial malalignment. A medial position indicates an external radial torsion, whereas a lateral position suggest an internal radial torsion.

Femur

The anatomic relationship between bone landmarks can also be reestablished in the femur, though it is more difficult.

Rotational alignment can be judged by palpation or by direct visualization of the greater trochanter and femoral trochlea through the proximal and distal approaches. The lateral aspect of the femoral trochlea can be palpated or observed through a stifle miniarthrotomy. The distal part of the femur is then held in a true lateral position. The position of the greater trochanter is then inspected through the proximal approach. If the femur is correctly aligned on the axial plane the greater trochanter should be slightly caudal compared with long axis of the bone. According to Dejardin and Guiot,[30] with the femur in a true lateral position, the midpoint of the greater trochanter should be slightly caudal to the coronal plane with the distal aspect of the line of origin of the vastus lateralis muscle aligned with the coronal plane.

Furthermore, in a correctly aligned femur, the surgeon can perform a 90° external and 45° internal rotation of the hip. This method is recommended only if the plate has been temporarily secured to the bone.

Humerus

The anatomic landmarks used for clinical evaluation are the humeral epicondyles, the greater tubercle, and the bicipital groove. These landmarks can be used to roughly evaluate humeral axial alignment. When holding the humeral epicondyles in a true mediolateral position, it should be possible to palpate the greater tubercle cranially and the bicipital groove medially.

Intraoperative Diagnostic Imaging

As previously stated, reliance on intraoperative diagnostic imaging is mandatory in the case of proximal limb fractures but generally suggested for all bone segments.

The anatomic details and relationship with the adjacent bones are evaluated through two orthogonal projections. These must include the whole bone segment and the proximal and distal joints. Comparison with the contralateral unaffected limb is also useful, if the required projections have been previously obtained.

Intraoperative fluoroscopy enables several quick spot projections of all the above-mentioned structures and is, therefore, the most useful method of assessing bone alignment.

SUMMARY

Indirect fracture reduction is used to align diaphyseal fractures in small animals when using minimally-invasive fracture repair. Indirect reduction achieves functional fracture reduction without opening the fracture site. The limb is restored to its previous length and spatial alignment is achieved to ensure proper angular and rotational alignment. Fracture reduction can be accomplished using a variety of techniques and devices, including hanging the limb, manual traction, distraction table, external fixators, and a fracture distractor.

REFERENCES

1. Hudson CC, Pozzi A, Lewis DD. Minimally invasive plate osteosynthesis: applications and techniques in dogs and cats. Vet Comp Orthop Traumatol 2009;22: 175–82.
2. Luenig M, Hertel R, Siebenrock KA, et al. The evolution of indirect reduction techniques for the treatment of fractures. Clin Orthop Relat Res 2000;375:7–14.
3. Bone L. Indirect fracture reduction: a technique for minimizing surgical trauma. J Am Acad Orthop Surg 1994;2:247–54.
4. Reems MR, Beale B, Hulse DA. Use of plate and rod constructs and principles of biological osteosynthesis for repair of diaphyseal fractures in dogs and cats: 47 cases (1994–2001). J Am Vet Med Assoc 2003;223(3):330–5.
5. King KF, Rush J. Closed intramedullary nailing of femoral shaft fractures. A review of one hundred and twelve cases treated by the Kuntscher technique. J Bone Joint Surg Am 1981;63:1319–23.
6. Wu CC. An improved surgical technique to treat femoral shaft malunion: revised reamed intramedullary nailing technique. Arch Orthop Trauma Surg 2001;121: 265–70.
7. Rovesti GL, Margini A, Cappellari G, et al. Intraoperative skeletal traction in the dog. A cadaveric study. Vet Comp Orthop Traumatol 2006;19:9–13.
8. Rovesti GL, Margini A, Cappellari G, et al. Clinical application of intraoperative skeletal traction in the dog. Vet Comp Orthop Traumatol 2006;19:14–9.
9. Johnson AL. Current concepts in fracture reduction. Vet Comp Orthop Traumatol 2003;16:59–66.
10. Piermattei DL, Flo G, DeCamp C. Fracture: Classification, Diagnosis and Treatment. In: Handbook of small animal orthopedics and fracture repair. 4th edition. Philadelphia: W.B. Sauders Company; 2006. p. 227–660.
11. Rudy RL. Principles of intramedullary pinning. Vet Clin North Am 1975;5:209–28.
12. Pozzi A, Lewis DD. Surgical approaches for minimally invasive plating osteosynthesis in dogs. Vet Comp Orthop Traumatol 2009;22(4):316–20.
13. Johnson AL, Hulse DA. Fracture reduction. In: Fossum TW, editor. Small animal surgery. 2nd edition. St. Louis (MO): Mosby Yearbook Inc; 2002. p. 889–93.
14. Dejardin L, Guiot L. "MIO in diaphyseal humeral fractures". Lectures abstracts booklet. Las Vegas (NV): Small Animal MIO Traumatology Course; 2011.

15. Witzberger TH, Hulse DA, Kerwin SC, et al. Minimally invasive application of a radial plate following placement of an ulnar rod in treating antebrachial fractures. Vet Comp Orthop Traumatol 2010;23:459–67.
16. Edgerton BC, An KN, Morrey BF. Torsional strength reduction due to cortical defects in bone. J Orthop Res 1990;8:851–5.
17. Jackson M, Topliss CJ, Atkins RM. Technical tricks: fine wire frame assisted intramedullary nailing of the tibia. J Orthop Trauma 2003;17(3):222–4.
18. Marti JM, Miller A. Delimitation of safe corridors for the insertion of external fixator pins in the dog 2: Forelimb. JSAP 1994;35:78–85.
19. Ferretti A. The application of the Ilizarov technique to veterinary medicine. In: Maiocchi AB, Aronson J, editors. Operative principles of Ilizarov. Baltimore (MD): Williams & Wilkins; 1991. p. 551–70.
20. Rovesti GL, Bosio A, Marcellin-Little DJ. Management of 49 antebrachial and crural fractures in dogs using circular external fixators. JSAP 2007;48:194–200.
21. Guiot LP, Dejardin LM. Prospective evaluation of minimally invasive plate osteosynthesis in 36 nonarticular tibial fractures in dogs and cats. Vet Surg 2011;40: 171–82.
22. Eidelman M, Ghrayeb N, Katzman A, et al. Submuscular plating of femoral fractures in children: the importance of anatomic plate precontouring. J Pediatr Orthop B 2010;19:424–7.
23. Schmokel HG, Hurter K, Schawalder P. Percutaneous plating of tibial fractures in two dogs. Vet Comp Orthop Traumatol 2003;16:191–5.
24. Sanders R, Haidukewych GJ, Milne T, et al. Minimal versus maximal plate fixation techniques of the ulna: the biomechanical effect of number of screws and plate length. J Orthop Trauma 2002;16:166–71.
25. Miller DL, Goswami T. A review of locking compression plate biomechanics and their advantages as internal fixators in fracture healing. Clin Biomech 2007;22: 1049–62.
26. Wagner M. General principles for the clinical use of the LCP. Injury 2003;34(2): B31–42.
27. On Tong G. Suthorn Bavonratanavech. AO manual of fracture management - Minimally Invasive Plate Osteosynthesis (MIPO). Davos Platz (Switzerland): AO publishing; 2007.
28. Haaland PJ, Sjöström L, Devor M, et al. Appendicular fracture repair in dogs using the locking compression plate system: 47 cases. Vet Comp Orthop Traumatol 2009;22:309–15.
29. Petazzoni M, Urizzi A, Verdonck B, et al. Fixin internal fixator: concept and technique. Vet Comp Orthop Traumatol 2010;23:250–3.
30. Dejardin L, Guiot L. "Limit and complications of MIO". Lectures abstracts booklet. Las Vegas (NV): Small Animal MIO Traumatology Course; 2011.

Perioperative Imaging in Minimally Invasive Osteosynthesis in Small Animals

Laurent P. Guiot, DVM[a], Loïc M. Déjardin, DVM, MS[a,b],*

KEYWORDS

- Minimally invasive osteosynthesis • Fluoroscopy • Surgical planning • Imaging

KEY POINTS

- The lack of intraoperative visualization associated with closed reduction and fixation techniques, makes preoperative planning even more critical in minimally invasive osteosynthesis.
- The main limitation associated with standard radiography is the inability to reproduce the three-dimensional (3D) configuration of structures examined.
- The use of 3D imaging helps in understanding such complex intraarticular fractures and improves preoperative planning.
- "He who fails to plan is planning to fail" Quote attributed to Sir Winston Churchill.

The lack of intraoperative visualization associated with closed reduction and fixation techniques, makes preoperative planning even more critical in minimally invasive osteosynthesis (MIO). Perioperative imaging begins with the acquisition and interpretation of high quality preoperative orthogonal radiographs of the affected segment plus, in some cases, additional projections such as oblique or stress views to obviate subtle lesions. Although not absolutely necessary, intraoperative imaging using fluoroscopy (C-arm) is often helpful. One must keep in mind, however, that the use of ionizing radiation may have long-term insidious health effects. Therefore, the benefits of this technology should be carefully weighed against potential health hazards, particularly for junior surgeons. Finally, postoperative imaging is essential to critically assess repair adequacy, including alignment and implant positioning. This step is essential to prognostication of clinical outcome and decision-making for revision, should it be necessary.

Neither author has any conflict of interest, financial or otherwise.
[a] Department of Small Animal Clinical Sciences, College of Veterinary Medicine, Michigan State University, East Lansing, MI 48824, USA; [b] Orthopaedic Surgery, Collaborative Orthopaedic Investigations Laboratory, Department of Small Animal Clinical Sciences, College of Veterinary Medicine—Michigan State University, East Lansing, MI 48824, USA
* Corresponding author.
E-mail address: Dejardin@cvm.msu.edu

PREOPERATIVE IMAGING

The goals of preoperative imaging include

1. To identify the nature, location, and extent of the fracture
2. To determine the ideal mode of fixation
3. To allow templating and preselecting of the surgical implants.

Passive restraint techniques are recommended over manual restraints

1. To improve personnel safety
2. To enhance image quality (suppression of motion artifacts)
3. To allow subtle position adjustments until accurate projections are acquired.

The inclusion of a calibration marker in every radiograph is paramount to adequate planning (**Fig. 1**). The marker may be spherical or linear and must be placed parallel to the bone of interest. This allows calculation of a magnification ratio, which in turn permits precise analog (acetate) or digital templating. Positioning of the marker closer to the x-ray beam source or to the cassette will induce an optical magnification of the marker greater or smaller than that of the bone, inducing under or over estimation of the bone size, respectively.

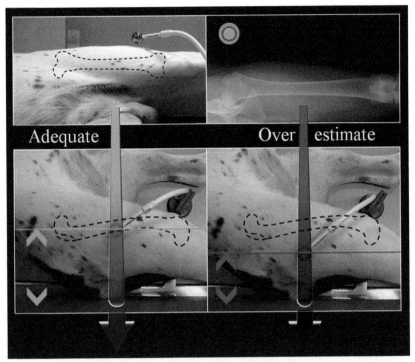

Fig. 1. The effect of placement of a magnification marker (spherical or linear) for a horizontal beam projection of the femur (the x-ray beam is directed from the top of the image (*arrows*). To avoid image distortion, the marker must be superimposed with the bone of interest (*left*). Only then will the magnification of the marker and the bone be identical on the radiographic image. Placement of the marker closer to or away from the x-ray generator will lead to misinterpretation of the magnification ratio in excess or default respectively (*right*). Similarly, the bone of interest should be parallel to the radiographic cassette.

Imaging of the contralateral segment is highly recommended in MIO as it is used

1. To optimize preoperative implant selection (type [plate/interlocking nail] and length)
2. To compare with the fractured segment to identify normal versus abnormal structures
3. To accurately evaluate postoperative alignment.

The main limitation associated with standard radiography is the inability to reproduce the three-dimensional (3D) configuration of structures examined. It is, however, a relatively cost-effective modality that addresses preoperative needs in most instances.

Advanced imaging is indicated in cases with comminuted fractures involving the periarticular regions (**Fig. 2**A, B) or for the assessment of complex structures such as the sacroiliac region in the pelvis (see **Fig. 2**A). A CT scan is best suited in such cases and provides two-dimensional (2D) transverse images and a 3D reconstruction of the affected bones. Transverse images are used for precise assessment of fissure lines, which is essential in optimizing implant placement, particularly with periarticular fractures (see **Fig. 2**B). Coronal and parasagittal images also provide invaluable information in cases of sacroiliac luxation associated with comminuted sacral fractures (see **Fig. 2**A).

The use of 3D imaging helps in understanding such complex intraarticular fractures and improves preoperative planning. Furthermore, 3D reconstruction is beneficial in evaluating fragment distribution and can be used to guide reduction maneuvers. The main shortcoming associated with CT imaging is cost. However, because the benefits of accurate planning and subsequent avoidance of intraoperative

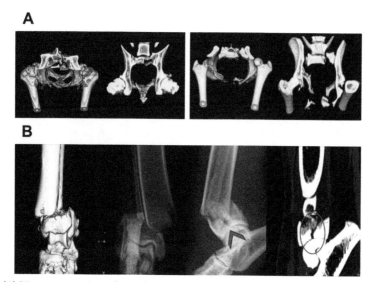

Fig. 2. (*A*) 3D reconstruction of two dogs with sacral fractures. In the first case (*left*), there is a comminuted fracture of the sacral body and left wing. Such lesion precludes fixation using a compression screw and should be treated conservatively to prevent iatrogenic neurologic lesions. Conversely, the simple parasagittal fracture in the second case (*right*) maybe treated surgically using MIO techniques with little risk of iatrogenic trauma. (*B*) Preoperative radiographs (*bottom center*) and CT scan (*bottom left* and *right*) of a periarticular distal tibial fracture. The radiographs were suggestive of a fissure extending in the frontal plane toward the talocrural joint. The 3D reconstruction (*left*) and coronal (*right*) CT images confirmed the presence of a complete fissure extending through the subchondral bone in the frontal plane.

complications likely overcomes this limitation, CT imaging should be considered an integral part of preoperative planning when using MIO. Alternative modalities, such as MRI and ultrasound are seldom used in veterinary orthopedic trauma. However, advanced applications for identifying stress fractures and musculotendinous lesions may prove these modalities beneficial in some instances.

The choice of a specific implant is then made based on fracture configuration, as identified with preoperative imaging, patient signalment, and surgeon's preferences. All systems described for conventional osteosynthesis may find MIO applications. Once a fixation system is selected, specific implant dimensions must be determined. Appropriate templating is mainly based on the preoperative radiographs of the contra-lateral intact side, corrected for magnification. Using premagnified (usually by 4% and 12%) acetate templates superimposed over the radiographs is a cost-effective, although fairly inaccurate, method. In contrast, digital templating can be performed using one of the dedicated software currently available. Most software will allow the surgeon to plan the entire procedure, including fracture reduction, planning of the location and magnitude of corrective osteotomies in angular limb deformity cases, implant selection and size, implant positioning and contouring (plates), as well as predetermination of plate screw or interlocking bolt lengths (**Fig. 3**). Considering the cost of this software, interested surgeons are encouraged to become familiar with

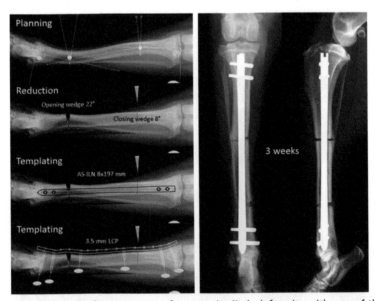

Fig. 3. Surgical planning for treatment of an angular limb deformity with one of the software currently available (OrthoView Veterinary Orthopedic Digital Planning software [Left– http://www.orthoview.com/]). Planning for the locations, types, and magnitudes of the wedges is based on the identification of the CORA (Center of Rotational Axis) of each deformity. Digital manipulation of the fragment using the reduction tool provided with the software, allows the surgeon to visualize realignment. In this case, an angle-stable nail was preferred over and LCP (Locking Compression Plate) because its intramedullary location greatly facilitates realignment. In contrast complex plate countering and use of MIPPO (Minimally Invasive Percutaneous Plate Osteosynthesis) technique make maintenance of alignment during fixation more challenging. Restoration of alignment and evidence of mild biologic activity are seen on the 3 week postoperative radiographs.

the system and ascertain that it is compatible with in-house picture archiving and communication systems (PACS) and that desired templates are available.

Implant position is based on a detailed evaluation of the fractured bone. The fracture pattern, including the presence and extent of fissures, as well as the spread of the fragments, should be carefully evaluated because it may influence the choice and/ or position of an implant.

INTRAOPERATIVE IMAGING
Indications

The most obvious limitation of MIO is the inability to assess the reduction status during surgery secondary to the lack of fracture site visualization. Indirectly, this greatly affects the evaluation of alignment and of structural abnormalities of the fractured bone (ie, presence of fissure lines). Intraoperative fluoroscopy reduces this relative blindness by providing live feedback on the reduction status, alignment restoration, and implant position.

The necessity of intraoperative fluoroscopy varies with segment and fracture pattern. In lower segments (ie, radius-ulna and tibia), readily palpable anatomic landmarks are available and may be used along with joint range-of-motion to assess fragment location and orientation. This allows for accurate assessment of the alignment, thus reducing the need for intraoperative fluoroscopy. In contrast, upper segments (ie, humerus, femur, and pelvis) are more difficult to assess owing to the presence of large soft-tissue envelopes and their proximity with the body wall. Fluoroscopy becomes helpful and sometimes necessary in these locations to assist with reduction maneuvers and improves intraoperative assessment of alignment.

Diverging from early AO (Arbeitsgemeinschaft für Osteosynthesefragen) principles, current recommendations in MIO include the use of bridging osteosynthesis in diaphyseal fractures repair.[1–3] The diaphysis is no longer reconstructed and the entire fracture site is spanned by the implants to create a construct that is semirigid to elastic. With bridging osteosynthesis, the longest possible implant expanding from joint to joint (adults) or physis to physis (immature animals) is selected. Accurate intraoperative imaging is then very useful to ascertain that screws or locking bolts are not violating these essential structures (**Fig. 4**). Because MIO entails that anatomic reconstruction of shaft fractures is unnecessary, there is no need to "see" the diaphyseal region; instead, adjacent joints alignment is solely taken into account. In fractures confined to the diaphysis, the use of a C-arm may facilitate the repair but is not paramount to success. In contrast, all principles of intraarticular fracture repair still hold true when using MIO. Fractures involving articular surfaces must be anatomically reduced and stabilized using rigid fixation and interfragmentary compression when possible. In these cases, proper assessment of the reduction status is critical and requires the use of intraoperative fluoroscopy. Finally, in nonarticular epiphyseal and metaphyseal fractures, the C-arm is used to ensure proper anchorage of the implants in the limited bone stock available for fixation. This guarantees optimal implant insertion and reduces risks of inadvertent joint penetration by the implants (see **Fig. 4**).

Equipment

Numerous necessary and optional items are involved in intraoperative imaging. Choices from the type of C-arm to the use of attenuating gloves and other safety equipment are made before surgery as part of the preoperative planning. These items may be categorized as required for those necessary for the safe acquisition of images or optional for those that may be used to improve personnel safety and image quality.

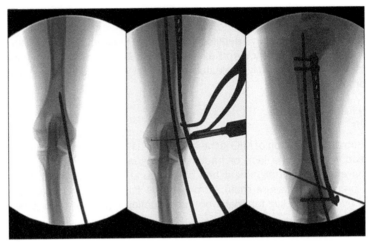

Fig. 4. Intraoperative fluoroscopy of a humeral fracture repaired using a plate rod combination. The rod is inserted normograde from the medial epicondyle for maximal anchorage (*left*). Following rod insertion, a plate is slid epiperiosteally along the medial cortex. The C-arm is used to ensure proper plate contouring and optimal insertion of the screws (*center* and *right*). Note the orientation of the two distal screws inserted above and below the supracondylar foramen. The distalmost screw was placed parallel to the elbow joint to maximize anchorage and prevent inadvertent joint penetration.

Required equipment includes

1. Intraoperative fluoroscopy unit (full-size or mini C-arm)
2. Lead gowns and thyroid shields (for all personnel in the OR)
3. Individual dosimeters
4. Radiolucent operating table (optional based on procedure and type of C-arm)
5. Warning signs of ionizing radiations use.

Optional equipment (recommended) includes

1. Attenuating gloves
2. Protective glasses
3. Sandbags and resting devices
4. Radiolucent operating table (optional based on procedure and type of C-arm).

Intraoperative fluoroscopy unit
Mini C-arms are mobile fluoroscopic systems that consist of an x-ray generator and an image intensifier mounted on a movable C-arm (**Fig. 5**). The x-ray tube and image intensifier are mounted coaxially at the opposite ends of the C-arm. The beam is collimated to the size of the image intensifier and focused on the screen to reduce radiation exposure and optimize image quality. The C-arm is attached via an articulated arm to, or directly mounted on, a wheeled base that facilitates maneuverability (mini or full-size C-arms, respectively). Four basic motions of the arm are enabled with various amplitudes and, based on individual models, can be remotely or manually operated. Motorized arms are available in full-size units only to improve mobility and allow memorization of specific positions to obtain identical images throughout a procedure. Computerized image processing coupled to position recognition is also used to create 3D rendering in advanced applications. The basic arm motions are

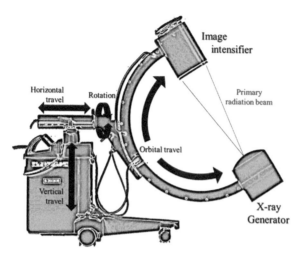

Fig. 5. Four basic motions of the full-size C-arm. Note the position of the x-ray generator downward compared with the image intensifier. This setting is preferred to selectively reduce scatter radiation toward the surgery crew. Alternatively, the x-ray generator may be placed high above the table with the image intensifier below the table, closer to the patient. Although this configuration may improve image definition, it also generates larger amount of harmful scattered radiation back to the surgical team and, therefore, should be discouraged.

1. Horizontal traveling (~ 200 mm)
2. Vertical travel (~ 460 mm)
3. Orbital travel ($\sim 115°$)
4. Rotation about horizontal axis ($\pm 210°$).

The arm unit is coupled to a workstation used for image display, manipulation, and storage. The workstation and C-arm may be independent, as in full-size C-arms, or part of a single unit, as with most mini C-arms. Numerous software have been developed for advanced applications ranging from digital subtractions to 3D image reconstructions. Basic functions allow image manipulation to modify contrast, reorient, and recall previous images. Current machines include compatibility programs to integrate the C-arm images to PACS using DICOM format. Alternatively, images maybe stored on the machine (not recommended), printed, or exported to various media, including USB flash drives, external hard disks, optical disk writer-rewriter, and DVD R/RW. Compatibility with the other systems in use in an institution should be taken into account before purchase to enhance work flow and minimize data loss.

The choice of particular equipment depends on the primary application purpose of the C-arm. The first choice to be considered is between a full-size and a mini C-arm. Both may be suitable for orthopedic procedures and should be considered. The final decision will be based on the availability of other equipment (such as a radiographic and fluoroscopy [R&F] room), the intended applications, and the budget allocated to the purchase of the equipment.

Full-size C-arms have a broad spectrum of applications extending beyond orthopedic surgery. Newer generations have 3D reconstruction capabilities, useful in periarticular trauma, and advanced cine mode that may be used in numerous interventional radiography procedures.[4] They are, however, more expensive and less mobile than mini C-arms. Although full-size C-arms are most often used as static units in veterinary applications, they may be mobilized intraoperatively by a dedicated radiology technician. In static mode, the machine is set up at the beginning of the procedure and left as is throughout the surgery. If necessary, the C-arm may be adjusted by an OR technician but, usually, the patient will be repositioned to obtain the desired projections. They are used through the surgery table as the broad C-arm allows enough clearance above the surgery site. One major drawback associated with this use may be the additional dose necessary to acquire images when compared with images obtained off the table. The increase in dose is directly correlated to the amount of attenuation produced by the table, which is a function of the tabletop material and thickness.

Mini C-arms are less costly but offer fewer options than full-size C-arms. Their major advantage is an improved mobility allowing more flexibility than full-size units do. They also produce lower levels of ionizing radiations, which helps reducing personnel exposure during surgical procedures.[5] With mini C-arms, the machine is maneuvered around the patient to produce orthogonal images. The "weaker" x-ray generator limits the use of these machines in cine mode and the subtraction modes are typically not available. The portability of mini C-arm is such that they are mainly surgeon operated and the need for an unscrubbed radiology technician is much reduced. The entire C-arm, including the generator and the image intensifier, is covered to be included in the sterile field, which facilitates manipulations and improve aseptic technique. Owing to the shorter distance between the generator and the amplifier, they are not commonly used through the operating table because they will not permit easy access to the surgery site. Their portability may allow easy in and out motion to circumvent this limitation, but the lower output from the generator will restrict this application to smaller patients and/or extremities.

Radiation safety equipment

Basic safety steps must be implemented during image acquisition by all personnel within range, typically the entire operating room (OR). These include individual lead aprons, thyroid shields, individual dosimeters, mobile shields, protective glasses, and attenuating gloves. In addition, adequate warning and labeling outside the OR must be posted to prevent inadvertent personnel exposure. Aprons are available in different protective strengths measured in lead equivalence (typically between 0.25 mm and 0.5 mm lead equivalence). Lower shielding capability is acceptable because the dosage necessary for image acquisition is smaller with image intensifiers when compared with radiographic acquisitions (0.1–0.6 mA compared with 20 to 60 mA for imaging identical structures, respectively). Light-weight, custom-fitted, and "zero fatigue" aprons are suitable to reduce upper back and extremities fatigue problems associated with extended and repetitive use.

In complement to standard aprons, thyroid shields must be used. Other protective equipment, including leaded glasses and attenuating gloves, should be considered. These specific shields are highly recommended to reduce incidence of thyroid carcinoma, cataract, and sarcomas associated with chronic, cumulative radiation exposure.[6–10]

Surgery table

The use of dedicated operative tables may be extremely valuable. The characteristics of the ideal table vary somewhat with the C-arm unit in use and the procedure to be performed. The different properties that should be taken into account include

1. Dimensions
2. Radiolucency

3. Motion or motorization
4. Position of the stands and/or wheels
5. Accessory rails and/or patient restraints.

It is advisable to use radiolucent tables to allow imaging through the table as needed. Although this is seldom necessary for the treatment of long-bone fractures when using a mini unit, it is required for the treatment of sacroiliac luxations or when using full-size C-arms. Radiolucent table have variable degrees of attenuation that may be expressed in aluminum equivalence. The attenuation depends the material in use and on the thickness at the site of exposure. Attenuation coefficient inferior to 0.5 mm–0.7 mm aluminum equivalence are ideal. Carbon fiber and some hard polymers are optimal for such applications and custom built boards using these materials may be adapted to a nonradiolucent table if necessary.

Motorized tables that allow progressive motion in all directions are valuable to adjust patient position before and during the procedure. Beside classic vertical motion, surgical tables may feature X-Y tabletop motion (head-to-toe and side-to-side float, respectively), Trendelenburg or reverse Trendelenburg longitudinal tilt (head-down or toes-up and head-up or toes-down, respectively) and lateral roll. The controls are foot or hand activated by an unscrubbed assistant or the surgeon.

The tabletop is mounted either on dual stands or in cantilever on a single stand. Tables on a cantilever are more "C-arm friendly" because the bottom of the table is clear for most its length. This allows unrestricted horizontal C-arm motion under the table. Their maximum weight capacity may be reduced when compared with similar size, dual stand tables and table specifications should be verified before use with larger sized patients.

Accessory rails and restraints are extremely valuable during MIO procedures. They are used to facilitate C-arm access to the area of interest, attach monitoring and anesthesia equipment (ie, endotracheal tube) and secure the patient to the table to prevent inadvertent motion during reduction maneuvers. The presence of accessory rails below (instead of on the edges of) the table is not recommended because it could interfere with proper visualization of the patient.

Intraoperative Radioprotection

Intraoperative fluoroscopy uses ionizing radiation comparable to that produced by conventional radiography. These emissions are known to produce deleterious effects on living organisms through production of free radicals and direct alteration of DNA sequences. In medical imaging applications, both the patient and the personnel are exposed and strict regulations are tied to the use of equipment producing ionizing radiation. These regulations are grouped under the concept of radiation protection or radiological protection. The system of radiation protection in medical radiology consists of justification of a practice involving radiation exposure, optimization of radiation protection, and monitoring of individual dose limits. The interested reader should consult the following document: *1990 Recommendations form the International Commission on Radiological Protection* (ICRP Publication 60); Ann ICRP, 1991, 21.

The terms ALARA (as low as reasonably achievable) or ALARP (as low as reasonably practicable; used in the UK) were introduced in the 1970s and refers to the principle of keeping radiation doses and release of radioactive material to the environment as low as possible, based on technologic and economic considerations.[11] The ALARA concept was integrated into the radiological protection protocols extending its application to the personnel at work and to the patient who is directly exposed to the radiation for diagnostic and treatment purposes.[12] The three pillars of ALRA in radiation safety are

1. Time (spend less time in radiation fields)
2. Distance (increase distance between radioactive sources and workers or population)
3. Shielding (use proper barriers to block or reduce ionizing radiation).

These mitigation methods are a practical and effective means of minimizing radiation effects. The reduction in time of exposure directly reduces acute and cumulative dose exposure; increasing distance reduces dose following the inverse square law; and shielding refers to a mass of absorbing material placed around a reactor, or other radioactive source, to reduce the radiation to a level safe for humans. The sievert (Sv) is a unit of dose equivalent radiation used to quantify the biologic effect of ionizing radiation.

Exposure time
Practically, in the OR set up, the first principle translates into complete avoidance of cine mode if possible and reducing the number of images to the minimum necessary for accurate diagnosis. In that regard, a recent study compared the exposure time and dose between senior (experienced) and junior (inexperienced) surgeons performing MIO. Senior surgeons used significantly less fluoroscopic time and, as a result, were exposed to markedly lower doses per operation than junior surgeons (4.43 minutes vs 6.95 minutes, respectively).[13]

OR personnel: radiation source distance
The surgeon and assistants should maintain the largest possible distance from the C-arm during image acquisition (**Fig. 6**). This can be achieved by using extended tools

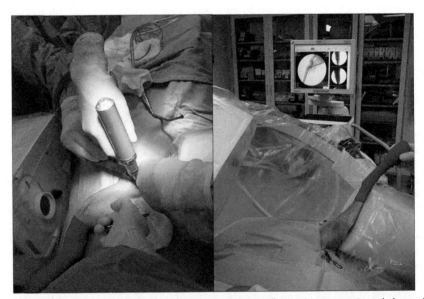

Fig. 6. Intraoperative photographs of MIO procedures. The main surgeon's and the assistant's hands are in the primary beam (*left*). In this situation configuration, C-arm images should not be taken because it will result in high exposure levels. All personnel are off the primary beam and the patient leg is held as far away as possible (*right*). This is an acceptable position to acquire images safely. Further improvement could include the use of a forceps placed at the leg extremity to further increase distance from the exposition field.

and instruments to hold the limb if necessary and avoiding facing the primary radiation beam. The inverse square law stipulates that the dose of radiation is reduced by the power of two of the distance to the x-ray source, making distance from the source of radiation the best protection. For example, when the distance between source and surgeon is doubled, the dose of radiation is reduced to a quarter of the initial dose.

$$I_2 = I_1 \frac{(D_1)^2}{(D_2)^2}$$ I_1 and I_2: radiation intensity at distances D_1 and D_2, respectively
D_1 and D_2: initial and final distance from the x-ray source

Note that the inverse square law only applies to primary beam electromagnetic radiations of x-rays but not to scatter radiation. Scattered radiation is radiation which arises from interactions of the primary radiation beam with the atoms in the object being imaged. Scatter radiation has random direction and poses the greatest radiation risk to occupational workers. Backscatter refers to those photons that return in the near direction from which they came, that is backward 180° toward the tube.[14] Forward scatter continues in the direction of the original photon with a few degrees of directional change; these photons are generally projected toward the image receptor and are the cause of image fog. It is that scatter which is propagated at angles between zero and 180° that is particularly harmful to the surgery crew. In particular, scatter is greatest between 90° and 180° with the lower kilovolt (peak) (kV[p]) settings used by C-arms. In addition, scatter is proportional to the amount of matter exposed to the primary beam. Therefore, when using full-size C-arms through the table for larger patients, the generator should be placed under the table to direct most of the scatter downwards, toward the OR floor, instead of upward, toward the surgery crew.

Shielding

The exposure level also varies considerably with the type of fluoroscopically assisted procedure and the radiation protection used by the OR personnel. As an example, a recent study showed that the effective dose to the surgeon during a routine hip or kyphoplasty was ~5 and 250 μSv, respectively, when a 0.5 mm lead-equivalent apron was used alone. This dose was significantly reduced to ~2.5 and 95 μSv, respectively, when an additional thyroid shield was worn.[15]

The use of shielding as a cardinal principle of radiation protection is required by both the National Council on Radiation Protection and Measurement (NCRP), the Nuclear Regulatory Commission (NRC), and various federal and state regulations. Shielding applies to the room in which ionizing radiation is in use, the personnel, and the patient.[16] Different materials are used for shielding, including lead and barium in aprons and attenuating gloves. The thickness of a shielding material ultimately determines how much radiation will be attenuated. Most shields are made of 0.25, 0.5, or 1.0 mm lead equivalent. Lead aprons of 0.5 mm lead will attenuate approximately 75% of a 100 kV(p) beam. However, most radiology, surgery, and orthopedic departments purchase 0.25 and 0.5 mm lead aprons, meaning that the exit radiation reaching the wearer can approach 25% to 50%. This is an important reason why, to optimize protection, shielding must be coupled to the other two cardinal principles of radiation protection, limited time of exposure to ionizing radiation and distance from it's source. Assuming that these principles are followed, exposure to radiation can remain very low, particularly when compared with other sources of radiations. The use of proper protective gears over a 6 months period has been shown to reduce cumulative radiation of surgeons by up to 45% (eg, thyroid: 0.51 mSv and 0.79 mSv with or without shield; waist: 0.48 mSv, 0.86 mSv with or without apron). These values were well within the NCRP safety guidelines.[17] In comparison, a chest radiograph or chest CT scan generates approximately 0.1 mSv or 12 mSv of dose equivalent radiation, respectively, while passengers in a transatlantic flight receive doses ranging from 0.001 to 0.01 mSv/h. It is currently recommended that the maximum dose to OR personnel does not exceed 10 mSv/y.[18]

Operative Technique

The layout of the OR is essential and should facilitate C-arm maneuvers while preventing interference with the surgical procedure (**Table 1**). The importance of this step is, however, often underestimated. Similarly, it should be emphasized that adequate patient positioning is critical to the smooth execution of the surgical procedure, from fracture reduction, to restoration of alignment, to suitable implant location. In particular, proper patient positioning will allow better full visualization of the joints adjacent to the fracture in two orthogonal planes. In turn, this will considerably limit the number of intraoperative images required to evaluate intraoperative realignment and, therefore, exposure of the surgical team to harmful radiation.

In each case, the patient position should be evaluated by both the anesthesiologist and the surgeon to prevent anesthetic complications while facilitating the surgical procedure. First and foremost, the position must not compromise patient safety. From an anesthesia standpoint, the final patient position should allow easy access to airways, prevent ventilation compromise, permit adequate monitoring, and allow use of an extracorporal warming apparatus. From a surgical standpoint, the patient should be positioned so as to facilitate all surgical phases, including approach and reduction maneuvers, as well as implant insertion and fixation. It must also permit unrestricted C-arm mobility around the patient so that intraoperative views of adjacent joints, in both sagittal and frontal planes, can be easily obtained throughout the surgical procedure (**Fig. 7**). One should bear in mind that poor positioning may result in circulatory compromise, perioperative pressure ulcers, and neurologic injury, even in routine surgical procedures. In addition, poor positioning will impair image accuracy, which in turn may lead to inadequate restoration of alignment and/or

Table 1 Recommended position for optimal use of a C-arm based on fractured segment and C-arm size		
	Static Full-Size C-arm—Through Table	**Mobile Mini C-arm—Table Top**
Humerus	Dorsal recumbency Leg extended caudally (CC view) Leg abducted (Lat view)	Lateral approach (interlocking nail) Lateral recumbency—surgery leg up Medial approach (plate or plate-rod) Dorsal recumbency—surgery leg abducted
Radius-ulna	Dorsal recumbency Leg extended caudally (CC view) Leg abducted (Lat view)	Dorsal recumbency Leg extended caudally (CC view) Leg abducted (Lat view)
Pelvis (SIL/F)	Lateral recumbency—surgery leg up Perfect lateral spine projection required	Optional, in conjunction with full-size C-arm to provide VD image (horizontal beam projection)
Femur	Lateral recumbency—surgery leg up Leg extended and abducted (CC view) Leg held horizontally (Lat view)	Lateral recumbency—surgery leg up Pelvis elevated to allow CC view Leg abducted (Lat view)
Tibia	Dorsal recumbency Leg extended caudally (CC view) Leg abducted (Lat view)	Lateral recumbency—surgery leg down to allow both CC and Lat views

Abbreviations: CC: craniocaudal or caudocranial; Lat: mediolateral or lateromedial; SIL/F: sacroiliac luxation/fracture; VD: ventrodorsal.

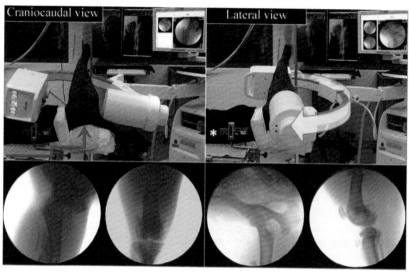

Fig. 7. Preoperative OR set up illustrating proper patient positioning and the use of restraining devices (*asterisk*) for the treatment of a femoral fracture. The pelvis has been elevated to allow unrestricted C-arm motion around the limb. This provides intraoperative views of the joints adjacent to the fracture in two orthogonal planes, facilitates restoration of alignment, and in turn reduces exposure to radiation.

improper fracture fixation. Once positioning is deemed adequate, the patient should be secured on the table using resting devices, sandbags, or tape to prevent inadvertent displacement during the surgery. Following completion of patient positioning, C-arm mobility is reassessed to ensure that orthogonal views of the joints proximal and distal to the fracture can be obtained (see **Fig. 7**). This ultimate preoperative assessment is made before final preparation to allow iteration of the patient position as necessary.

In-depth knowledge of the locoregional anatomy is paramount to a successful surgical outcome. Although this statement holds true in all surgical fields, this prerequisite is even more critical with MIO because direct visualization of the fracture site is not available to the surgeon. Although mini open approaches remote from the fracture site are most often used in MIO, in advanced applications, implants may be fed transcutaneously through large gauge needles used as cannulae. In such cases, the surgeon relies exclusively on percutaneous landmarks and on intraoperative fluoroscopy to achieve fracture reduction, to restore alignment, and to complete fixation. Because a comprehensive 3D understanding of the bone's anatomy is necessary to enable adequate implant contouring and fixation, using dry specimens in the OR in addition to CT scan reconstruction, is highly recommended.

Assessment of reduction status and implant position using the C-arm may be critical in MIO procedures. Similar to what is recommended with conventional radiographs, orthogonal views of the joints adjacent to the fracture site should be obtained. Further, the x-ray beam should consistently be perpendicular to the long axis of the bone and centered over the area of interest to minimize image distortion. Alignment is verified before final fixation using adequate landmarks in the frontal and sagittal planes for the joint proximal and distal to the fracture site. If both joints cannot be seen within one C-arm image, a first image is obtained from the proximal joint and then the C-arm is translated to take an image of the distal joint without changing the plan of imaging or the leg's position. The same procedure is repeated for the orthogonal projection.

POSTOPERATIVE IMAGING

Critical assessment of postoperative images is performed immediately postoperatively. The four "A" rules apply when performing a comprehensive radiographic reading and producing an accurate radiographic diagnosis.[19] The four "A" rules of radiographic evaluations follow.

Alignment

Alignment refers to the anatomic relationship between the joints adjacent to the fracture site. It includes axial alignment (ie, length) and alignment in the frontal (varus-valgus) and sagittal (procurvatum-retrocurvatum) planes. Ideally, postoperative alignment is directly compared with the intact contralateral limb. Severe malalignment should be immediately identified and corrected to avoid long-term consequences of aberrant transarticular forces that would result from such deformities.

Apposition

Apposition is the relationship between fracture fragments. In biological/bridging osteosynthesis, apposition is seldom used as an outcome measure because reconstruction of the bonny columns is not intended, nor desired.

Apparatus

Apparatus includes primary and secondary fixation devices. Assessment of apparatus aims at determining adequacy of the repair in terms of strength and compliance. It also aims at identifying inadvertent misplacement of implants (ie, joint penetration).

Activity

Activity refers to biologic activity as evaluated on follow-up images. These will be compared with the immediate postoperative images to identify progression of healing in terms of callus formation and remodeling. Reevaluation of alignment, apposition, and apparatus is also performed on each follow-up radiograph. Implant and/or bone failure should be addressed as needed.

SUMMARY

Perioperative imaging using various appropriate modalities is critical to the successful planning and performance of any orthopedic surgery. Although not an absolute prerequisite, the use of intraoperative imaging considerably facilitates the smooth and effective execution of MIO. One must keep in mind, however, that the risk of overexposure to radiation is real, particularly when considering its insidious effect over time. Therefore, the primary concern of the surgeon must be safety of the surgical team. If properly implemented, basic, simple steps will be effective in reducing radiation exposure, which in turn will make MIO a safe alternative to traditional open reduction and internal fixation. One should also remember that intraoperative imaging is in no way a substitute to fine surgical skills and in-depth knowledge of surgical anatomy.

REFERENCES

1. Johnson AL, Houlton JEF, Vannini R. AO principles of fracture management in the dog and cat. Stuttgart (Germany): Georg Thieme Verlag; 2005.
2. Perren SM. Evolution of the internal fixation of long bone fractures. The scientific basis of biological internal fixation: choosing a new balance between stability and biology. J Bone Joint Surg Br 2002;84:1093–110.

3. Tong GO, Bavonratanavech S. Minimally invasive plate osteosynthesis (MIPO). 1st edition. Davos (Switzerland): AO Publishing; 2007.
4. Stubig T, Kendoff D, Citak M, et al. Comparative study of different intraoperative 3-D image intensifiers in orthopedic trauma care. J Trauma 2009;66:821–30.
5. Athwal GS, Bueno RA Jr, Wolfe SW. Radiation exposure in hand surgery: mini versus standard C-arm. J Hand Surg Am 2005;30:1310–6.
6. Mrena S, Kivela T, Kurttio P, et al. Lens opacities among physicians occupationally exposed to ionizing radiation—a pilot study in Finland. Scand J Work Environ Health 2011;37:237–43.
7. Vano E, Kleiman NJ, Duran A, et al. Radiation cataract risk in interventional cardiology personnel. Radiat Res 2010;174:490–5.
8. Venneri L, Foffa I, Sicari R. Papillary thyroid carcinoma of an interventional cardiologist. A case report. Recenti Prog Med 2009;100:80–3 [in Italian].
9. Ainsbury EA, Bouffler SD, Dorr W, et al. Radiation cataractogenesis: a review of recent studies. Radiat Res 2009;172:1–9.
10. Furlan JC, Rosen IB. Prognostic relevance of previous exposure to ionizing radiation in well-differentiated thyroid cancer. Langenbecks Arch Surg 2004;389: 198–203.
11. Risk management: ALARP at a glance, in executive LHaS (ed) Health and safety at work etc. Act 1974. 2011. Available at: http://www.hse.gov.uk/risk/theory/alarpglance.htm. Accessed January 16, 2012.
12. Willis CE, Slovis TL. The ALARA concept in radiographic dose reduction. Radiol Technol 2004;76:150–2.
13. Blattert TR, Fill UA, Kunz E, et al. Skill dependence of radiation exposure for the orthopaedic surgeon during interlocking nailing of long-bone shaft fractures: a clinical study. Arch Orthop Trauma Surg 2004;124:659–64.
14. North D. Pattern of scattered exposure from portable radiographs. Health Phys 1985;49:92–3.
15. Theocharopoulos N, Perisinakis K, Damilakis J, et al. Occupational exposure from common fluoroscopic projections used in orthopaedic surgery. J Bone Joint Surg Am 2003;85:1698–703.
16. Christodoulou EG, Goodsitt MM, Larson SC, et al. Evaluation of the transmitted exposure through lead equivalent aprons used in a radiology department, including the contribution from backscatter. Med Phys 2003;30:1033–8.
17. Lo NN, Goh PS, Khong KS. Radiation dosage from use of the image intensifier in orthopaedic surgery. Singapore Med J 1996;37:69–71.
18. Kirousis G, Delis H, Megas P, et al. Dosimetry during intramedullary nailing of the tibia. Acta Orthop 2009;80:568–72.
19. Piermattei DL, Flo GL, DeCamp CE. Fractures: classification, diagnosis, and treatment. In: Farthman L, editor. Handbook of small animal orthopedics and fracture repair, vol. 1. St Louis (MO): Saunders Elsevier; 2006. p. 25–159.

External Fixators and Minimally Invasive Osteosynthesis in Small Animal Veterinary Medicine

Ross H. Palmer, DVM, MS

KEYWORDS

- External skeletal fixation • Minimally invasive osteosynthesis • Fracture fixation
- External fixator

KEY POINTS

- Many of the minimally invasive plate osteosynthesis (MIPO) implant systems and techniques were, consciously or not, developed in order to ascribe to internal fixation the many inherent advantages of external fixators.
- ESF principles, categorized as general, implant selection, application technique and decision-making/frame design, are essential to follow in order to reduce the risk of ESF complications.
- Inexperienced orthopedists often determine fracture treatment by matching patient radiographs to textbook illustrations. Use of the Fracture Case Assessment Score (FCAS) will help veterinarians overcome this disregard for pertinent patient-specific biological, mechanical and clinical factors that should influence the treatment plan.
- Timely staged-disassembly of ESF to encourage callus remodeling is an advantage over other MIO fixation systems.

External fixation, also called external skeletal fixation, ESF, or Ex-Fix, was introduced to veterinary medicine in the 1930s and 1940s, but it was not really popularized until the 1990s when advanced techniques, instrumentation, and training opportunities permitted applications with predictably low patient morbidity.[1] Despite a history of high morbidity, ESF quickly earned a new reputation as a biologically friendly means to treat a growing scope of fractures and osteotomies. As the mantra of internal fixation morphed from anatomic reduction and rigid fixation to incorporation of more BIO-logical methods, the awareness of the limitations of existing internal fixation implants and techniques grew. The principles of BIO-logical fixation were use of indirect reduction techniques, minimal soft tissue stripping, bridging osteosynthesis and relative

Financial disclosures and/or conflicts of interest: None to disclose.
Department of Clinical Sciences, College of Veterinary Medicine & Biomedical Sciences, Colorado State University, 300 West Drake Road, Fort Collins, CO 80523, USA
E-mail address: ross.palmer@colostate.edu

Vet Clin Small Anim 42 (2012) 913–934
http://dx.doi.org/10.1016/j.cvsm.2012.06.001
0195-5616/12/$ – see front matter Published by Elsevier Inc.

vetsmall.theclinics.com

(rather than absolute) stability. Many of the minimally invasive plate osteosynthesis (MIPO) implant systems and techniques described within this issue and elsewhere were, consciously or not, developed to ascribe to internal fixation the many inherent advantages of external fixators. Nowhere is this more evident than in the description of locking plate/screw devices as internal fixators.

INDICATIONS

Minimally invasive osteosynthesis (MIO) application of ESFs is primarily indicated for fixation of long bone fractures and osteotomies, but it can also be very useful for treatment of spinal and pelvic fractures.[2,3] The intraoperative adjustability of ESFs, in addition to the potential for MIO application, makes them very useful for stabilization of corrective osteotomies. Additionally, they are well suited to distraction osteogenesis for limb lengthening as well as the filling of bone defects left behind following bony resections.[4–7]

TYPES OF ESFs

Early in the clinical application of ESF, the Kirschner-Ehmer (KE) device was so predominant in veterinary medicine that the term KE was nearly synonymous with external fixator. Now, veterinarians have a wide array of ESF devices available to them. These modern ESF devices can be classified as linear, acrylic, circular, or hybrid. Linear ESFs use pin-gripping clamps to secure fixation pins to linear connecting rods made of metal or carbon fiber. Acrylic frame ESFs use various acrylic compounds molded into free-form connecting columns that are bonded to the fixation pins. The acrylic, therefore, replaces the linear connecting rods and the pin-gripping clamps used in linear ESF. Circular ESF (CESF) typically uses fine nonthreaded fixation wires secured under tension to ring platforms. These ring platforms are connected to one another by several threaded connecting rods. Variations to CESF can include the use of incomplete rings or arches or the use of traditional fixation pins in lieu of the tensioned wires. Use of arches and fixation pins has been described for the MIO treatment of various spinal fractures and luxations, as well as other long bone fractures.[1] Finally, various types of ESF devices can be mixed to form a hybrid ESF. The most common ESF hybrid is the use of linear fixator components applied to a long bony segment and a single ring CESF applied to a smaller juxta-articular segment.[8,9]

EXTERNAL FIXATOR CONFIGURATIONS

The connecting rod(s), fixation pins, and clamps define an ESF frame (**Figs. 1** and **2**). Frame configuration is described by the number of distinct sides of the limb from which it protrudes (unilateral or bilateral) as well as the number of planes it occupies (uniplanar or biplanar):

- Unilateral–uniplanar (type 1a) frames protrude from just 1 side of the limb and are restricted to 1 plane. type 1a frames (see **Fig. 2** left) are formed by connecting 1 or more half-pins of each main fracture segment.
- Bilateral–uniplanar (type 2) frames protrude from 2 distinct sides of the limb (180° to each other), but are restricted to just 1 plane (typically the mediolateral plane). Type 2 frames (see **Fig. 2** right) are formed by connecting 1 or more full pins of each main fracture segment. When the frames are comprised entirely of full pins, they are called maximal type 2 frames. A minimal type 2 frame is comprised of 1 full-pin in the proximal main fracture segment and 1 full pin in the distal segment, and the remaining positions are filled in with half-pins.

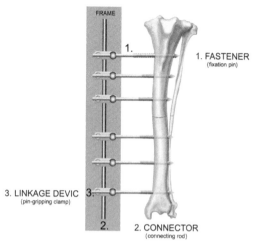

Fig. 1. A linear Ex-Fix frame is comprised of 3 elements: (1) fixation pin, (2) connecting rod, and (3) pin-gripping clamp.

- Bilateral–biplanar (type 3) frames protrude from 2 distinct sides of the limb and occupy 2 planes. Type 3 frames are formed when both a type 1a and a type 2 frame are applied to a bone.
- Unilateral–biplanar (type 1b) frames occupy 2 planes, but because these frames do not protrude from 2 distinct sides of the limb (the frames are <180° to each

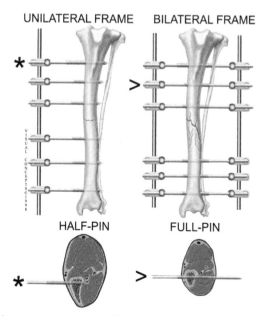

Fig. 2. Unilateral frames are comprised of half-pins that penetrate the near skin surface and both the near and far cortex of the bone. Bilateral frames are defined by at least 1 full pin on each side of the fracture. Full pins penetrate both the near and far skin and bone surfaces. The bilateral frame shown is a maximal type 2, because it is comprised exclusively of full pins.

other), they are thought of as unilateral. A type 1b frame (**Fig. 3**) is formed when 2 type 1a frames are applied to a bone.

This frame classification system fosters accurate communication between colleagues but also provides a basic sense of frame stiffness under axial loading (type 3 > type 2 > type 1).[10-12]

Combination of 2 or more frames in different planes is sometimes referred to as a montage. These multiplanar frames are typically interconnected to form a stiffer construct. These interconnections between frames can be made either as articulations or diagonals:

- Articulations do not span the fracture zone as the frames are interconnected (see **Fig. 3**A).
- Diagonals span the fracture zone as the frames are interconnected (see **Fig. 3**B).

Clinical Variations in Frame Configuration

Femur/humerus

The presence of the body wall adjacent to the proximal half of these bones precludes the use of type 2 and type 3 frames. Additionally, the large soft tissue envelope surrounding these bones means that a larger moment is acting upon the longer fixation pins, and connecting rods are subjected to great bending loads. Incorporation of an intramedullary pin as a tie-in to the ESF is often a useful strategy for these bones in particular.[13,14] Type 1a frames may be suitable for reconstructed fractures, but more sophisticated enhanced 2-frame and 3-frame type 1b configurations are often indicated for the non-reconstructable fractures for which MIO is so valuable (**Fig. 4**).

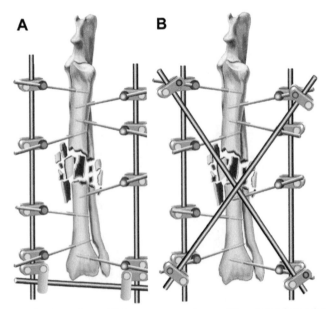

A   **B**

Fig. 3. Unilateral–biplanar (type 1b) frames are made up of 2 unilateral–uniplanar (type 1a) frames. On the radius, the type 1a frames are typically applied in the craniomedial and craniolateral planes in order avoid skewering the extensor tendons and to maximize purchase of the dorsopalmar flattened radius. (*A*) Use of an articulation to interconnect the 2 frames. (*B*) Use of diagonals to interconnect the 2 frames.

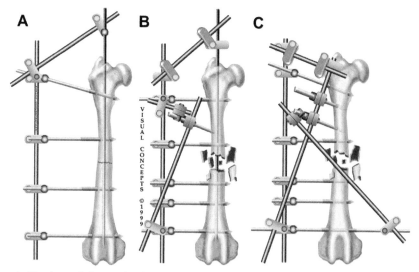

Fig. 4. Fixation of femur (and humerus) fractures is challenging because of the large surrounding soft tissue mass and the position of the body wall. Frequently employed strategies include (*A*) the use of intramedullary pin/ESF tie-in configurations, the use of modified type 1b frames such (*B*) as enhanced 2-frame type 1b, and (*C*) enhanced 3-frame type 1b configurations.

Radius

Uniplanar frames are most able to resist bending forces that are applied in the plane of the frame (versus those in the plane perpendicular to the frame). As an example, a frame occupying the mediolateral plane is less able to resist bending forces in the craniocaudal plane. Application of multiplanar frames, therefore, imparts better multiplanar stiffness. In theory, this is best accomplished by placing the frames 90° to one another. Clinical practicality, however, dictates that frames be applied as regional soft tissue anatomy and bony cross-sectional structure warrant. As an example, type 1b frames applied to the radius typically consist of a frame in the craniomedial plane and a second frame in the craniolateral plane (see **Fig. 3**).

EXTERNAL FIXATOR PRINCIPLES

Despite the numerous advantages of the ESF system, it also has some inherent disadvantages that must be addressed to consistently obtain positive outcomes. Most obvious is that the fixation pins penetrate the skin and soft tissue envelope. This breach of the normal physical defense barriers, combined with the potential for entrapment and irritation of regional soft tissues, puts pin tracts at risk for infection and painful inflammation. Additionally, the connecting rods are distant from the mechanically advantageous position within the central axis of the bone. This eccentric position of the connecting rods means that there are large moments acting on the fixation pins. As a result of these disadvantages, premature pin loosening and pin tract inflammation are the most common complications with ESF.[3,15] The principles described herein minimize the risk of these complications. These principles can be categorized as: (1) general, (2) implant selection, (3) application technique, (4) and decision-making/frame design.

General Principles

Obtain high-quality orthogonal radiographs

Failure to identify subtle fissure lines or other pathology can lead to preoperative treatment planning that may necessitate significant intraoperative alteration. Paradoxically, the fewer fracture fixation systems (eg, bone plating, ESF, interlocking nail) available to the surgeon, the more important it is to have detailed radiographic images on which to base preoperative planning.

Strict adherence to aseptic surgical techniques
Any tendency to minimize the importance of aseptic technique when MIO methods are used must be avoided.

Implant Selection Principles

Use threaded fixation pins
Threaded ESF pins should always be used with linear and acrylic ESFs and linear portions of hybrid ESFs, because nonthreaded pins rapidly loosen in the bone and become very painful.[16–19] Conventional end-threaded pins (**Fig. 5** Top) have a negative thread profile, in which the threads are cut into the pin stock, and the abrupt change in pin diameter at the thread–shaft junction predisposes them to fatigue failure (breakage).[20] Positive-profile pins, introduced to the veterinary market in the 1990s, are more resistant to breakage and have excellent holding power within the bone.[16–18] Positive profile pins are available in end-threaded designs (see **Fig. 5**) for use as half-pins and centrally-threaded designs for use as full-pins. Additionally, they are available in cancellous thread forms for application in regions of thin cortical bone and abundant soft cancellous bone. Cancellous thread forms are typically reserved for use in the proximal tibia, but are occasionally used in the distal femur and proximal humerus. In 2010, a negative-profile pin featuring a tapered thread runout (DuraFace pin, IMEX Veterinary, Incorporated, Longview, Texas) that mitigates the stress–riser effect at the thread–shaft junction was introduced to the veterinary market (see **Fig. 5**).[21]

Pin diameter should be approximately 25% of the bone diameter
Since the bending stiffness of fixation pins is proportional to their radius raised to the 4th power, small incremental increases in pin diameter have dramatic improvements in stiffness. Conversely, proportionate loss of bone strength occurs with incremental increases in circular cortical defect size greater than 20% of the bone diameter.[22] Duraface pins are often useful, as they have improved stiffness, ultimate strength, and cycles to failure when compared with positive profile pins of the same thread diameter.[21] These pins may be particularly advantageous when used in clinical situations involving short fracture segments, nonload-sharing fixations, and fractures of the

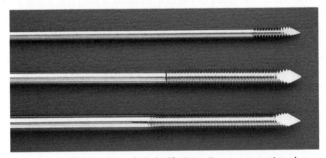

Fig. 5. Commercially available threaded half-pins. *Top*—conventional negative thread profile (SCAT pin, IMEX Veterinary, Incorporated, Longview, Texas). The abrupt thread–shaft junction is stress-concentrator that predisposes them to breakage. *Middle*—positive thread profile (Interface pin, IMEX Veterinary, Incorporated). These pins have good holding power and resistance to breakage. *Bottom*—negative thread profile (Duraface pin, IMEX Veterinary, Incorporated) with a tapered runout that imparts resistance to pin breakage.

femur or humerus, where the thickness of the surrounding tissue envelope requires use of longer fixation pin working lengths.

Use fixation wires with single-lip cutting point with CESF

Circular ESFs are typically applied with 1.6 mm nonthreaded fixation wires under tension. These fine wires may be either smooth or olive (or stopper) wires that have a small tear drop-shaped stopper that can be applied against the outer bony cortex. While Kirschner wires with a standard trocar tip can be used as fixation wires, purpose-specific fixation wires with a single-lip cutting point are preferred, because they cut much more smoothly across the cortex and are less prone to deviating from their intended directional path. Either tensioned wires or fixation pins can be used with CESFs and hybrids, but it is generally recommended to avoid using combinations of pins and wires as fixation elements of any single bone segment. Use of fine wires is advantageous for fixation of very short juxta-articular segments.

Use modern ESF devices

The KE device is primarily of historical significance, since modern ESF devices are mechanically superior and more user-friendly.[12] The morbidity experienced with these modern devices and frame complexity have been dramatically reduced as compared with the KE era.

Application Technique Principles

Use the hanging limb position for spatial alignment of extremity fractures

Just as a hanging limb position is used for the aseptic preparation and draping of most long bone fractures, this limb suspension is maintained throughout ESF/MIO application to the extremities (tibia, radius, metacarpal, and metatarsal bones).[23,24] The affected limb is clipped from body wall to the digits. Adhesive tape is firmly applied to the paw, but must not cover the carpus or tarsus. The surgical table height is set. Tape or another suspending element is attached to a ceiling-mounted suspension apparatus (much easier than working around an intravenous stand) centered directly over the limb axis. The limb is hoisted taut, raising the patient partially from the table. The surgical table height can be adjusted to increase or decrease limb traction as needed. Traction on the limb provides some spatial alignment of the fractured bone within the surrounding soft tissue envelope. The limb is surgically prepared in the usual manner. Drapes are applied proximal to the elbow (or knee), and a sterile, impervious wrap is applied distal to the carpus (or tarsus). During fracture fixation, fine-tuning of spatial alignment is often necessary. The surgeon can, by temporarily raising the table height, flex/extend joints adjacent to the fracture to assess transverse (rotational) and frontal (varus/valgus) plane alignment in the limb. Suspension from a pointed bone-holding forcep anchored to the tuber calcis, rather than a tape stirrup on the foot, often improves sagittal plane alignment of the tibia. The hanging limb position is not suitable for the treatment of fractures of the humerus or femur.

Use an intramedullary pin for spatial alignment of upper limb fractures

An intramedullary pin approximately 25% the diameter of the bone is often used to maintain approximate axial alignment of femur or humerus fractures while the ESF device is applied.[23,24] This usually allows ESF application with less manipulation of the fracture zone. Normograde pin placement is preferred, when technically feasible, because it induces less disruption of the fracture gap. This alignment pin may be a temporary fracture treatment aid that is removed during application of the ESF, or it may be incorporated into the ESF as a tie-in configuration (see **Fig. 4**A, B).

Use safe zones for placement of fixation pins

A thorough knowledge of the cross-sectional anatomy of the limb is required so that critical neurovascular bundles, large muscle masses, and gliding muscle groups can be avoided with the fixation pins or fine wires.[25,26] This cross-sectional anatomy and description of safe, hazardous, and unsafe zones for ESF have been well described in the canine.[25,26] In general, placement of fixation elements is never advised in the caudal surface of any long bone because of the large muscle mass overlying these surfaces. Other generalizations can be made:

- Tibia: placement of pins in the medial and cranial surfaces is safe. Moderate morbidity is associated with fixation pins placed in the lateral surface owing to the larger muscle mass surrounding that surface. Pins placed in the soft bone of the proximal metaphyseal region are prone to premature loosening.
- Radius: low morbidity is associated with pin insertion in the craniomedial surface of the distal half of the bone, and moderate morbidity is anticipated with placement of pins in the cranio-lateral surfaces. Pins in the mediolateral plane are not preferable due to the dorso-palmar flattened shape of the radius (25% bone diameter in this plane is a very small pin).
- Femur: placement of pins through the lateral surface is safe, although the high motion of the knee joint and the weeping of joint fluid through the pin tract generate moderate morbidity when pins are placed in the femoral condyle. ESF pins can be placed in the cranial surface of the femur provided they are in the proximal approximately 25% of the bone; pins placed distal to this will restrict the normal gliding motion of the quadriceps muscle group relative to the femur and are associated with high morbidity. Pins should not be placed proximal to the supracondylar region on the medial surface due to the location of the body wall and critical underlying neurovascular structures.
- Humerus: pins can be safely placed through the lateral surface, although caution must be used to identify and avoid the radial nerve in the distal 1/3 of the diaphysis. Pins can be safely inserted through the cranial surface of the proximal 1/2 of the humerus. Pins should not be placed proximal to the supracondylar region on the medial surface due to the location of the body wall and critical underlying neurovascular structures. Transcondylar pins are technically difficult to place because of the surrounding joint surfaces, but tend to be low morbidity pins when properly placed. Humeral condylar bone is very hard; predrilling technique must be used and cancellous pins avoided.

Make wide soft tissue corridors for ESF pin placement

Soft tissue tension on fixation pins during patient movement is a source of ongoing irritation and results in large ulcerative pin tracts. In contrast, when soft tissue tension is relieved via wide corridors around fixation pins, there is no soft tissue irritation, and the pin tract incisions will contract and epithelialize around the pin. This is typically performed by making an approximately 2 to 3 cm longitudinal incision over the identified safe zone, and a hemostat is then used to make a grid approach down to the bone. Often, retraction of the soft tissues from the pin implantation site can be maintained by placing one tip of the hemostat on each side of the bone, because soft tissue tension against the hemostat will maintain its position. Although wide corridors are not critical around the fine fixation wires used with CESF, relief of soft tissue tension is still important. In contrast to some early ESF recommendations, fixation wires and pins can be placed through the primary surgical approach incision, as may occur with open but do not touch (OBDNT) methods, when this position is free of soft tissue tension.

Fixation pins should be placed using the predrill method

Direct pin insertion using a hand chuck should also be avoided, because the inherent hand wobble during insertion fosters premature pin loosening.[27–29] In order to avoid excessive heat production and bony microtrauma associated with direct power drill insertion of pins, ESF pins should be placed into a predrilled bony channel. A sharp drill bit that is approximately 0.1 mm smaller than the core diameter of the threaded portion is typically used. Drill bits that have a special fine-point (eg, Stick-Tite, IMEX Veterinary Inc, Longview, TX, USA) are helpful as they are resistant to walking along the cortical surface as drilling is started. The fine fixation wires used with CESF can be inserted directly into bone, but new wires with sharp tips are preferred for obvious reasons.

Use of the clamp-in position is mechanically advantageous

When linear ESF is used, the fixation clamp should be positioned on the connecting rod such that the pin-gripping portion is toward the skin in order to reduce the working length of the fixation pin (the distance between the near cortex of bone and the pin-gripping portion of the clamp).[30] While orientation of the pin-gripping channel toward the bone is important, the position of the pin-gripping portion of the clamp on either the cranial or caudal side of the connect bar should also be considered. Typically the clamp is positioned such that the fixation pin will be oriented to traverse desired cross-sectional soft tissue and bony anatomy. In some cases, it is anatomically feasible and mechanically advantageous to have some pins affixed to clamps oriented cranial to the connecting rod and in others affixed to clamps oriented caudal to it.[31]

Distribute fixation pins/wires through each main fracture segment

Fixation pins or wires are normally distributed throughout each main fracture segment.[30] While it is mechanically advantageous to have fixation elements close to the proximal and distal joint surface, it is prudent to avoid penetrating a joint capsule (eg, distal femur) as well as areas of high soft tissue motion (proximal radial neck region) when possible. Similarly, while it is mechanically advantageous to place fixation elements close to the fracture zone (to shorten the working length of the connecting rod), pins are typically placed no closer than 1 bone diameter from the fracture zone in order to avoid areas of unrecognized bony microfracture and fissure formation. In general, fine fixation wires can be placed closer to the joint surfaces and fracture zones than larger fixation pins; thus, linear-circular ESF hybrids are often used for treatment of juxta-articular fractures and osteotomies.

Connecting bars should be placed approximately 1 finger's breadth from the skin

Minimizing the working length of each fixation pin decreases pin–bone interface stress and the likelihood of premature pin loosening.[3,30] However, placing the fixation clamps and connecting bars too close to the skin may cause tissue impingement and ulceration.

Decision-Making/Frame Design Principles

Absolute stability in the early postoperative period

With any form of osteosynthesis, there exists a race between fracture zone healing and the onset of patient morbidity. Due to inherent mechanical and biologic limitations of the ESF system, it is not intended for chronic duration use, because patient morbidity is certain to arise. Instead, the ESF system should be applied such that the patient can begin controlled limb use in the first postoperative days, and fracture zone healing can rapidly progress through the debridement stage and enter into the stage of proliferation. In general, insufficient early fracture zone stability is associated with poor limb use (morbidity), persistence of the debridement stage, and delayed callus formation.

In these instances, it is difficult for the clinician to adequately alter the fixation to help the fracture zone and patient to catch up. Instead, since the ESF system lends itself to staged disassembly, it is advantageous to err toward absolute (rather than relative) stability in the early postoperative period. This approach assumes that the clinician will be attentive to the earliest appropriate opportunity for staged disassembly.

Use of the fracture case assessment score (FCAS) to custom fit the treatment plan to the patient needs

Inexperienced orthopedists often determine fracture treatment by matching patient radiographs to textbook illustrations to find the best fit treatment plan.[32] This disregard for pertinent, patient-specific biologic factors such as age and soft tissue health, mechanical factors such as patient size, feasibility of fracture reconstruction, and concurrent mobility dysfunction, and clinical factors such as patient/owner compliance elevates the risk of undue patient morbidity. The FCAS is a simple 1 to 10 scoring system that is determined by evaluating the pertinent biologic, mechanical, and clinical factors to determine the relative priorities in fracture treatment (**Table 1**). A well-reasoned FCAS gives the veterinarian an accurate understanding of the overall challenge posed by each individual case. Since bone healing requires both suitable biologic and mechanical environments, analysis of the FCAS allows the clinician to custom fit the treatment plan to the specific fracture healing needs in each individual patient. Thus, when the biologic FCAS is lower than the other scores, treatment strategies that preserve fracture zone viability (such as MIO and other strategies discussed in subsequent sections of this article) are a priority (**Table 2**). In contrast, when the

Table 1
Fracture-case assessment score [a]

	1 ☹	☺	☺ 10
Mechanical Factors	Marked instability Nonload sharing Large patient size Multilimb dysfunction Femur	Moderate instability Partial load sharing Medium patient Moderate multilimb Humerus Radius	Mild instability Ideal load sharing Small patient size Single limb dysfunction Tibia

Clinical Factors
Owner
Patient
	Unwilling to follow-up
	Unable to restrict
	  activity
	Intolerant of activity
	  restrict
	Rambunctious
	Intolerant of
	  treatments
		Questionable follow-
		  up
		Willing to try
		Somewhat tolerant
		Active, but responsive
		Difficult to treat
			Willing/able to
			  follow-up
			Able to restrict activity
			Tolerant of restriction
			Calm
			Easy to treat

Biologic Factors Local Factors	Severe tissue injury Comminuted Open Fx–type 3 Marked instability Previous radiation Tx	Moderate tissue injury Transverse/oblique Type 2, type 1 Moderate instability	Minimal tissue injury Spiral/greenstick Closed fracture Mild instability
Systemic Factors	Geriatric Debilitated/ill Second-hand smoke?	Mature adult Compensated illness	Immature patient Healthy

[a] Factors not included on this list can and should be incorporated into the FCAS, because the score will be that much more representative of reality. If, for instance, one notes marked bruising and weeping of blood through the skin, add each of these to the local biology score.

combined mechanical and clinical FCAS are lower than the biologic score, then treatment strategies that restore rigid fracture zone stability (such as increased numbers of pins and frames discussed in subsequent sections of this article) are a priority (**Table 3**). When all of the FCAS categories (biologic, mechanical and clinical) are low, then the balance between treatment strategies becomes especially delicate. Conversely, when all FCAS categories are high, there is a great deal more latitude in the relative balance of treatment strategies while retaining a high likelihood for success. ESF/MIO is most often indicated for fractures that are classified as non-reconstructable or fractures with a moderate-to-low biologic FCAS.

BIOLOGIC CONSIDERATIONS

MIO is a collection of biologic strategies that can be employed for treatment of non-reconstructable fractures or when preoperative FCAS indicates the need to maximize bone healing through the preservation of fracture zone viability. The essence of MIO includes using minimally traumatic surgical approaches, using fixation systems that minimize the vascular insult to bone and periosteum, and augmenting bone healing through minimally invasive bone grafting methods when indicated.

Minimally Traumatic Surgical Approaches

Closed alignment and application of stabilizing hardware is one of the most powerful biologic strategies that a surgeon can employ.[23,24,33] ESF is unique in its ability to span the fracture zone without any insult to the fracture zone, because the connecting elements (connecting rods) are extracorporeal. Closed alignment and stabilization are realistic goals with many fractures of the radius and tibia because of the relatively small soft tissue envelope surrounding these bones. Use of the hanging limb position

Table 2 ESF treatments based upon biologic FCAS	1 ☹	☺	☺ 10
Fixation Priorities	Spatial alignment, preservation of fx zone viability, fixation capable of withstanding loads for estimated fx healing period	As dictated by fracture configuration (reconstructable vs non-reconstructable)	
Surgical Approach	Closed or OBDNT	Miniopen if it will aid load-sharing fixation	Open or personal preference
Graft Open Approaches?	Yes	Usually	Not in immature pets
Fixation pin position	Keep out of soft tissue fracture zone		Tolerant of pins in soft tissue fracture zone
Surgical Time	<2 h	2–3 h	>3 h
Tolerance for Surgical Trauma	Intolerant	Moderate	Tolerant
Supplemental Fixation in Fracture Zone	None	Minimal–moderate if mechanically indicated	Tolerant and can be used if mechanically indicated

Table 3
ESF treatments based upon total mechanical FCAS

	1 ☹	☺	☺ 10
Frame	3-frame type 1b	2-frame type 1b	Type 1a + IM pin
Femur and	(+ IM pin tie-in if	(+ IM pin tie-in if	tie-in
Humerus[a]	possible)	possible)	
Radius	Type 1b	Type 1b	Type 1a
Tibia	Minimal type 3 or	Type 2 or type 1b	Type 1a
	Type Ib		
Pin Distribution	3 + 4 or 4 + 4	3 + 3	2 + 2 (1 + 1 or 1 + 2 only with IM pin tie-in)
Pin Position	Strive to minimize working length of connecting bar	Minimizing working length of connecting bar is valuable	Working length of connecting bar not a critical issue
Use of DuraFace or positive profile pins[b]	Critical; in all pin positions	Important; most pins	Ideal (not critical); most pins
Supplemental Fixation	Strong supplemental fixation highly desirable (when biofeasible)	Moderate supplemental fixation (when biofeasible)	Mild supplemental fixation (if feasible) Not critical
Articulations	Double diagonal	Single diagonal	Horizontal (though seldom applicable due to uniplanar frame use)
Load Sharing	Ideal (but seldom advisable with these cases due to non-reconstructable configuration)	Valuable (only if is a reconstructable fracture configuration)	Optional

[a] The general goal with the femur and humerus is to attain maximal rigidity while striving to limit to 3–4 fixation pins per bone segment because of the large regional muscle bulk. The safe zones for pin placement are quite specific for these bones to minimize interference with sliding muscle movement, neurovascular structures, and joint motion.
[b] IMEX-SK, Securos ESF, and APEF devices all simplify the use of modern threaded pin designs compared with the KE device such that there is little reason to use anything, but positive-profile pins or DuraFace pins with these modern ESF devices.

simplifies closed ESF application to these bones. Closed fracture alignment and fixation are more difficult with fractures of the humerus and femur, but they can be accomplished in some instances. If the surgeon deems that adequate alignment cannot be achieved with closed methods, then he or she may opt for an OBDNT approach. The OBDNT approach can be employed with most any fixation system except interfragmentary compression techniques using cerclage wire or lag screw fixation. The objective of OBDNT is to achieve adequate spatial alignment of the bony column with minimal disruption of the fracture zone. A skin incision is made followed by dissection between pertinent muscle bellies only as far as necessary to accomplish spatial alignment and application of the fixation system. Manipulations to the bony column (application of bone holding forceps, etc) take place peripheral to the fracture zone. The surgeon does not expose or handle cortical (butterfly) bone fragments. The surgeon only removes cortical fragments that are entirely devoid of soft tissue attachment. In this way, the attached cortical fragments remain viable and function as a vascularized graft. Sequestration is uncommon because of the soft tissue attachments and the relatively low-strain environment afforded by comminuted fracture patterns. Use of the previously described intramedullary *"alignment pin"* simplifies the achievement of spatial alignment of many humerus and femur fractures whether using a closed or OBDNT approach. In rare instances, it may be advantageous to employ a "mini-open" approach in which a small approach to the fracture allows for restoration of load-sharing but preserves soft tissue attachments to the bony segments.

Use Fixation Systems that Minimize Vascular Insult to Bone & Periosteum

Recent years have seen a strong shift in internal fixation toward surgical methods and bone plate designs that minimize the periosteal "footprint" and compression.[33] The advancement of locking plate/screw technology has permitted the use of bone plates as "internal fixators" with minimal/no periosteal footprint or compression. These recent bone plate advances are the inherent essence of ESF because the connecting rod(s) that span the fracture zone are positioned outside of the body.

Minimally Invasive Bone Grafting

In some instances, surgeons may opt to enhance bone healing through the use of autogenous cancellous bone grafting. Autogenous grafting is traditionally performed through open exposure of the fracture zone. The benefit of bone grafting relative to the biologic insult of an open surgical approach to the fracture can be debated. Methods to place the graft percutaneously have, therefore, been developed. One method involves the traditional harvest of autogenous cancellous bone chips and associated blood. This coagulum is then placed into a 1 to 3 cc syringe in which the end has been cut off (**Fig. 6**). The syringe is used to deliver the graft through a keyhole incision, and the plunger deploys the graft into the fracture zone. The use of percutaneous bone marrow aspiration and subsequent fracture zone injection has also been described.[34] This technique involves standard bone marrow aspiration and immediate delivery via injection into the fracture zone. This method is attractive whenever delayed grafting is desirable, as it can easily be performed as an outpatient procedure under heavy sedation or short anesthetic episode.

MECHANICAL CONSIDERATIONS

Each and every orthopedic patient is different. While the mechanical effects of many ESF construct variables are well described, the specific strategies to employ are a function of the preoperative FCAS (see **Table 1**). When preoperative FCAS indicates the need to maximize fracture zone stability and pin–bone interface longevity, most if not all of the following strategies can be used (see **Table 3**). In other instances, fewer of these strategies may be indicated, especially if they interfere with important biologic priorities in a given patient.

Load Sharing

Load sharing refers to the relative amount of loading shared between the bony column and the applied fixation.[3] For instance, in some fractures it is reasonable and feasible to anatomically reconstruct the bony column to reduce the mechanical demand placed upon the fixation system. Some degree of load sharing can be an achievable goal in reconstructable (also called reducible) fractures. These are transverse

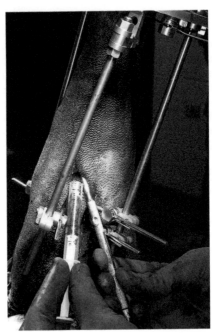

Fig. 6. Percutaneous delivery of an autogenous cancellous bone graft to a comminuted fracture zone.

fractures, long oblique or spiral fractures, or fractures with a large cortical butterfly fragment. In such instances, it may be feasible to reconstruct the bony column such that some of the weight-bearing loads are transmitted from one main bone segment to the other main bone segment directly through the reconstructed bony column. However, bony column reconstruction via interfragmentary cerclage wire or lag screw fixation by definition requires invasion of the fracture zone and cannot be regarded as MIO. It is also often difficult to achieve ideal load sharing of transverse fractures with traditional linear or acrylic ESF because of their inability to compress the ends of the major bone segments against one another. Use of linear motors within CESFs and advanced linear ESFs can help achieve load sharing of transverse fractures and osteotomies even when MIO techniques are used. Load sharing should not be a treatment goal for non-reconstructable (also called nonreducible) fractures. Multiple, small cortical fragments characterize these fractures. Invariably, exhaustive attempts to reconstruct the bony column of these fractures result in an incompletely reconstructed bony column that is devoid of significant soft tissue attachments. The treatment priority in these non-reconstructable fractures should instead shift to MIO goals of restoration of spatial alignment (rather than anatomic reconstruction) and preservation of fracture zone viability.

Pin Number

Increasing the number of fixation pins per bone segment (up to 4 pins per segment) increases the stiffness of the construct, decreases the cyclic stress applied to each pin, and reduces the incidence of premature pin loosening.[30,35] In practicality, 3 or 4 pins per bone segment are often used, because additional pins offer little mechanical advantage while increasing the potential for soft tissue entrapment and introduction of contaminating bacteria. This practice not only reduces the incidence of pin loosening, but also affords simple removal of a single prematurely loose fixation pin should it occur. Conversely, if too few fixation pins are used, multiple loose pins often require removal and replacement in different implantation sites. The only time it is suitable to use 1 pin per bone segment is in combination with an intramedullary pin tie-in configuration, and even then, only when very rapid bone healing is anticipated.

Frame Configuration

Frame stiffness should be maximized when the combined mechanical and clinical FCAS is low or when an extended fracture healing time is anticipated. In general, bilateral frames are stiffer than unilateral frames, and biplanar frames are stiffer than uniplanar frames.[10–12,30,35] Modern linear ESF devices such as the SK use larger-diameter connecting bars that are considerably stiffer than the KE device.[12] As a result, frame configuration with the IMEX SK device is typically simpler than would have been required in previous years with the KE device. While the author still tends to err toward use of slightly stiffer frames than one initially thinks may be necessary, careful attention must be paid to early identification of callus formation such that timely staged disassembly of the ESF is performed.

Articulations and Diagonals

Multi-planar frames are used in mechanically challenging scenarios as dictated by the combined mechanical and clinical FCAS. Multiplanar frames are typically interconnected to form a stiffer construct. In general, use of diagonals is the most efficient way to add fracture zone stiffness with a minimum of extra frame bulk.

CLINICAL APPLICATION

External skeletal fixation is an extremely versatile system for MIO of fractures and osteotomies. However, its versatility represents a complex array of decisions that must be made by the clinician in order for the treatment to be successful. The principles of external fixation, including implant selection, application technique, and decision making have been described within this article. The single most important and commonly overlooked step in clinical application is the thoughtful development of a biologic, mechanical, and clinical FCAS for each clinical case. This process guides the clinician's decision making with regard to device selection, frame configuration, number of pins used, surgical approach (closed, OBDNT, miniopen, open), use of diagonals versus articulations, and bone grafting.

ASSESSMENT OF BONE HEALING AND OUTCOME

The most important goal of fracture treatment is early and sustained return of limb function. That is to say, evidence of radiographic bone healing is of little value if the patient cannot comfortably use the limb. During slow paced walks on a short leash, the animal should be using the limb on every step within 3 to 7 days after surgery. If the animal is not bearing weight on the limb within 7 days of the surgery, close radiographic and physical examination scrutiny is warranted to determine the cause. Insufficient fracture stability, pin penetration into a joint space, and transfixation of a critical sliding muscle group are common reasons for poor limb use following surgery. Animals that display good limb use in the immediate postoperative period may develop a progressive lameness and discomfort later in the convalescent period. In these animals, observant physical examination will often reveal increased pin tract drainage, irritation, and pain that correspond with the radiographic appearance of lysis surrounding one or more of the fixation pins. Management of this complication will be discussed in the postoperative care section of this article.

The mechanisms of bone healing are determined by the biologic and mechanical environments of the fracture zone and, as such, are not unique to external skeletal fixation.[3,33] Most minimally invasive fracture treatments using ESF are applied to non-reconstructable fractures in a closed or OBDNT fashion. In these instances, the indirect (callus) healing pathway is typical.

Indirect bone healing is characterized by a progression from hematoma/granulation tissue to fibrous connective tissue to fibrocartilage to cancellous bone to cortical remodeling.[3,33] Traumatic fracture disrupts bone matrix and induces hemorrhage. Cytokines from the bone matrix and platelets create a chemoattraction for mesenchymal stem cells. These cells then proliferate and follow a fibroblastic, chondroblastic, or osteoblastic lineage according to the local fracture environment. The mechanical environment has a strong influence upon this progression. Motion in the fracture zone causes a change in the width of the gap between fragments. Strain is the ratio between the change in gap width in relation to the original gap width.[33] A given tissue will not proliferate under strain conditions that exceed its deformation limits. Sequential formation of stiffer tissues within the fracture zone allows for decreasing fracture gap motion and, thereby, strain. Hematoma and granulation tissue have a high strain tolerance and can proliferate in the unstable fracture zone with strains up to 100%. As granulation fills the fracture zone, there is less motion and, thereby, less fracture gap strain. This reduced strain allows for proliferation of fibrous connective tissue that can tolerate 20% strain and then proliferation of fibrocartilage with a 10% strain tolerance. This progression to stiffer tissues continues until fracture gap strain approaches 2%, a mechanical environment in which lamellar bone can form. As the fracture zone stabilizes, mineralization of the cartilage begins at the periosteal periphery of the large callus cuff and continues toward the center of the gap. This large periosteal callus cuff imparts good resistance to bending and torsional forces as the area moment of inertia and polar moment of inertia are related to the callus radius raised to the 4th power. The callus volume is a function of patient age (young animals tend to form more callus), fracture zone stability (more callus is formed with less rigid fixations), fracture configuration (less callus is produced in transverse fractures as compared with oblique and comminuted fractures), and species (cats tend to produce less callus than dogs). The combined structural and material properties of the mineralized callus allow for continued trabecular bone formation that is progressively remodeled down to cortical bone.

Bone healing can be assessed by palpation and radiography. Indirect bone healing is often palpably evident as a soft callus (especially in young animals) before there is radiographic evidence of healing. In the heavily sedated animal, the ESF connecting bars can be removed such that palpable relative stability is evident upon gentle rotation or bending of the fracture zone.[24] Radiographically, fracture gap width often increases as a function of bone resorption early in the process. Indirect bone union is first radiographically evident as proliferation of endosteal and periosteal new bone at the ends each fracture segment. The periosteal component starts as thin cuff distant from the fracture ends and enlarges as it approaches the fracture gap. The fracture gap becomes less distinct as the newly formed mineralized callus replaces the soft fibrocartilaginous and fibrous tissue callus. Fracture gap stability is achieved once the fracture is bridged by cancellous bone callus and cortical remodeling can begin. Radiographically, this appears as a decrease in callus bone density within the intramedullary canal and evidence of cortical bone reconstruction at the fracture site.

The time to ESF removal is variable depending upon patient age, soft tissue damage, fracture location, and fracture fixation. Average time ESF to removal is approximately 12 weeks (range from 4 to 32 or more weeks) for canine tibial and radial fractures.[36] There is a balance between too much and too little fracture zone stability. When fractures are provided absolute stability, the healing process can be delayed, but limb use is better than with relative stability. In order to restore early limb use, it the author's experience that it is desirable to begin with absolute stability. There is some evidence that staged disassembly of the ESF frame, when performed at the appropriate time, may mitigate the tendency for absolute stability to slow the healing process.[37–39] Studies have shown that exposure of the healing fracture zone to increased loading at approximately 6 to 8 weeks after operation may be beneficial in the skeletally mature dog.[37–39] It is likely that there exists a critical window of opportunity with regard to the timing and form of destabilization needed and that if missed, the benefits of staged disassembly are minimal.[40] This window of opportunity may be as early as 3 to 4 weeks after surgery in skeletally immature dogs. Cats appear to heal more slowly than dogs,[41] and staged disassembly is often deemed appropriate 8 to 10 weeks after surgery in the adult feline. Use of excessively rigid type 2 ESF was associated with tibial nonunions in cats and suggests the importance of timely pursuit of staged disassembly strategies in the feline.[42]

POSTOPERATIVE PATIENT MANAGEMENT

The need for attentive postoperative care is often regarded as the most significant disadvantage of ESF use. Conversely, the need for this level of care may be beneficial as it prevents the pet owner from slipping into a "out of sight, out of mind" mentality with regard to convalescent care. Recommended postoperative care is usually comprised of patient activity restriction, pin tract cleansing, and bandaging. Most pet owners can be trained to properly perform these functions at home. The goals of this care are to encourage early restoration of limb use, promote bone healing, to maintain pin–bone interface stability, and to minimize pin tract drainage and discomfort.

Slow, controlled walking on a very short leash is instituted the day following surgery as a means to encourage early use of the limb. Usually it is helpful if the dog walker walks on the side opposite the injury in order to lean into the pet to encourage weight bearing. Excessive gait speed commonly results in a nonweight-bearing gait.

Pin tract care begins immediately following ESF application with the goals of minimizing pin tract contamination and impingement/motion of the soft tissues upon the fixation pins. Before anesthetic recovery, the limb is passed through a full range of motion, and a #11 blade is used to relieve all detected soft tissue tension/motion upon fixation elements. Several sterile gauze squares are incised halfway across, and the split dressing is applied around each fixation pin. Packing of gauze squares or laundered and sterilized foam scrub sponges can be placed between the connecting bar and the sterile gauze dressing to immobilize the soft tissue zone around each fixation pin. Bumper padding can be applied over the tops of fixation pins and bars, and outer elastic wrap is applied around the frame to keep all of the bandaging material in place. This bandage with sterile gauze pin tract dressing is typically changed 2 to 3 times in the first 5 to 10 postoperative days depending upon the amount of drainage, regional soft tissue health, and other factors. Patient sedation is often necessary for the first few bandage changes, and the pet owner can be trained how to perform the pin tract care and bandage change by approximately 10 days after surgery. Once the pin tracts are filling with granulation tissue, the frequency of the bandage changes can be reduced to every 3 to 5 days. The owner is instructed to use gauze soaked in an antiseptic solution in a shoe shine fashion to remove any accumulated crusts and scabs from around each pin in order to promote free drainage of any pin

---

Box 1
Assessment for staged ESF disassembly

- Examine the patient for any pin tract morbidity (active wound around pins, pin tract drainage, sensitivity to manipulation of pin tract or fixation pin).
- Heavy sedation
  - Radiographs—examine for early callus formation in the fracture zone as well as for lucency around any pins. Patients with complex, multiconnecting rod frames may require oblique radiographic views or temporary removal of a connecting rod to allow assessment of fracture zone healing (radiographic ease is an advantage of composite carbon fiber connecting rods).
  - Palpation of fracture zone—if mineralized callus formation is not evident on radiographs, the connecting rods are temporarily removed, and the fracture zone is palpated for relative stability imparted by early soft callus formation.
- Decision making
  - Neither radiographs nor fracture zone palpation reveals early callus formation—reapply connecting rods and consider interventions that may accelerate healing.
  - If radiographs and/or palpation reveal early callus formation—begin staged disassembly strategies.

---

tract exudate. Pet owners are cautioned that excessive limb use and infrequent pin tract care are common contributors to increased pin tract drainage, lameness, and pain that may be encountered 4 to 8 weeks after surgery as the owner's attention to ESF care begins to wane. Owners are encouraged to remain vigilant in their

---

Box 2
Guidelines for staged disassembly of linear ESF devices

1. Base disassembly strategy upon removal of any pins that are causing patient morbidity (eg, pain, drainage, irritation, loosening)
2. Removal of a frame is preferable to removal of healthy pins when feasible
   a. Type 3 frames → type 2, type 1b or even a type 1a depending on the amount of fracture zone callus present
   b. Type II → type 1a
   c. Type 1b → disassemble to type 1a or remove articulations/diagonals (if frame removal is too aggressive)
   d. Type 1a → removal of pins closest to fracture to reduce construct stiffness (increased working length of connecting rod)
   e. Intramedullary (IM) pin tie-in—progressive removal of fixation frames (modified type 1b frames) or removal of fixation pins (type 1a frames) until the IM pin and its tie-in are the last elements to be removed (the IM pin provides excellent protection against disruptive bending forces). If, however, there is significant morbidity involved with the IM pin site, the IM pin is removed, and the ESF is left in place
3. Decrease the size of the connecting rods when feasible. Some of the fixation pin sizes are compatible with 2 different sizes of fixation clamps and connecting rods of certain devices (eg, IMEX SK). When such pins are used, the ESF construct is initially built with the larger size of clamps and connecting rods for greater rigidity. At the time of staged disassembly, the larger size of clamps and rods are removed and they are replaced with smaller clamps and rods
4. Changing from a metallic connecting rod to a carbon fiber rod will decrease construct stiffness with certain ESF devices (eg, IMEX SK)

Table 4
Common complications with external skeletal fixation

Complication	Common Causes	Treatment
Pin loosening	Nonthreaded pins; incorrect pin insertion technique; too few pins/segment; inadequate frame stiffness; excessive patient activity; inadequate pin tract care at home	Identify and correct cause(s); single loose pin can be removed as a component of staged disassembly if adequate radiographic callus or relative stability is detected
Pin tract drainage	As listed above + soft tissue tension/motion on pin(s); pin tract infection	Identify and correct cause(s); single morbid pin can be removed as a component of staged disassembly if adequate radiographic callus or relative stability is detected. Systemic and/or topical antimicrobials may be indicated, but are not a substitute for correction of predisposing cause(s)
Poor limb use	As listed above + impingement of gliding muscle group with fixation pin; nerve injury; pin penetrating or very near a joint	Identify and correct cause(s)
Delayed union	As listed above + inadequate preservation of biologic healing potential	Identify and correct cause(s); may need liberal application of bone grafting

aftercare, as premature pin tract irritation and pin loosening may necessitate revision surgical procedures that can add significantly to the overall treatment cost.

Timely staged disassembly of ESF to encourage callus remodeling is an advantage ESF has over other MIO fixation systems. Staged disassembly is more commonly pursued with linear ESF than circular ESF devices. Patients are assessed for the suitability of staged disassembly according to the following general guidelines: adult dogs at 6 to 8 weeks, adult cats at 8 to 10 weeks, skeletally immature dogs and cats as early as 3 to 4 weeks. In general, patients are assessed for disassembly as detailed in **Box 1**. If staged disassembly is deemed appropriate, there are a variety of strategies that may be pursued. Prioritized guidelines for staged disassembly of linear ESF devices are summarized in **Box 2**.

Major complications with ESF/MIO are rare with proper preoperative planning, device application, and postoperative care. Complications such as pin tract drainage/sepsis, pin loosening, poor limb use, delayed union, and fixation failures are all inter-related. Early signs of pin tract drainage may lead to pin sepsis and loosening, followed by increased lameness/pain, and, ultimately, delayed union and fixation failure. Common complications, their causes, and possible treatments are summarized in **Table 4**.

SUMMARY

Modern ESF is a very versatile system that is well suited to the ideals of MIO. It provides variable angle, locked fixation that can be applied with minimal/no disruption of the fracture zone. Rigid bilateral or multiplanar frames are relatively simple to apply in instances of nonload-sharing fixation of non-reconstructable fractures, but timely staged disassembly allows for a gradual shift of loading from the frame to the healing bone column. Hybrid ESF is ideally suited for the treatment of many juxta-articular fractures. Adherence to the principles of ESF and postoperative care detailed in this article is essential to overcome the various disadvantages inherent to ESF.

ACKNOWLEDGMENTS

I offer my sincere thanks and gratitude to my many mentors and colleagues (you know who you are) without whom I would never have developed an interest, knowledge, or skill set in ESF.

REFERENCES

1. Palmer RH, Hulse DA, Hyman WA, et al. Principles of bone healing and biomechanics of external skeletal fixation. Vet Clin North Am Small Anim Pract 1992; 22:45–68.
2. Wheeler JL, Lewis DA, Cross AR, et al. Closed fluoroscopic-assisted spinal arch external skeletal fixation for the stabilization of vertebral column injuries in five dogs. Vet Surg 2007;36:442–8.
3. Fitzpatrick N, Lewis D, Cross A. A biomechanical comparison of external skeletal fixation and plating for the stabilization of ilial osteotomies in dogs. Vet Comp Orthop Traumatol 2008;21:349–57.
4. Yanoff SR, Hulse DA, Palmer RH, et al. Distraction osteogenesis using modified external fixation devices in five dogs. Vet Surg 1992;21:480–7.
5. Petazzoni M, Palmer RH. Femoral angular correction and lengthening in a large-breed puppy using a dynamic unilateral external fixator. Vet Surg 2012;41(4): 507–14.
6. Fox SM, Bray JC, Guerin SR, et al. Antebrachial deformities in the dog: treatment with external fixation. J Small Anim Pract 1995;36:315–20.
7. Marcellin-Little DJ, Ferretti A, Roe SC, et al. Hinged Ilizarov external fixation for correction of antebrachial deformities. Vet Surg 1998;27:231–45.
8. Farese JP, Lewis DD, Cross AR, et al. Use of IMEX SK-Circular external fixator hybrid constructs for fracture stabilization in dogs and cats. J Am Anim Hosp Assoc 2002;38:279–89.
9. Anderson GM, Lewis DD, Radasch RM, et al. Circular external skeletal fixation stabilization of antebrachial and crural fractures in 25 dogs. J Am Anim Hosp Assoc 2003;39:479–98.
10. Egger EL. Static strength evaluation of six external skeletal fixation configurations. Vet Surg 1983;12:130–6.
11. White DT, Bronson DG, Welch RD. A mechanical comparison of veterinary linear external fixation systems. Vet Surg 2003;32:507–14.
12. Bronson DG, Ross JD, Toombs JP, et al. Influence of the connecting rod on the biomechanical properties of five external skeletal fixation configurations. Vet Comp Orthop Traumatol 2003;16:82–7.
13. Dewey CW, Aron DN, Foutz TL, et al. Static strength evaluation of two modified unilateral external skeletal fixators. J Small Anim Pract 1994;35:211–5.
14. Radke H, Aron DN, Applewhite A, et al. Biomechanical analysis of unilateral external skeletal fixators combined with IM-pin and without IM-pin using finite-element method. Vet Surg 2006;35:15–23.
15. Guerin SR, Lewis DD, Lanz OI, et al. Comminuted supracondylar humeral fractures repaired with a modified type I external skeletal fixator construct. J Small Anim Pract 1998;39:525–32.

16. Palmer RH, Hulse DA, Pollo FE, et al. Pin loosening in external skeletal fixation: the effect of pin design and implantation site. Vet Surg 1991;20:343.

17. Aron DN, Toombs JP, Hollingsworth SC. Primary treatment of severe fractures by external skeletal fixation: threaded pins compared to smooth pins. J Am Anim Hosp Assoc 1986;22:659–70.

18. Anderson MA, Mann FA, Wagner-Mann C, et al. Comparison of nonthreaded, enhanced threaded and Ellis fixation pins used in type I external skeletal fixators in dogs. Vet Surg 1993;22:482–9.

19. Anderson MA, Palmer RH, Aron DN. Improving pin selection and insertion technique for external skeletal fixation. Comp Contin Educ Pract Vet 1997;19: 485–93.

20. Palmer RH, Aron DN. Ellis pin complications in seven dogs. Vet Surg 1990;19: 440–5.

21. Griffin H, Toombs JP, Bronson DG, et al. Mechanical evaluation of a tapered thread-run-out half-pin designed for external skeletal fixation in small animals. Vet Comp Orthop Traumatol 2011;24:257–61.

22. Edgerton BC, An KN, Morrey BF. Torsional strength reduction due to cortical defects in bone. J Orthop Res 1990;8:851–5.

23. Palmer RH. Biological osteosynthesis. Vet Clin North Am Small Anim Pract 1999; 29:1171–85.

24. Aron DN, Johnson AL, Palmer RH. Biologic strategies and a balanced concept for repair of highly comminuted long bone fractures. Comp Contin Educ Pract Vet 1995;17:35–49.

25. Marti JM, Miller A. Delimitation of safe corridors for the insertion of external fixator pins in the dog 1: hindlimb. J Small Anim Pract 1994;35:16–23.

26. Marti JM, Miller A. Delimitation of safe corridors for the insertion of external fixator pins in the dog 2: forelimb. J Small Anim Pract 1994;35:78–85.

27. Egger EL, Histand MB, Blass CE, et al. Effect of fixation pin insertion on the pin–bone interface. Vet Surg 1986;15:246–52.

28. McDonald DE, Palmer RH, Hulse DA, et al. Holding power of threaded external skeletal fixation pins in the near and far cortices of cadaveric canine tibiae. Vet Surg 1994;23:488–93.

29. Clary EM, Roe SC. In vitro biomechanical and histological assessment of pilot hole diameter for positive-profile external skeletal fixation pins in canine tibiae. Vet Surg 1996;25:453–62.

30. Bouvy BM, Markel MD, Chelikani S, et al. Ex vivo biomechanics of Kirschner-Ehmer external skeletal fixation applied to canine tibiae. Vet Surg 1993;22:194–207.

31. Reaugh HF, Rochat MC, Bruce CW, et al. Stiffness of modified type Ia linear external skeletal fixators. Vet Comp Orthop Traumatol 2007;20:264–8.

32. Palmer RH. Fracture-patient assessment score (FPAS): a new decision-making tool for orthopedists and teachers. Proc Am Coll Vet Surg Conf 1996;155–7.

33. Perren SM. Review article: evolution of the internal fixation of long bone fractures—the scientific basis of biological internal fixation: choosing a new balance between stability and biology. J Bone Joint Surg Br 2002;84(8):1093–110.

34. Goel A, Sangwan SS, Siwach RC, et al. Percutaneous bone marrow grafting for the treatment of tibial non-union. Injury 2005;36:203–6.

35. Brinker WO, Verstraete MC, Soutas-Little RW. Stiffness studies on various configurations and types of external fixators. J Am Anim Hosp 1985;21:801–8.

36. Johnson AL, Kneller SK, Weigel RM. Radial and tibial fracture repair with external skeletal fixation—effects of fracture type, reduction and complications on healing. Vet Surg 1989;18:367–72.

37. Egger EL, Histand MB, Norrdin RW, et al. Canine osteotomy healing when stabilized with decreasingly rigid fixation compared to constantly rigid fixation. Vet Comp Orthop Traumatol 1993;6:182–7.
38. Egger EL, Gottsauner-Wolf F, Palmer J, et al. Effects of axial dynamization on bone healing. J Trauma 1993;34:185–92.
39. Larsson S, Wookcheol K, Caja VL, et al. Effect of early axial dynamization on tibial bone healing: a study in dogs. Clin Orthop Relat Res 2001;388:240–51.
40. Auger J, Dupuis J, Boudreault F, et al. Comparison of multistage versus one-stage destabilization of a type II external fixator used to stabilize an oblique tibial osteotomy in dogs. Vet Surg 2002;31:10–22.
41. Risselada M, Kramer M, De Rooster H, et al. Ultrasonographic and radiographic assessment of uncomplicated secondary fracture healing of long bones in dogs and cats. Vet Surg 2005;34:99–107.
42. Nolte DM, Fusco JV, Petersen ME. Incidence of and predisposing factors for nonunion of fracture involving the appendicular skeleton in cats: 18 cases (1998-2002). J Am Vet Med Assoc 2005;226:77–82.

Interlocking Nails and Minimally Invasive Osteosynthesis

Loïc M. Déjardin, DVM, MS[a],*, Laurent P. Guiot, DVM[a],
Dirsko J.F. von Pfeil, DVM[b]

KEYWORDS

- Interlocking nail • Angle-stable interlocking nail • Bone healing • Fracture model
- Traumatology • Minimally invasive osteosynthesis
- Minimally invasive nail osteosynthesis • Small animals

KEY POINTS

- Ongoing reviews of clinical outcomes led to a radical paradigm shift toward further emphasizing the biologic component of fracture healing; this became the foundation of a new philosophic approach known as minimally invasive osteosynthesis.
- With the recent paradigm shift toward biologic osteosynthesis, interlocking nails have emerged as an attractive alternative to bone plating and, to some surgeons, the method of choice for the repair of most comminuted diaphyseal and metaphyseal fractures in human and veterinary patients.
- Interlocking nails have common characteristics: they are solid intramedullary rods featuring transverse holes (cannulations) at both extremities and sometimes along the whole length of the nail. Various locking devices such as screws, bolts or blades are used to lock the nail within the medullary cavity.
- Orthogonal radiographs of the fractured and contralateral intact bone of interest are essential to accurate planning. Imaging of the affected bone is used for evaluation of the fracture location, configuration, and identification of fissures that could extend in the metaphyses.
- As intramedullary devices, interlocking nails can only be used in long bones that provide a non-articular entry point for the nail (which excludes the radius).

Some of the work presented here was supported by the Michigan State University Companion Animal Fund (grants CAF 81-2156-D, 81-2625-D, 31-1086-D, and 81-1086) as well as by implant donations by BioMedtrix.

Loïc M. Déjardin is the inventor of 1 of the nails described in this article and receives honoraria for teaching interlocking nailing on behalf of BioMedtrix.

[a] Department of Small Animal Clinical Sciences, College of Veterinary Medicine, Michigan State University, East Lansing, MI 48824, USA; [b] Veterinary Specialists of Alaska, PC, 3330 Fairbanks Street, Anchorage, AK 99503, USA

* Corresponding author. Orthopaedic Surgery, Collaborative Orthopaedic Investigations Laboratory, Department of Small Animal Clinical Sciences, College of Veterinary Medicine, Michigan State University, East Lansing, MI 48824.

E-mail address: Dejardin@cvm.msu.edu

INTRODUCTION

In an effort to improve on the poor functional outcomes associated with external fixation or coaptation and/or long-term patient immobilization, starting in the late 1950s, open reduction and internal fixation (ORIF) became the modus operandi recommended by the Arbeitsgemeinschaft für Osteosynthesefragen (AO) Foundation for the treatment of long bone fractures.[1] Although strict adhesion to ORIF principles of anatomic reduction and rigid fixation allowed the restoration of absolute mechanical stability, it came with a hefty biologic price inherent to extensive iatrogenic surgical trauma, including disturbance of the fracture hematoma and inevitable damage to the local soft tissues and blood supply. As a result, despite improved outcomes compared with earlier techniques, ORIF was accompanied by the rise of new complications, such as delayed or nonunion, implant failure, and osteomyelitis. As an example, humeral and tibial fractures in dogs treated with conventional techniques have a complication rate of up to 40% and 18%, respectively.[2,3] Such observations led to the reiteration of the early AO principles of preservation of blood supply, gentle soft tissue handling, and early mobilization and, in practical terms, to a biologically friendlier "Open But Do Not Touch" (OBDNT) approach to osteosynthesis. Nonetheless, OBDNT techniques, which still favor manipulation of the bone fragments (albeit remotely), continued to put an emphasis on mechanical rigidity of the repaired bone as illustrated by the extensive use of the plate-rod combination (PRC) in the treatment of comminuted fractures.[1]

During the past 2 decades, the ongoing review of clinical outcomes by the AO led to a radical paradigm shift toward further emphasizing the biologic component of fracture healing.[1] This became the foundation of a new philosophic approach known as minimally invasive osteosynthesis (MIO).[4–8] With MIO, the fracture site is not exposed, which in turn preserves the fracture hematoma and promotes earlier fracture healing. Rather, indirect reduction techniques through gentle manipulation of the main bone fragments and small approaches remote to the fracture site are used to introduce the implant in an epiperiosteal (plate) or intramedullary (interlocking nail [ILN]) manner. In addition, quasi-abandonment of interfragmentary screws, cerclage wires, or bone grafts and anatomic reduction became the hallmarks of MIO.[9] This evolution favors the preservation of a biologic environment essential to bone healing. From a mechanical perspective, emphasis is put on restoration of alignment rather than anatomy and on achieving optimal construct stability rather than rigid interfragmentary stability. This is accomplished through several iterations of traditional osteosynthesis techniques such as increased reliance on longer, more compliant bridging implants that bypass the fracture site altogether. Today, biologic osteosynthesis principles and MIO are readily implemented in human orthopedics and are slowly gaining momentum and acceptance in veterinary medicine.[5,6,10] While numerous acronyms have been used to describe specific implant related minimally invasive surgical techniques, adherence to these new principles is collectively known as MIO. This article will address the use of minimally invasive nail osteosynthesis (MINO) in the treatment of long bone fractures in companion animals.

HISTORY OF ILN USE

The ILN concept in the treatment of long bone fractures evolved from the original intramedullary nail and later "detensor" nail designed by Küntscher[11] (Germany) in the 1940s and late 1960s. The first true ILN was developed in the 1970s by Huckstep[12] (Australia) to treat femoral fractures in people. Following the successful experimental and clinical use of modified Huckstep nails in animals by Johnson and Huckstep[13] and then Muir and colleagues,[14–16] several dedicated veterinary systems were independently designed in the early 1990s by Dueland and Johnson[17] (United States), Duhautois and van Tilburg[18] (France), Durall and Diaz[19] (Spain), and Nagaoka and colleagues[20] (Japan). These systems are not compatible with each other. Recently, in an effort to address some of the limitations of currently available designs, a new angle-stable (AS)-ILN was developed at Michigan State University.[21–24] Currently, 2 systems are available in the United States. The Original Interlocking Nail System is a standard nail system commercialized by Innovative Animal Products (IAP; Rochester, MN, USA), and the I-Loc, an AS-ILN commercialized by BioMedtrix (Booton, NJ, USA). Throughout the remainder of the text, IAP and I-Loc may be used to refer to standard and AS nails, respectively.

ILN DESIGNS

Regardless of their designs, ILNs have common characteristics. They are solid intramedullary rods (IMRs) featuring transverse holes (cannulations) at both extremities and sometimes along the whole length of the nail (Durall system). The nail is locked in place via bone screws or partially treaded bolts that engage the *cis*- and *trans*-cortices in addition to the nail. The proximal nail extremity features keying flanges for rigid linkage between the nail and an alignment guide via extension rods. The distal end of the nail presents a dull or trocar point to facilitate insertion.

Standard Nail Design and Instrumentation (IAP)

Implants
To accommodate dogs and cats of various sizes, nails are available in several diameters (4, 4.7, 6, 8, and 10 mm) and lengths (68–230 mm). Each nail extremity features 1 or 2 smooth cannulations that accommodate locking screws or bolts of different size (2.0, 2.7, 3.5, and 4.5 mm) depending on nail diameter (**Fig. 1**). To improve the versatility of the device, particularly with regard to its use in the treatment of metaphyseal fractures, cannulations are either 11 or 22 mm apart. The smaller spacing is more suitable for metaphyseal fractures when limited bone stock is available for the placement of 2 interlocking bolts.

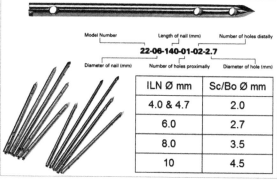
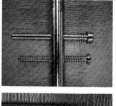
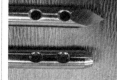

ILN Ø mm	Sc/Bo Ø mm
4.0 & 4.7	2.0
6.0	2.7
8.0	3.5
10	4.5

Model Number — Length of nail (mm) — Number of holes distally
22-06-140-01-02-2.7
Diameter of nail (mm) — Number of holes proximally — Diameter of hole (mm)

Fig. 1. Standard nails from IAP (Rochester, MN, USA) come in various sizes (diameter and length) to accommodate dogs and cats. The nails can be locked using partially threaded solid bolts (preferred) or standard cortical bone screws. The nail extremities feature proximal keying flanges for coupling of the nail to an insertion handle or an alignment guide and a trocar or dull tip distally.

Instrumentation

The use of the standard nails from IAP requires dedicated instrumentation consisting of (1) an insertion handle, (2) a drill jig featuring a series of holes whose location matches that of the nail cannulations, (3) extension rods for attachment of the nail to the insertion handle or to a drill jig, (4) a set of drilling (and tapping) sleeves and size-matched drill bits and taps, and (5) a dedicated depth gage (**Fig. 2**). Once the drill guide is rigidly secured to the nail via the extension rod, accurate transcortical insertion of the locking devices is possible.

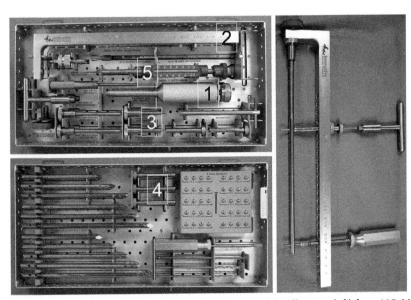

Fig. 2. Interlocking instrument (*top left*) and implant modules (*bottom left*) from IAP. Most currently available ILN systems rely on specific instrumentations for their implantation including (1) an insertion handle, (2) a drill jig, (3) extensions linking nail and drill jig, (4) drilling and tapping sleeves, and (5) a dedicated depth gage. Assembled nail (*right*) illustrating the matching locations of the nail and alignment guide cannulations.

AS Nail Design and Instrumentation (BioMedtrix)

Implants

In an effort to improve construct stability, facilitate surgical procedures and adherence to MIO principles of bridging osteosynthesis, the I-Loc nail was designed as an AS, compliant implant. Compared to standard nails, the main differences relate to the design of the locking mechanism, the profile of the nail, and the implantation technique.[21,25]

Locking mechanism

Each nail cannulation (2 at each extremity) features a self-centering and self-locking mechanism consisting of a threaded Morse taper. The locking bolt main characteristic is its threaded conical central section that matches both taper and thread of the nail cannulations. This creates an AS rigid linkage between bolt and nail. The bolts also feature a solid triangular end-section designed to drive the bolt through the *cis*-cortex into the nail and a thinner cylindrical end-section meant to engage the *trans*-cortex. Both end-sections are free of threads (**Figs. 3**). Although the diameters of the locking

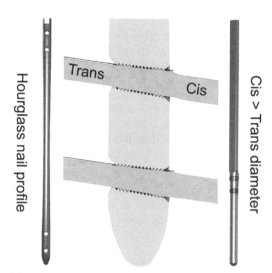

Fig. 3. Schematic of the I-Loc AS-ILN locking mechanism from BioMedtrix (*center*). Each nail hole features a threaded cone with dimensions that match those of the central section of locking bolt. Once tightened, the bolt is rigidly locked into the nail, thus creating an AS link between nail and bolt. The nail hourglass profile is intended to reduce iatrogenic endosteal damages, optimize revascularization of the medullary cavity, and increase overall construct compliance (*left*). Because of the fixed nail/bolt relationship, cortical threads on the end-sections of the bolt are unnecessary (*right*).

bolt sections are nail specific, the length of each end-section is common to all bolts and can be cut to size as appropriate.

Nail profile
The AS-ILN features an hourglass profile designed to limit iatrogenic damage to the endocortices and medullary blood supply and to increase overall construct compliance (compliance is the inverse of stiffness). Furthermore, the thinner core diameter of the nail facilitates its insertion and virtually eliminates the need for reaming of the medullary cavity (see **Fig. 3**). Because of the conical geometry of the nail cannulations and matching central bolt section, proximal asymmetric keying flanges are used to guarantee proper nail orientation and accurate connection of the nail to a customized alignment guide via a single dedicated extension. Finally, an oblong bullet-shaped distal tip was designed to optimize fracture reduction, particularly with regard to restoration of bone length, while limiting the risk of joint violation (see **Fig. 3**). Currently, this AS-ILN is available in 3 diameters (6, 7, and 8 mm) and lengths ranging from 122 to 203 mm.

Implantation technique
An important modification of the surgical technique is the use of temporary smooth locking posts to create a rigid frame between the nail and alignment guide. These posts are systematically inserted in a proximal to distal sequence, rather than alternating from distal to proximal as with standard nails. This step progressively reduces the alignment guide lever arm and therefore its potential deviation from the nail axis, which in turn further limits the risk of off-site distal bolt insertion.

Instrumentation

As with most veterinary nail systems, an alignment guide is necessary for accurate bolt insertion. In addition to typical nailing equipment, instrumentation specific to this system includes (1) a cutting awl and a trial nail used to open the medullary cavity proximally and the distal metaphysis, respectively; (2) smooth locking posts used to temporarily link nail and alignment guide; (3) a dedicated depth gage for simultaneous measurement of the *cis*- and *trans*-bolt end-sections; and (4) a dedicated bolt shearing tool (**Figs. 4**). To simplify surgical steps throughout the procedure, system components are linked using cam-based quick couplings.

BIOMECHANICAL PROPERTIES OF ILNS

With the recent paradigm shift toward biologic osteosynthesis, ILNs have emerged as an attractive alternative to bone plating and, to some surgeons, the method of choice for the repair of most comminuted diaphyseal and metaphyseal fractures in human and veterinary patients.

General Considerations

The efficacy of ILNs rests on several mechanical and biologic advantages inherent to the fixation method. Like any intramedullary devices, ILNs are placed near the neutral axis of the fractured bone and consequently are shielded against deleterious cyclic bending. Throughout physiologic activity, bones are subjected to various forces that create tensile and compressive loads on opposite cortices and, as a net result, bending moments along the entire bone. The neutral axis of a bone is a concept that describes the location where tensile and compressive loads are virtually

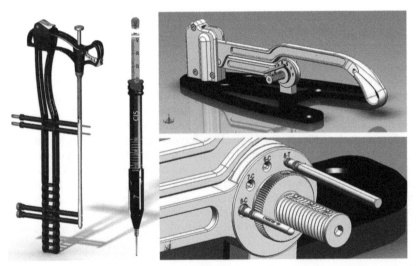

Fig. 4. Schematic representation of an assembled I-Loc nail and dedicated instrumentation used for implantation (*left*). The position of the alignment guide can be adjusted along the insertion handle to accommodate patients of various sizes. Temporary smooth locking bolts (*proximal 2 holes*) are used to rigidify the frame during fixation, thus reducing the risk of distal off-site bolt insertion. Cam-shaped quick couplings are used to consecutively link the insertion handle to an awl and a trial nail (not shown) and to the nail and alignment guide. A dedicated depth gage (*center*) is used to concomitantly measure the lengths of the bolt end-sections, which are then cut using a custom shearing bolt (*right*).

eliminated along with their resultant bending moment.[26] As a consequence, the farther away an implant is positioned from the bone neutral axis, the more susceptible it is to fatigue failure from cyclic bending.[27,28] Although the exact position of the neutral axis is unknown, and likely varies during activity, it is assumed that it is located near or within the medullary cavity. From a mechanical standpoint, this makes an ILN superior to a bone plate or an external fixator, particularly when anatomic reconstruction is not pursued, as it is with MIO. In addition, most ILNs are made of cold worked 316L stainless steel[21,29] and have a relatively larger and more homogeneous area moment of inertia (AMI) than comparable bone plates.[30,31] Both features account for their intrinsic high resistance to bending. The AMI of an implant characterizes material distribution with respect to the plane or axis of deformation and is proportional to the implant bending or torsional stiffness. The AMI is proportional to the fourth power of the ILN diameter and to the third power of a plate thickness. Consequently, although the AMI of the solid section of a plate varies considerably based on the plate orientation, it is constant regardless of the direction of applied loads in nails. As an example, the AMI of the solid section of a 3.5-mm broad dynamic compression plate bent along its flat surface is only 25% that of an 8-mm ILN but approximately 3 times greater if the same plate is bent on edge.[31]

Finally, unlike solid intramedullary pins, ILNs can resist torsional, compressive, and shear forces by using screws or bolts passing through both bone cortices and nail cannulations (locking effect).[21,29] However, nail holes act as stress concentrators, promoting nail failure through the holes.[32,33] Because screws or bolts do not rigidly interact with the nail, filling the nail holes, as found with bone plates, does not reduce local stresses. Furthermore, assuming that in most cases the locking devices are oriented perpendicular to the sagittal plan of the limb, ILNs are structurally weaker in mediolateral bending because the nail AMI is smaller in a bending plane parallel to the nail hole.[30,34]

Interlocking nails also have biologic advantages.[5,35,36] Following fracture, severe disruption of the intramedullary vascularization occurs. As a result, the extraosseous blood supply becomes a critical component of bone healing. When applied remotely to the fracture site via limited approaches, ILNs preserve soft tissues and extraosseous blood supply. Indeed, to reduce disruption of the fracture environment, ILNs can be placed in a normograde fashion. This less invasive approach reduces postoperative morbidity and promotes fracture healing and functional recovery.

Standard Nail Biomechanics

Early generations of standard nails featured relatively large cannulations, which weakened the nail and make them prone to fatigue failure through the nail hole.[29,32] To address this drawback, the 6-mm and 8-mm IAP nail hole diameters were reduced in current designs to accommodate 2.7-mm and 3.5-mm locking screws or bolts, instead of the previous 3.5-mm and 4.5-mm sizes. Although such changes resulted in a 52- and 8-fold increase in the nail fatigue life, respectively, screw failure became predominant over nail failure.[32] Indeed, screw size reduction results in an approximately 40% decrease in the screw AMI, which translates into a similar decrease in bending yield strength. To limit the incidence of screw failure, partially threaded solid bolts featuring a self-tapping thread at the level of the *cis*-cortex have been devised and are currently recommended (**Fig. 5**).[37,38] A recent study demonstrated that, under axial loads, metaphyseal insertion of the bolts further expends their fatigue life and decreases the incidence of catastrophic failure. Yet another theoretical advantage of metaphyseal, rather than diaphyseal, bolt location is the subsequent increase in construct working length and therefore compliance.

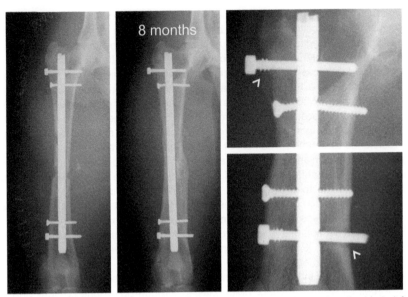

Fig. 5. Immediate (*left*) and 8-month (*center*) postoperative radiographs of a healed fractured femur. The femur was treated using MIO with an 8-mm standard nail locked with two 3.5-mm solid bolts and two 3.5-mm cortical screws. The relative strength of the locking devices is illustrated by the plastic deformation of the proximal screw (*top right*). Delayed healing was observed in that case, presumably as a result of postoperative instability as suggested by the backing of the proximal bolt and by the osteolysis around the distal bolt (*arrows*).

Despite overall favorable clinical outcomes, the reliability of standard ILN designs in ensuring fracture repair stability has been challenged in human and veterinary orthopedics. In an original mechanical study, torsional and bending angular deformations were significantly greater with standard nail constructs than in those treated with a PRC, a fixation method often used in the treatment of comminuted fractures.[39] Importantly, IAP nail constructs experienced up to 28° of acute rotational instability, or slack, and showed an overall angular deformation (AD) of up to 40°. In contrast, PRC constructs maximum AD was 11° and occurred without slack. Construct instability was attributed to the inherent mismatch between locking screws and nail cannulations, which precludes rigid locking, as well as to structural damage to the screw threads and nail hole.[39]

Although veterinary clinical studies have reported that 12% to 14% of diaphyseal fractures treated with standard ILNs required additional fixation to overcome perioperative instability,[40,41] other studies showed that torsional and bending instability significantly reduced bone healing and functional recovery[42,43] when a standard ILN was compared with an external fixator. These studies suggest that current human and veterinary ILN systems do not counteract torsional and bending forces as much as initially anticipated. This, in turn, could contribute to complications such as delayed or nonunions. To improve construct stability and reduce the risk of bolt failure, reaming, which allows for the implantation of larger nails and locking devices, has been recommended. Although potentially beneficial from a mechanical standpoint, reaming severely impairs the medullary blood supply and has been associated with a higher incidence of infection and fat embolism, and therefore should be avoided.[44] In contrast, the use of smaller, unreamed ILNs better preserves the endosteal and medullary blood supply, which, from a biologic standpoint, may be preferable. From a mechanical standpoint, however, the postoperative stability of unreamed ILNs relies primarily on the efficacy of the locking mechanism.[22]

AS Nail Biomechanics

The main impetus behind an AS-ILN design was the realization that the lack of rigid interaction between nail and locking devices in standard nails resulted in acute angular instability (slack). During the past few years, several in vitro studies, using a tibial diaphyseal gap fracture model, have compared the mechanical behavior of 6- and 8-mm screwed or bolted standard nails to that of an AS-ILN prototype (8-mm extremities – 6 mm midshaft core diameter).[21–23,34] These studies showed that constructs treated with an AS-ILN sustained significantly less AD in bending and torsion than those treated with IAP nails. More important, although AD of the AS-ILN constructs occurred without slack, constructs treated with screwed standard nails sustained nearly 10° and 20° of bending and torsional acute instability, respectively.[21–23,34] The use of locking bolts instead of than screws reduced but did not eliminate construct slack in standard nails. Assuming continuous construct deformation, ILNs effectively resist torsional, and presumably bending moments, through a recoil mechanism known as "spring back" effect.[45] In standard nails, construct slack has been misinterpreted as a spring back effect.[46] One must keep in mind, however, that these 2 mechanisms are very different and may have opposite effects on bone healing. Optimization of the spring back mechanism requires that construct AD occurs without slack and that the nail be somewhat compliant. This was achieved in early human models by the use of slotted nails. Although ideal construct compliance for optimal bone healing is unknown, one can speculate that overly compliant or stiff systems may promote either deleterious local shear stresses or stress shielding. Construct compliance in the AS-ILN was between that of the 6- and 8-mm standard nails.[22]

The high 25% complication rate seen in human tibial metaphyseal fractures treated with standard ILNs has been attributed to increased (up to 20°) construct slack due to the lack of interference between nail and endocortices in relatively wider metaphyseal regions.[6,47–49] These clinical reports underscore the shortcoming of the current locking mechanism and agree with the authors' experience that approximately 40% of canine tibial fractures treated with standard ILNs require additional fixation to control intraoperative or acute postoperative instability, particularly in comminuted metaphyseal and submetaphyseal fractures. In a subsequent mechanical study, our group demonstrated that an AS-ILN maintained construct bending stability ($\sim$4° of AD) regardless of the fracture configuration. In contrast, standard nail AD doubled from up to 11° to up to 22° between transverse and metaphyseal fracture patterns. This strongly suggests that contrary to AS-ILNs, the intrinsic slack of standard ILNs jeopardized construct stability particularly in a fracture configuration involving the metaphyses.[23]

In a subsequent in vivo study,[24] a 7- $\times$ 5.25-mm (extremities and core diameters, respectively) AS-ILN was compared with a 6-mm bolted standard nail using a canine mid diaphyseal tibial gap fracture model. Dogs treated with standard nails showed tibial rotational slack up to 2 weeks postoperatively and, from 4 to 8 weeks after surgery, were significantly lamer than dogs treated with an AS-ILN. Radiographic clinical union started at 8 weeks and was completed in all AS-ILN dogs at 10 weeks postoperatively. In contrast, bone healing was significantly slower in the dogs treated with the IAP nails, as only 50% of them reached clinical union by 18 weeks (**Fig. 6**). Mechanical testing of the calluses at 18 weeks showed that failure torque and energy

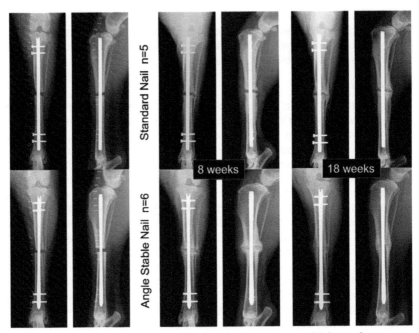

Fig. 6. Radiographic follow-up showing callus progression in a tibial gap fracture model stabilized with either a 6-mm bolted IAP standard nail (*top row*) or a 7- × 5.25-mm AS-ILN (*bottom row*). Clinical union, defined as bridging of 3 of 4 cortices, was completed in all AS-ILN dogs by 10 weeks postoperatively. In contrast, at 18 weeks, only 3 of the 5 dogs treated with an IAP nail had reached clinical union. By then, callus remodeling had occurred in the AS-ILN group.

were significantly greater in the AS-ILN than in the standard nail specimens. In addition, contralateral intact tibiae (controls) and AS-ILN–treated tibiae consistently failed via acute spiral fractures along the tibial diaphysis, whereas tibiae treated with an standard IAP nail failed progressively via transverse fracture through the initial gap (**Fig. 7**).[24]

From a mechanical standpoint, these studies suggest that through reengineering of the locking mechanism and nail profile, the new hourglass AS-ILN system can eliminate bending and torsional instability associated with the use of current ILNs. Considering the deleterious effect of acute deformation on bone healing, compared with current ILNs, an AS-ILN may represent a mechanically more effective fixation method for the treatment of diaphyseal and metaphyseal fractures.[21–23,34] Similarly, from a biologic standpoint, the use of an AS-ILN, rather than a standard nail, seems to yield faster functional recovery and bone healing as evidenced by the presence of a stronger and more mature callus.[24]

INDICATIONS FOR INTERLOCKING NAILING
General Considerations

As intramedullary devices, ILNs can only be used in long bones that provide a nonarticular entry point for the nail (which excludes the radius). Although conventional ILNs have traditionally been used to treat diaphyseal fractures of the humerus, femur, and tibia, in recent years, their range of application has been considerably and successfully expanded thanks in part to the use of MINO techniques and to the introduction

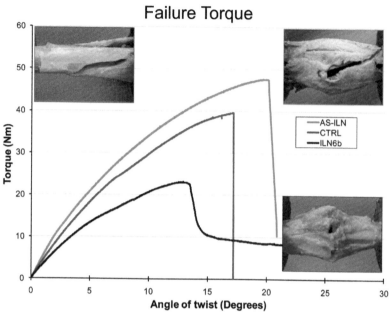

Fig. 7. Representative 18-weeks torque/deformation curves generated during mechanical testing of the bony callus of AS-ILN and standard 6-mm bolted nail (ILN6b) groups, as well as intact contralateral tibia (CTRL). Failure torque was greatest in the AS-ILN group ($P<.05$). Calluses were significantly weaker in the standard ILN6b group than in both the control and AS-ILN groups. Failure occurred as an acute spiral fracture in the control and AS-ILN specimens (*top inserts*) and a progressive transverse fracture through the original gap in the standard nail specimens (*bottom insert*).

of an AS locking design. The combined effect of MINO and elimination of perioperative slack with subsequent improvement in construct stability likely contribute to enhancing bone healing even in more challenging cases, including periarticular and transverse fractures, corrective osteotomies, and revision surgeries. The added strength of the locking mechanism in AS-ILNs in addition to the nail intramedullary location allowed the authors to stabilize pathologic humeral and femoral fractures rather than resort to amputation.

Common Indications

Because of established unique biomechanical advantages, ILN osteosynthesis is the treatment of choice for most long bone diaphyseal fractures in people. During the past 20 years, because of the work of such pioneer surgeons as Johnson,[13] Dueland,[17] Duhautois,[18] Durall,[50] Basinger,[51] Nagaoka,[20] and others, interlocking nailing has gained increasing acceptance in veterinary orthopedics as a reliable osteosynthesis method. Although ILNs are often placed through open approaches, the recent use of minimally invasive techniques further amplifies the biologic benefits of interlocking nailing (**Fig. 8**).

Early ILNs were mostly used for the treatment of closed diaphyseal canine fractures of the femur, tibia, and, to a lesser extent, humerus. Current indications, particularly since the recent availability of an AS-ILN, include open contaminated fractures, such as from gunshot injuries (see **Fig. 8**), as well as infected and nonunion fractures. A case report describes the successful use of an ulnar nail in the treatment of a severely

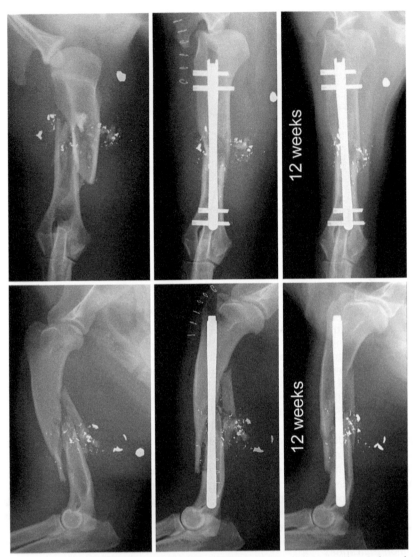

Fig. 8. Radiographs of a gunshot humeral fracture in a 4-year-old intact male mix-breed dog (preoperative [*left*], immediate postoperative [*center*]). The fracture was treated with a 7-mm AS-ILN using MINO. The fracture site was not approached surgically, in an attempt to limit further soft tissue trauma. The dog was weight bearing immediately after surgery, and recovery was uneventful. Clinical union was achieved by 12 weeks postoperative (*right*).

comminuted proximal radioulnar gunshot fracture in a dog.[52] Once reserved for midsize and large dogs, the introduction of smaller nail models has made interlocking nailing suitable for the treatment of feline diaphyseal fractures, regardless of fracture pattern.

Extended Indications

Alternative to PRC

While the acceptance of MIO is gaining momentum, the treatment of long bone diaphyseal fractures using ORIF with a PRC technique remains widespread among veterinary orthopedic surgeons. The popularity of this technique likely stems from the perception that the IMR facilitates fracture reduction and that it provides added strength to the repair compared with plate fixation alone. From a mechanical standpoint, a PRC is conceptually analogous to an ILN, although the technique requires at least 2 implants, rather than 1, to effectively control all fracture forces. From a surgical perspective, the PRC may be challenging due to the difficulty of screw placement around the IMR. Consequently, despite the plate-sparing effect of the IMR, the eccentric location of the plate remains a concern when surgical constraints preclude the use of an appropriately sized IMR (**Fig. 9**). Finally, from a biologic

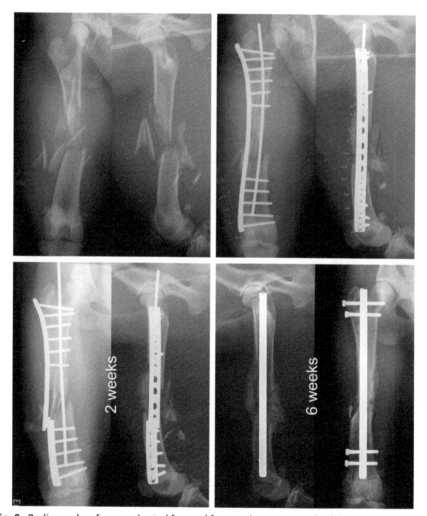

Fig. 9. Radiographs of a comminuted femoral fracture in an 11-month-old Labrador (*top left*). The initial repair consisted of a PRC applied using ORIF technique (*top right*). Although the IMR filled ~30% of the medullary cavity, plate failure occurred 2 weeks postoperatively, presumably due to the relative small size of the IMR (*bottom left*). Successful revision was achieved using minimally invasive techniques to remove the implants followed by MINO with a standard ILN. One can speculate that primary repair with an ILN is a valid alternative to PRC.

standpoint, PRC inherently induces more extensive damage to the main blood supplies to the fractured bone, namely its endosteal/medullary, and, to a greater extent, periosteal blood supplies than an ILN. Presumably, the hourglass profile of the AS-ILN also contributes to limiting iatrogenic damage to the endosteal and medullary blood supply because reaming is unnecessary. Furthermore, the narrow central core diameter of the AS-ILN likely facilitates revascularization of the medullary cavity, which in turn may enhance bone healing and functional recovery. Based on these observations, the authors surmise that everything else being equal, from biologic and surgical standpoints, an ILN is an implant that is as effective as, if not superior to, a PRC (**Fig. 10**). From a mechanical standpoint, although direct comparison between PRC and AS-ILN is not available, a recent study showed that an AS-ILN sustains less angular deformation than a size-matched dynamic compression plate.[22]

Angular limb deformities—patellar luxation

Yet another theoretical argument in favor of ILNs over PRC is that restoration of axial alignment is technically facilitated by the use of an intramedullary device. Indeed,

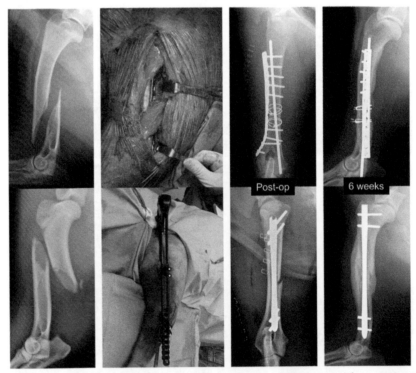

Fig. 10. Radiographs and intraoperative photographs of 2 similar humeral fractures in a 12- and a 9-month midsize dog (*top* and *bottom row*, respectively). Note the presence of a long distal fissure in the second patient. Anatomic reduction and traditional ORIF with cerclage wires and a PRC was achieved in the first case. In contrast, MINO with an AS-ILN was performed in second case to achieve realignment without attempting anatomic reduction. Although both patients eventually healed, delayed union was observed when osteosynthesis consisted of ORIF with a PRC. Note that the limited callus formation and presence of discernible fracture line remain at 6 weeks in the PRC case. In contrast, callus remodeling is well under way in the fracture treated with MINO and an AS-ILN.

using an epiperiosteal plate often requires complex contouring, particularly in the presence of a callus in cases of revision surgery. This argument holds true in the treatment of angular limb deformities specifically for those involving multiple corrections. Similarly, correction of distal femoral varus or valgus associated with medial or lateral patellar luxation, respectively, can be facilitated by the use of an ILN rather than a plate (**Fig. 11**).

Revision surgery—nonunion

In the authors' experience, MINO is of particular interest in the revision of failed pin, plate, and/or PRC osteosyntheses of diaphyseal fractures (see **Fig. 9**). In such cases, implant removal can be performed through periarticular incision remote to the fracture site. The same approaches can be used for nail insertion and stabilization, often without the need to further disturb the fracture site. Similarly, the treatment of nonunions using MINO has proved beneficial (**Fig. 12**). Following implant removal as appropriate, a reamer is used to reopen the medullary cavity. Furthermore, because the fracture is not exposed, the bone fragments generated during reaming remain in the vicinity of the nonunion site, acting as an autogenous graft. Further grafting may be performed as appropriate under fluoroscopic guidance using a Michel trephine to percutaneously inject a mixture of marrow and corticocancellous material.

Metaphyseal and epiphyseal fractures

Presumably because of the limited bone stock available for locking and the inherent instability of current locking mechanisms, a traditionally reported limitation of interlocking nailing is the treatment of metaphyseal and epiphyseal fractures. In people, up to 58% of valgus malalignment[49] and up to 20° of acute, uncontrolled motion at the fracture site have been documented in ILN-treated tibial metaphyseal fractures.[47] These reports agree with the authors' experience that approximately 40% of canine comminuted metaphyseal and submetaphyseal tibial fractures treated with standard ILNs

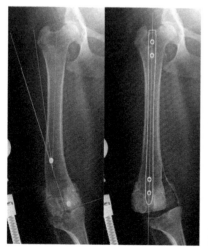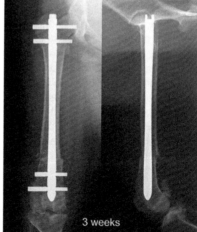

Fig. 11. A distal femoral corrective osteotomy was used for the treatment of a medially luxating patella (grade II/IV). The procedure was planned using OrthoView Veterinary Orthopedic Digital Planning software (*left,* http://www.orthoview.com/) and consisted of a 20° lateral closing wedge and an abrasion sulcoplasty. The use of an AS-ILN simplified realignment without need for extensive soft tissue dissection and complex implant contouring required with plate fixation.

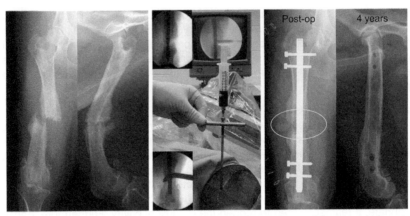

Fig. 12. Three consecutive surgical attempts at repairing a femoral fracture with a single IMR resulted in a chronic, 4-month highly unstable nonunion. Several biomechanical factors were carefully evaluated during preoperative planning: (1) multiple previous surgical traumas, (2) extensive muscle atrophy and fibrous adhesions, (3) challenging plate contouring in the presence of a bony callus, and (4) poor bone quality due to extensive disuse osteopenia. Accordingly, MINO with a standard nail and percutaneous injection of a bone marrow/cancellous autograft mixture (*center*) was selected over plate fixation as the optimal option for revision. Oversize reaming was performed to open the medullary cavity and locally release bone material (*central inserts*). The graft is clearly visible on the immediate postoperative anteroposterior radiograph (*right*). Clinical union was obtained at 12 weeks (not shown). Bone remodeling can be appreciated after implant removal due to the presence of a distal seroma, 4 years postoperatively.

require additional fixation to control perioperative instability. Various supplemental fixation techniques, including external skeletal fixator, stack pins, and additional plating, have been advocated to circumvent construct instability.[40,51,53] However, these methods may not conclusively achieve optimal stability without additional surgical trauma, which offsets the biomechanical benefits of MINO.

In contrast, the reliance on the rigid locking mechanism of the AS-ILN proved effective in eliminating construct slack in a submetaphyseal comminuted fracture model.[23] Several clinical cases recently performed at Michigan State University have thus far confirmed that an AS-ILN can be used effectively and reliably in the treatment of metaphyseal and epiphyseal fractures. In these cases, the distal nail tip may be customlathed to optimize deep nail seating against the subchondral bone plate. In turn, this allowed for the safe use of the locking bolts despite the limited available bone stock and the presence of metaphyseal fissures (**Fig. 13**). The surgeon should keep in mind that although, in most cases, the locking bolts are inserted in the frontal plane, this plane can be reoriented to avoid fissures. This property, unique to ILNs, considerably increases the versatility of this fixation method in metaphyseal and epiphyseal fractures.

CLINICAL USE OF ILNS
Preoperative Planning

Orthogonal radiographs of the fractured and contralateral intact bone of interest are essential to accurate planning. Imaging of the affected bone is used for evaluation of the fracture location, configuration, and identification of fissures that could extend into the metaphyses. In such cases, a computed tomography scan with 3-dimensional reconstruction may prove beneficial. Radiographs of the intact contralateral bone

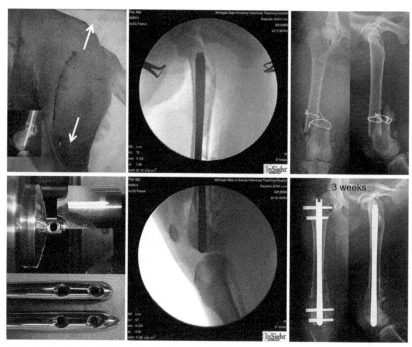

Fig. 13. Proximal and distal rod migration (*top left, arrows*) occurred 2 weeks after repair of a distal metaphyseal femoral fracture with 2 IMRs and cerclage wires (*top left, insert*). The choice of a plate for revision seemed ill-advised due to the presence of iatrogenic fissures extending toward the lateral fabella, which considerably limited bone stock availability for reliable screw fixation (*top right*). In contrast, based on a previous study form our laboratory, the use of an AS-ILN seemed to be a valid alternative. The nail tip was custom-lathed to allow deeper seating in the distal epiphysis, thus avoiding the distal fissures (*bottom left*). Care was taken to ensure that the subtle protrusion of the rounded nail tip, immediately proximal to the origin of the caudal cruciate ligament, did not interfere with patellar tracking. Robust callus formation was noticed 3 weeks after revision.

should take into account magnification and distortion. Therefore, the proper use of a linear or spherical calibration marker placed over the bone of interest is critical. Similarly, to avoid image distortion, the bone diaphysis should be parallel to the plane of the film. Horizontal beam projections are particularly helpful for that purpose.

Selection of the appropriate nail can be performed using premagnified (usually by 4% and 12%) acetate templates superimposed over the radiographs. This cost-effective method is, however, fairly inaccurate. In contrast, digital templating can be performed using one of the dedicated software products currently available. Most software will allow the surgeon to plan the entire procedure (**Fig. 14**). Valuable steps include fracture reduction, planning of the location and magnitude of corrective osteotomies in angular limb deformity cases, implant selection and positioning, and predetermination of the locking bolt lengths. Considering the cost of this software, interested surgeons are encouraged to become familiar with the system and ascertain that it is compatible with in-house picture archiving and communication system and that desired templates are available.

Traditionally, selection of the largest possible nail fitting the isthmus of the medullary has been recommended.[1] To achieve this, however, reaming is often necessary. The

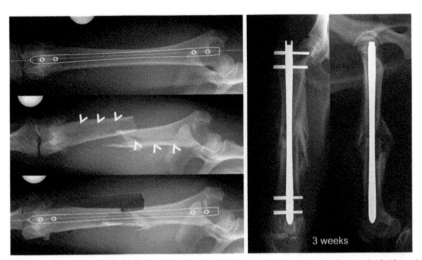

Fig. 14. Preoperative planning using OrthoView Veterinary Orthopedic Digital Planning software (*left,* http://www.orthoview.com/). Selection of an appropriately sized nail is based on digital templating of the intact contralateral bone (*top left*). In this young animal, care is taken to ensure that the locking bolts are not bridging the growth plates. Note that the presence of extensive fissures (*arrows*) is *not* a contraindication for interlocking nailing and does *not* require further stabilization (*center left*) as long as 1 locking bolt is placed in healthy bone (*bottom left*). Through an increase in construct compliance, bridging osteosynthesis combined with the use of an hourglass AS-ILN provides beneficial controlled micromotion at the fracture site. Along with adherence to MINO principles, these techniques enhance bone healing as demonstrated by robust callus formation and clinical union by 3 weeks postoperative (*right*). The hourglass profile of the AS-ILN also promotes revascularization of the medullary cavity and reduces the need for overreduction.

rationale for this recommendation is 2-fold: (1) larger nails can accommodate relatively larger, hence stronger, locking bolts and (2) the inherent slack of standard nails may be attenuated (in bending) by direct nail bone impingement. Although this may be true for standard nails, it becomes obsolete with the AS-ILN. Considering the biologic disadvantages of reaming and mechanical advantages of compliant systems, the authors recommend that, when using an AS-ILN, the nail largest diameter (extremities) be approximately 75% of the medullary cavity at its narrowest point. Similarly, the longest possible nail should be selected to optimize construct compliance. Seating the nail extremities in the epiphyses, flushed with the subchondral plates (or physes in immature dogs), provides added benefits, including (1) improved bending stability, (2) increased fatigue life of the locking bolts, and (3) easier nail capture if explantation becomes necessary.

General Techniques

Although ILNs can be applied using an OBDNT approach, MINO implies that the nail is inserted through small incisions remote from the fracture site. The size of the incisions varies with the bone of interest and the skills of the surgeon. A common mistake early on is *not to open wide enough* to allow for easy fracture realignment and to ensure that placement of the alignment guide and drill sleeves will not be hindered by soft tissues. As an example, the approach to the proximal femur may expand from the level of the acetabulum to subtrochanteric region initially. This will facilitate normograde nail insertion through the intertrochanteric fossa and provide access to the trochanter for interlocking. With experience, the nail is inserted blindly through a proximal stab incision and blunt dissection through the superficial gluteal; the trochanter is exposed through a smaller distal and lateral incision followed by caudal and cranial retraction of the biceps and vastus lateralis muscles, respectively.

Although not absolutely necessary, intraoperative fluoroscopy is often beneficial with MINO to ascertain proper restoration of rotational alignment. One of the benefits of interlocking nailing is that alignment in the sagittal and frontal planes is easily restored by the mere intramedullary location of the implant. The surgeon should verify before initiating surgery that complete, unobstructed visualization of the adjacent joints in both craniocaudal and lateromedial planes are obtainable throughout the procedure.

Preservation of the fracture site during reduction is a hallmark of MINO. However, the use of hanging leg techniques or traction tables is inappropriate for MINO because the resulting extension of the limb precludes nail insertion in any bone segment. In contrast, the use of small bone reduction forceps applied at the level of the epiphyses/metaphyses is acceptable. Alternatively, the application of toothed reduction handles; Also known as joysticks (Synthes, Paoli, PA, USA) specially designed for MIO may be preferred, particularly for realignment of tibial fractures (**Fig. 15**). Successful reduction should lead to restoration of alignment in the sagittal, frontal, and transverse planes. Multiple unsuccessful attempts should be discouraged because they will induce iatrogenic trauma. Conversion to an open approach must be considered when atraumatic restoration of alignment cannot be completed using MINO techniques. The use of small portals over the facture and the use of bone graft during primary osteosynthesis should be regarded as invasive surgical acts unsuited for MINO and therefore should be avoided.

In MINO, the only acceptable nail insertion technique is normograde. The medullary cavity is first opened using intramedullary pins of increasing diameter or a dedicated awl. The nail is coupled to an insertion handle via an extension, then carefully impacted intramedullary with a hammer until deeply seated in the distal epiphysis. Leverage on the nail during insertion *must* be avoided because it may result in structural damage to the couplings and *will* lead to loss of alignment between the nail and drill guide and thus off-site placement of the locking bolts. For these same reasons, the nail *must not* be used for fracture reduction.

Following proper nail insertion, placement of the locking bolts is achieved through the use of an alignment guide coupled to the nail. System specific instruments (sleeves, drill bits, temporary locking bolts, depth gages, etc) are used for that purpose. Depending on the distribution of the locking bolts on either side of the fracture, ILNs can be used in a static (bolts above and below the fracture) or dynamic mode (bolts on 1 side of the fracture only). Although dynamic locking is occasionally performed in people,[54] full ILN biomechanical potential is only achieved in static mode, which remains the sole viable option when bridging osteosynthesis is desirable. Dynamic nailing can be achieved at a later date to stimulate bone remodeling once sufficient continuity and strength of the bone column have been restored.[55] Accurate placement of the distal bolts has been challenging with off-site insertion reported in up to 28% of the cases treated with standard nails.[41,50,56] Resting the leg on a Mayo stand, which adds stability, and using proper drilling techniques are simple surgical steps that may be used to limit this drawback. Light and steady pressure pulse drilling without leaning on the alignment guide in particular is very effective. Similarly, the use of sharp drill bits featuring a StickTite(TM) like design (Imex(TM) Veterinary, Inc, Longview, TX) helps prevent skidding of the drill bit. Accurate bolt insertion is further facilitated by the use of (1) an adjustable alignment guide than can moved closer to the

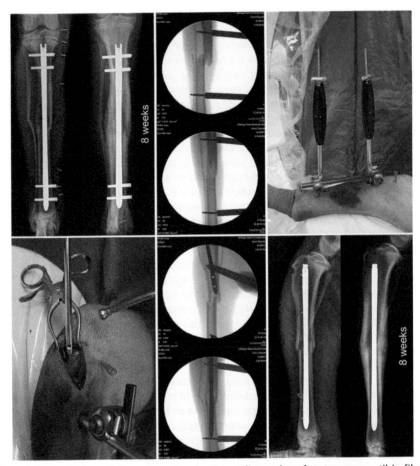

Fig. 15. Immediate and 8-week postoperative radiographs of a transverse tibia-fibula fracture in a 7-month-old Labrador treated using MINO with an AS-ILN (*top left* and *bottom right*). Note the continuous bone growth without loss of alignment. Toothed reduction handles, also known as joysticks (Synthes, Paoli, PA, USA) were used to realign the bone fragments. Following reduction, a temporary dedicated Snap-on external fixator was used to connect the joysticks and maintain stability during normograde nail insertion (*top right* and *bottom left*). The procedure was conducted under fluoroscopic guidance (*center column*).

bone, (2) extended smooth locking bolts that temporarily link the nail to the alignment guide, and (3) self-centering conical bolts. Using these devices, the rate of off-site placement of the AS-ILN locking bolts was reduced to 0.7% in a series of 41 consecutive cases (internal observations).

Specific Application

It is beyond the scope of this article to describe specific techniques that are the objects of specialized courses. The interested reader is encouraged to visit the following Web sites, http://www.innovativeanimalproducts.com/ and http://www.biomedtrix.com/, as well as the AO Foundation, http://www.aovet.org/, for course availability on specific nail systems and MIO techniques.

Humeral fractures

Because approximately 55% of all humeral fractures affect the center and/or the distal thirrd of the diaphysis, nailing of humeral fractures may be challenging. Preoperative planning is paramount to ensure that there is enough bone stock available for distal locking. In particular, fracture pattern (eg, distal fissures) and location in relation to the supratrochlear foramen may limit, and even preclude, deep seating of the nail. The use of a single distal bolt has been recommended in such cases. Alternatively, to circumvent this potential limitation, the tip of the nail may be lathed down and allowed to slightly protrude through the roof of the foramen (see **Fig. 8**).

With the affected leg up and the animal in lateral recumbency, normograde nail insertion is performed via a limited craniolateral approach centered over at the crest of the greater tubercle. A distal incision immediately above the lateral epicondyle and cranial retraction of the brachialis muscle allow exposure of the distal 25% of the diaphysis while avoiding the radial nerve.[57] We found that orienting the locking plane approximately 45° from the frontal plane in a slightly more craniocaudal direction facilitates bolt insertion and improves anchorage in the medial epicondylar ridge (see **Fig. 10**).

Radioulnar fractures

To the authors' knowledge, only one case report describes the successful use of an ulnar standard nail to treat a highly comminuted fracture of the proximal *radius and ulna*.[52] The relative size of the nail and ulnar medullary cavity remains a limiting factor in the treatment of such factures.

Femoral fractures

The approaches and nail insertion techniques have been described earlier ("General techniques" section). Because of the natural femoral procurvatum, overreduction, particularly in distal femoral fractures, is necessary when using bridge interlocking nailing (**Fig. 16**). The subsequent subtle loss of anatomic alignment in the sagittal plane, however, is clinically irrelevant. Conversely, this technique allows deep nail penetration in the distal epiphysis without jeopardizing the integrity of the femoral trochlea. By moving the bolts away caudal to the edges of the trochlea, the technique also improves distal bone purchase by the bolts while limiting soft tissue irritation during flexion/extension. Distal normograde nail insertion has been described in distal metaphyseal fractures. This technique, which destroys the articular surface of the distal trochlea, is, however, more invasive and may be avoided by using lathed-down nails and overreduction of the fracture, as shown in **Fig. 13**.

Tibial fractures

The limited soft tissue coverage of the tibia makes this bone well suited for closed interlocking nailing even without fluoroscopic assistance. Through a small medial par-apatellar incision, the nail is inserted immediately cranial to the footprint of the cranial cruciate ligament insertion.[58] Care should be taken to preserve the cranial cruciate and intermeniscal ligaments. The nail should be aiming at the talocrural joint between the malleoli to avoid premature exit through the caudal or lateral tibial cortices. Traditionally, unless reaming is performed, relatively smaller nails are used in the tibia to account for the sigmoid shape of its diaphysis (**Fig. 17**). Because of its hourglass profile, the AS-ILN can be used without reaming.

Clinical Outcome and Complications

Although postoperative recommendation may vary based on the specifics of a case, our patients are usually sent home within 48 hours following surgery without

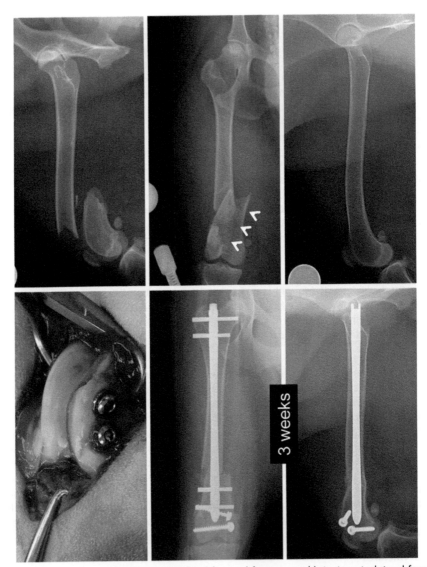

Fig. 16. Preoperative radiographs of a distal femoral fracture and intact contralateral femur in a middle-age Labrador (*top row*). Note the presence of distal fissures through the trochlea (*arrowheads*) and the natural procurvatum of the distal femur. The trochlear fracture was stabilized with 2 lag screws (*bottom left*), whereas the distal femoral fracture was reduced with a slight retrocurvatum and then stabilized with an AS-ILN (*bottom right*). As noted previously, fissures do *not* preclude interlocking nailing as long as 1 locking bolt is placed in healthy bone. The hourglass profile of the AS-ILN facilitates nail insertion in curvilinear bones such as the femur and tibia.

bandages, other than superficial dressings over the skin incisions. Low-impact activity is recommended until there is radiographic evidence of sufficient (subjective assessment) callus formation (typically 3 weeks). The success rate of interlocking nailing using traditional nailing techniques and standard nails varies from 83% to 96%, with healing times ranging from 13 to 17 weeks.[19,41,56,59]

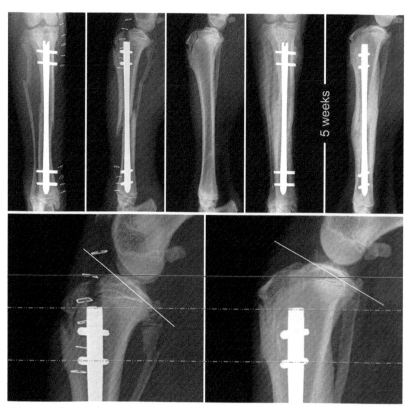

Fig. 17. Immediate and 5-week postoperative radiographs of a mid-shaft tibial fracture and intact contralateral tibia in a 6-month-old German shepherd (*top row*). The postoperative tibial plateau angle (TPA) was similar to that of the contralateral tibia. Bridging osteosynthesis was achieved by selecting the longest possible nail extending within the constraints of the tibial physes. Observed at 5 weeks, bony union was associated with a mild reduction in TPA (*yellow lines*), likely due to partial closure of the cranial aspect of the proximal tibial physis. The reduced TPA may have a sparing effect on the cranial cruciate ligament later in life. Conversely, there was no growth disturbance in this case (*red line*). Note that the magnification between preoperative and postoperative radiographs (*bottom row, green lines*) is identical.

Complications have been reported in up to 17% of cases treated with standard nails.[56] Although most complications are related to poor indications (eg, metaphyseal fractures with insufficient bone for screw insertion) or technical errors (eg, empty screw hole near a fracture site), some may be attributed to the limitation of the current nail designs including implant fracture, missed screw holes, and delayed unions or nonunions. Catastrophic nail fractures in early designs are now rare occurrences. Complications such as delayed unions or nonunions may be related to torsional and bending slack in standard nails, which may be accentuated by structural failure and/ or off-site placement of the locking screws. Although the use of solid bolts may limit the incidence of implant failure, it has little to no effect on construct stability.[22] The use of additional implants such as type I external fixator has been reported in 12% of the cases to provide adequate construct rigidity.[40] Other nonspecific complications include infection, sciatic neuropraxia, coxofemoral luxation (immature dogs), and joint violation.[40,56,60]

Stress shielding has not been a clinical issue with standard nails and is even more unlikely with the compliant AS-ILN design (**Fig. 18**). Accordingly, unless motivated by a complication, ILN removal is unnecessary. Nonetheless, a perceived problem is that explantation may be challenging due to difficulties in recapturing the nail. Simple effective strategies may be used to circumvent this potential drawback. Bone wax capping the nail flanges may be used to prevent bone ingrowth. Choosing the longest possible implant, as recommended for semirigid fixation, also places the nail tip near the proximal subchondral plate (in adults). In turn, this facilitates nail identification, coupling to the extension and handle, and, finally, extraction following removal of the locking devices. The hourglass shape of the AS-ILN has not been a factor preventing nail explantation. In a recent in vivo study,[24] using a twisting and pulling motion, all nails were extracted in less than 30 seconds at loads smaller than 300 N, even though explantation was performed 18 weeks postoperatively, before callus remodeling.

Although no objective clinical data are currently available on the efficacy of MINO and new nail designs, the comparative outcome of standard versus angle stable nails in an experimental in vivo study demonstrated the biomechanical superiority of the AS-ILN over standard nails.[24] Similarly, an internal (unpublished) review of 13 femoral and tibial fractures treated with and AS-ILN using MINO showed a mean healing time

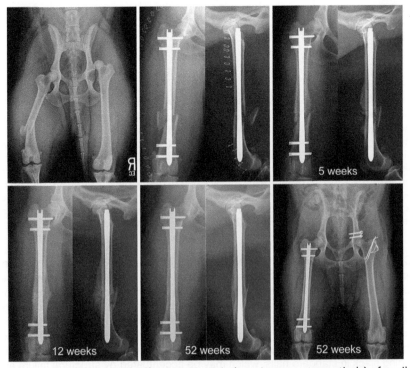

Fig. 18. Sequential radiographs (from preoperatively to 1 year postoperatively) of a mildly comminuted diaphyseal femoral fracture and concurrent contralateral hip luxation in a 1-year-old Labrador. The fracture was treated using MINO with an AS-ILN. Note the large callus at 12 weeks, as well as its complete resorption with restoration of the normal femoral shape at one year. This suggests that this compliant nail does not shield the repaired bone from physiologic loads and allow normal bone remodeling to occur unhindered. Also note the absence of OA in the reduced hip at 1 year.

of 36 ± 9.3 days (21–45 days). This was shorter than that previously reported with standard nails (90–120 days).[56] To date, the AS-ILN has been successfully used in 41 consecutive cases. These involved femoral (24), tibial (9), and humeral (5) fractures, as well as 3 corrections of distal varus angular deformities of the femur (2) and tibia (1). Anecdotally, major complications have not been observed in this limited series, which compares favorably with 17% of complication requiring revision surgery reported in a series of 134 cases treated with ORIF using standard nails.[56] Atraumatic reduction, preservation of the soft tissue envelope surrounding the fracture site, and MIO techniques as well as the use of an AS-ILN, may explain both findings.

SUMMARY

Interlocking nailing of long bone fractures has long been considered the gold standard osteosynthesis technique in people. Because of improvements in the locking mechanism design and nail profile, a recently developed veterinary angle stable nail has become the first true intramedullary fixator providing accurate and consistent repair stability while allowing semirigid fixation. As a result, indications for interlocking nailing have expanded to include treatment of periarticular fractures, corrections on angular deformities, and revisions of failed plate osteosyntheses. Perfectly suited for MIO, interlocking nailing is an attractive and effective alternative to plate and plate-rod osteosynthesis.

REFERENCES

1. Johnson AL, Houlton JE, Vannini R. AO principles of fracture management in the dog and cat. Stuttgart (Germany)/New York: AO Publishing & Thieme; 2005.
2. Kirkby KA, Lewis DD, Lafuente MP, et al. Management of humeral and femoral fractures in dogs and cats with linear-circular hybrid external skeletal fixators. J Am Vet Med Assoc 2008;44(4):180–97.
3. Dudley M, Johnson AL, Olmstead M, et al. Open reduction and bone plate stabilization, compared with closed reduction and external fixation, for treatment of comminuted tibial fractures: 47 cases (1980-1995) in dogs. J Am Vet Med Assoc 1997;211(8):1008–12.
4. Tong GO, Bavonratanavech S. Minimally invasive plate osteosynthesis (MIPO). Davos (Switzerland): AO Publishing; 2007.
5. Gerber C, Mast JW, Ganz R. Biological internal fixation of fractures. Arch Orthop Trauma Surg 1990;109(6):295–303.
6. Gerber A, Ganz R. Combined internal and external osteosynthesis a biological approach to the treatment of complex fractures of the proximal tibia. Injury 1998;29(Suppl 3):C22–8.
7. Gautier E, Sommer C. Guidelines for the clinical application of the LCP. Injury 2003;34(Suppl 2):B63–76.
8. Perren SM. Evolution of the internal fixation of long bone fractures. The scientific basis of biological internal fixation: choosing a new balance between stability and biology. J Bone Joint Surg Br 2002;84(8):1093–110.
9. Rozbruch SR, Muller U, Gautier E, et al. The evolution of femoral shaft plating technique. Clin Orthop Relat Res 1998;(354):195–208.
10. Guiot LP, Dejardin LM. Prospective evaluation of minimally invasive plate osteosynthesis in 36 nonarticular tibial fractures in dogs and cats. Vet Surg 2011; 40(2):171–82.
11. Küntscher G. Die Behandlung von Knochenbrüchen bei Tieren durch Marknagelung. Archiv für Wissensch Prakt Tierheil 1940;75:262.

12. Huckstep RL. Proceedings: an intramedullary nail for rigid fixation and compression of fractures of the femur. J Bone Joint Surg Br 1975;57(2):253.

13. Johnson KA, Huckstep RL. Bone remodeling in canine femora after internal-fixation with the huckstep nail. Vet Radiol 1986;27(1):20–3.

14. Muir P, Johnson KA. Tibial intercalary allograft incorporation: comparison of fixation with locked intramedullary nail and dynamic compression plate. J Orthop Res 1995;13(1):132–7.

15. Muir P, Johnson KA. Interlocking intramedullary nail stabilization of a femoral fracture in a dog with osteomyelitis. J Am Vet Med Assoc 1996;209(7): 1262–4.

16. Muir P, Parker RB, Goldsmid SE, et al. Interlocking intramedullary nail stabilisation of a diaphyseal tibial fracture. J Small Anim Pract 1993;34(1):26–30.

17. Dueland RT, Johnson KA. Interlocking nail fixation of diaphyseal fractures in the dog: a multi-center study of 1991-1992 cases. Vet Surg 1993;22(5):377.

18. Duhautois B, vanTilburg J. Veterinary bolted pinning or interlocking nail: clinical study of 45 cases. Vet Q 1996;18:S21.

19. Durall I, Diaz MC. Early experience with the use of an interlocking nail for the repair of canine femoral shaft fractures. Vet Surg 1996;25(5):397–406.

20. Endo K, Nakamura K, Maeda H, et al. Interlocking intramedullary nail method for the treatment of femoral and tibial fractures in cats and small dogs. J Vet Med Sci 1998;60(1):119–22.

21. Dejardin LM, Lansdowne JL, Sinnott MT, et al. In vitro mechanical evaluation of torsional loading in simulated canine tibiae for a novel hourglass-shaped interlocking nail with a self-tapping tapered locking design. Am J Vet Res 2006; 67(4):678–85.

22. Lansdowne JL, Sinnott MT, Dejardin LM, et al. In vitro mechanical comparison of screwed, bolted, and novel interlocking nail systems to buttress plate fixation in torsion and mediolateral bending. Vet Surg 2007;36(4):368–77.

23. Ting D, Cabassu JB, Guillou RP, et al. In vitro evaluation of the effect of fracture configuration on the mechanical properties of standard and novel interlocking nail systems in bending. Vet Surg 2009;38(7):881–7.

24. Cabassu JB, Villwock M, Guillou RP, et al. In vivo biomechanical evaluation of a novel angle-stable interlocking nail design in a canine tibial gap fracture model. Breckenridge (CO): Veterinary Orthopaedic Society; 2010.

25. Dejardin LM, Cabassu J, Guillou RP, et al. In vivo biomechanical evaluation of a novel angle-stable interlocking nail design in a canine tibial gap fracture model. Bologna (Italy): World Veterinary Orthopaedic Congress; 2010.

26. Hulse D, Hyman B. Biomechanics of fracture fixation failure. Vet Clin North Am Small Anim Pract 1991;21(4):647–67.

27. Hulse D, Hyman W, Nori M, et al. Reduction in plate strain by addition of an intramedullary pin. Vet Surg 1997;26(6):451–9.

28. Hulse D, Ferry K, Fawcett A, et al. Effect of intramedullary pin size on reducing bone plate strain. Vet Comp Orthop Traumatol 2000;13(4):185–90.

29. Dueland RT, Berglund L, Vanderby R, et al. Structural properties of interlocking nails, canine femora, and femur-interlocking nail constructs. Vet Surg 1996; 25(5):386–96.

30. Muir P, Johnson KA, Markel MD. Area moment of inertia for comparison of implant cross-sectional geometry and bending stiffness. Vet Comp Orthop Traumatol 1995;8:146–52.

31. Roe SC. Biomechanics principles of interlocking nails fixation. 8th Annual American College of Veterinary Surgeons Symposium; October 8–11, 1998; Chicago.

32. Dueland RT, Vanderby R Jr, McCabe RP. Fatigue study of six and eight mm diameter interlocking nails with screw holes of variable size and number. Vet Comp Orthop Traumatol 1997;10:194–9.

33. Bucholz RW, Ross SE, Lawrence KL. Fatigue fracture of the interlocking nail in the treatment of fractures of the distal part of the femoral shaft. J Bone Joint Surg Am 1987;69(9):1391–9.

34. Dejardin LM, Guillou RP, Ting D, et al. Effect of bending direction on the mechanical behaviour of interlocking nail systems. Vet Comp Orthop Traumatol 2009; 22(4):264–9.

35. Broos PL, Sermon A. From unstable internal fixation to biological osteosynthesis. A historical overview of operative fracture treatment. Acta Chir Belg 2004;104(4): 396–400.

36. Wheeler JL, Lewis DD, Cross AR, et al. Intramedullary interlocking nail fixation in dogs and cats: clinical applications. Comp Cont Educ Pract 2004;26(7): 531–43.

37. Aper RL, Litsky AS, Roe SC, et al. Fatigue life and push-out strength of a 2.7 mm locking bolt for use in a 6mm interlocking nails. 13th Annual American College of Veterinary Surgeons Symposium, October 9-12, 2003. Washington, DC; 2003.

38. Dueland RT, Vanderby R, McCabe RP. Comparison of interlocking nail screws and bolts: insertion torque, push-out strength, and mode of failure. 13th Annual American College of Veterinary Surgeons Symposium, October 9-12, 2003. Washington, DC; 2003.

39. von Pfeil DJ, Déjardin LM, DeCamp CE, et al. In vitro biomechanical comparison of plate-rod combination-construct and an interlocking nail-constructs for experimentally induced gap fractures in canine tibiae. Am J Vet Res 2005;66(9): 1536–43.

40. Basinger RR, Suber JT. Two techniques for supplementing interlocking nail repair of fractures of the humerus, femur, and tibia: results in 12 dogs and cats. Vet Surg 2004;33(6):673–80.

41. Duhautois B. Use of veterinary interlocking nails for diaphyseal fractures in dogs and cats: 121 cases. Vet Surg 2003;32(1):8–20.

42. Schandelmaier P, Krettek C, Tscherne H. Biomechanical study of nine different tibia locking nails. J Orthop Trauma 1996;10(1):37–44.

43. Kaspar K, Schell H, Seebeck P, et al. Angle stable locking reduces interfragmentary movements and promotes healing after unreamed nailing. Study of a displaced osteotomy model in sheep tibiae. J Bone Joint Surg Am 2005;87(9): 2028–37.

44. Klein MP, Rahn BA, Frigg R, et al. Reaming versus non-reaming in medullary nailing - interference with cortical circulation of the canine tibia. Arch Orthop Trauma Surg 1990;109(6):314–6.

45. Wheeler JL, Stubbs PW, Lewis DD, et al. Intramedullary interlocking nail fixation in dogs and cats: biomechanics and instrumentation. Comp Cont Educ Pract Vet 2004;26(7):519–29.

46. Tarr RR, Wiss DA. The mechanics and biology of intramedullary fracture fixation. Clin Orthop Relat Res 1986;(212):10–7.

47. Lang GJ, Cohen BE, Bosse MJ, et al. Proximal third tibial shaft fractures. Should they be nailed? Clin Orthop Relat Res 1995;(315):64–74.

48. Freedman EL, Johnson EE. Radiographic analysis of tibial fracture malalignment following intramedullary nailing. Clin Orthop Relat Res 1995;(315):25–33.

49. Buehler KC, Green J, Woll TS, et al. A technique for intramedullary nailing of proximal third tibia fractures. J Orthop Trauma 1997;11(3):218–23.

50. Durall I, Diaz-Bertrana MC, Morales I. Interlocking nail stabilization of humeral fractures: initial experiences in seven clinical cases. Vet Comp Orthop Traumatol 1994;7:3–8.
51. Basinger RR, Suber JT. Supplemental fixation of fractures repaired with interlocking nails: 14 cases. 29th Annual Veterinary Orthopedic Society Conference. The Canyons (UT); 2002.
52. Gatineau M, Plante J. Ulnar interlocking intramedullary nail stabilization of a proximal radio-ulnar fracture in a dog. Vet Surg 2010;39(8):1025–9.
53. Goett SD, Sinnott MT, Ting D, et al. Mechanical comparison of an interlocking nail locked with conventional bolts to extended bolts connected with a type-IA external skeletal fixator in a tibial fracture model. Vet Surg 2007;36(3):279–86.
54. Tigani D, Fravisini M, Stagni C, et al. Interlocking nail for femoral shaft fractures: is dynamization always necessary? Int Orthop 2005;29(2):101–4.
55. Durall I, Falcon C, Diaz-Bertrana MC, et al. Effects of static fixation and dynamization after interlocking femoral nailing locked with an external fixator: an experimental study in dogs. Vet Surg 2004;33(4):323–32.
56. Dueland RT, Johnson KA, Roe SC, et al. Interlocking nail treatment of diaphyseal long-bone fractures in dogs. J Am Vet Med Assoc 1999;214(1):59–66.
57. Piermattei DL, Johnson KA. An atlas of surgical approaches to the bones and joints of the dog and cat. 4th edition. Philadelphia: Saunders; 2004.
58. Pardo AD. Relationship of tibial intramedullary pins to canine stifle joint structures: a comparison of normograde and retrograde insertion. J Am Anim Hosp Assoc 1994;30(4):369–74.
59. Diaz-Bertrana MC, Durall I, Puchol JL, et al. Interlocking nail treatment of long-bone fractures in cats: 33 cases (1995-2004). Vet Comp Orthop Traumatol 2005;18(3):119–26.
60. Durall I, Diaz MC, Puchol JL, et al. Radiographic findings related to interlocking nailing: windshield-wiper effect, and locking screw failure. Vet Comp Orthop Traumatol 2003;16(4):217–22.

Percutaneous Pinning for Fracture Repair in Dogs and Cats

Stanley E. Kim, BVSc, MS*, Caleb C. Hudson, DMV, MS,
Antonio Pozzi, DMV, MS

KEYWORDS

- Growth plate fracture • Pinning • Percutaneous • Minimally invasive

KEY POINTS

- Pinning is the treatment of choice for the surgical repair of physeal fractures.
- All traditional principles of intramedullary or cross-pinning apply when considering the use of percutaneous pinning.
- Fractures should ideally be minimally displaced with a signification portion of bridging periosteum remaining intact.
- A thorough physical and orthopedic examination should be performed to identify any serious concomitant injury.
- For closed reduction of physeal fractures, the precise technique depends on the direction and degree of displacement of the epiphysis.

INTRODUCTION

Steinman pins or Kirschner wires (herein referred to as pins) can be used to stabilize a variety of different fracture configurations in the dog and cat.[1–3] Traditional pinning of fractures has been typically described with an open approach in order to achieve direct reduction and facilitate accurate placement of implants. When this method of fracture fixation is performed in a minimally invasive fashion, the procedure is known as percutaneous pinning. Placement of pins in a minimally invasive fashion through small stab incisions may offer significant advantages when compared with traditional open pinning, such as less postoperative pain, accelerated healing, and less iatrogenic trauma to important structures such as the physes and joint capsule.[4] Juxta-articular pediatric fractures in humans are frequently treated in this manner.[4–8] Percutaneous pinning has been used at the authors' institution with a high success rate; however, appropriate case selection, fluoroscopic guidance, and surgeon experience is required if it is attempted. The purpose of this article is to describe the optimal selection of cases, surgical technique, and anticipated outcomes for percutaneous pinning in the dog and cat.

Department of Small Animal Clinical Sciences, College of Veterinary Medicine, University of Florida, 2015 Southwest 16th Avenue, PO Box 100126, Gainesville, FL 32610-0126, USA
* Corresponding author.
E-mail address: stankim@ufl.edu

Vet Clin Small Anim 42 (2012) 963–974
http://dx.doi.org/10.1016/j.cvsm.2012.07.002
0195-5616/12/$ – see front matter Published by Elsevier Inc.

vetsmall.theclinics.com

SURGICAL TECHNIQUE
Case Selection

All traditional principles of intramedullary or cross-pinning apply when considering the use of percutaneous pinning. Salter-Harris type I and II physeal fractures are the most amenable to this form of fracture fixation, for several reasons. Pins mainly serve to counteract bending forces, whereas rotational and compressive forces are poorly neutralized, even when multiple pins are used. As such, juxta-articular, noncomminuted fracture configurations with some inherent stability after reduction are suitable for stabilization by use of pins alone. Because pins have limited ability to sustain long-term stability in all 3 planes when compared with other forms of fixation, pinning alone is generally used in young animals with rapid capacity for bone healing. As pins cannot provide interfragmentary compression, intra-articular fractures should not be treated with pins alone.

Candidates for percutaneous pinning must meet additional criteria to those already described. Fractures should ideally be minimally displaced with a signification portion of bridging periosteum remaining intact. Intact periosteum has the potential to further contribute to stability by acting as a tension band if combined with appropriately positioned pins.[9] Percutaneous pinning may still be possible in moderately displaced fractures, as long as the interval between trauma and surgical intervention is short. Closed reduction will not be possible in fractures that are not immediately treated (more than 24–48 hours after trauma), because of muscular contraction and adhesions from callus formation. Very small fracture fragments can be difficult to palpate, manipulate, or identify with intraoperative fluoroscopy, hence an open approach is more suitable in these cases. Fracture fragments that are covered with large amounts of soft tissue may also be more difficult to align with indirect methods, which may preclude the use of percutaneous pinning.

The authors have successfully performed percutaneous pinning for Salter-Harris type I and II fractures of the distal femoral, femoral capital, proximal tibial, tibial apophyseal, distal tibial, distal radial, and proximal humeral physes.

Preoperative Management and Planning

Preoperative planning for fracture repair must begin with appropriate case selection, as already described. A thorough physical and orthopedic examination should be performed to identify any serious concomitant injury. At a minimum, thoracic radiographs and orthogonal-view radiographs of the affected bone are acquired. Radiographs typically require moderate sedation or anesthesia to achieve optimal positioning and projections. It is strongly recommended to obtain radiographs of the contralateral bone. Comparing contralateral radiographs can help accurately discriminate minimally displaced physeal fractures from normal physeal anatomy. Rarely, stress radiographs are necessary to demonstrate location and degree of instability of a physeal fracture. Radiographic tracings of the fracture fragments in normal alignment, or digital templating is required to plan pin insertion site, size, and trajectory. Implant size and positioning is often more accurate when planned from the normal contralateral radiographs, because it is not uncommon for fracture segments to be rotated out of plane.

As manipulation of the affected limb may not be well tolerated, sedation for radiographs presents an opportunity to carefully palpate the fracture site. Thorough palpation of the fracture is particularly crucial when considering percutaneous pinning. Occasionally, minimally displaced fractures that retain extensive soft-tissue integrity may be stable enough to treat conservatively with cage rest with or without external coaptation. At the other end of the spectrum, physeal fractures that are several days old may have already developed soft-tissue callus and muscle contractions that preclude indirect reduction. Reduction may be attempted at the time of radiography, but this requires heavy sedation or anesthesia. As limb immobilization for humeral and femoral fractures are difficult to attain with bandages, the main goal of initial manipulation of these fractures is assessing fracture instability rather than obtaining better alignment. Radial and tibial physeal fractures should be temporarily immobilized with a Robert-Jones bandage or an appropriate splint to prevent further displacement of the fracture segments and decrease discomfort associated with motion at the fracture site. Parenteral opioids should be administered for analgesia.

Preparation and Patient Positioning

At the time of surgery, the entire affected limb must be aseptically prepared to enable adequate intraoperative maneuvering required for closed reduction and percutaneous placement of the implants. A full limb preparation is also required to allow conversion to a traditional open approach if needed. The hanging limb preparation is useful to fatigue contracted muscles and facilitate closed reduction. For hind-limb fractures at the level of the distal femur and below, patients are positioned in dorsal recumbency; proximal femoral and humeral physeal fractures are approached with the patients in lateral recumbency. Before final aseptic limb preparation, trial images with the fluoroscope should be acquired to ensure that the fractured bone can be imaged. Use of towel clamps should be minimized, as they can hinder optimal visualization of the fracture segments during intraoperative imaging; drapes can be sutured into place. Adhesive dressings (Ioban, Opsite) can become wrapped up by the pin during insertion, and are thus generally avoided. A radiolucent operating table, or Plexiglas support for small dogs and cats, is advantageous but not essential.

Surgical Approach

Figs. 1–7 depict preoperative and postoperative radiographs, as well as intraoperative procedures for percutaneous pinning of a distal femoral physeal fracture in a dog. **Figs. 8–12** depict intraoperative fluoroscopic images from percutaneous pinning of a distal tibial physeal fracture in a cat.

For closed reduction of physeal fractures, the precise technique depends on the direction and degree of displacement of the epiphysis. The first principle in reduction is to minimize harm to the physis. To achieve this, the maneuver should generally be 90% traction and 10% leverage.[9] Initial traction may slightly increase the deformity; the epiphysis is then translated into alignment while maintaining traction; reduction is complete by realignment of the angular deformity. Audible or palpable grinding of the physeal cartilage should be avoided. Assessment of reduction is performed with intraoperative fluoroscopy.

Although rarely used in the authors' institution, reduction can be facilitated by use of a traction device, temporary external skeletal fixation, or a traction table. Temporary pins for skeletal traction should not be placed directly through the epiphysis because of the risk of iatrogenic fracture and interference with definitive pin placement; site of the traction and countertraction pins should be placed well above and below the epiphysis. In addition, traction instruments can be cumbersome and bulky, so these devices are not recommended for routine use with percutaneous pinning. Manual reduction is sufficient in most cases. Alternatively, temporary half pins can be safely placed in the diaphysis of the affected bone and used to facilitate manual control of the larger fracture segment; the epiphyseal segment is indirectly controlled by manipulating the long bones distal to the fracture site.

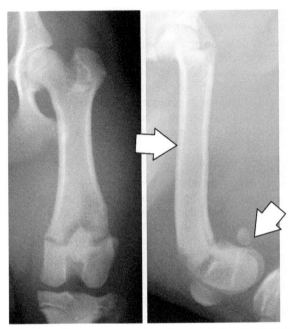

Fig. 1. Orthogonal-view radiographs of a distal femoral Salter-Harris type I fracture. This injury is amenable to repair by percutaneous pinning, as the fracture segments are minimally displaced. *Arrows* indicate direction of force applied on the fracture segments for closed reduction.

Following reduction, small (10 mm) approaches are made over the proposed pin-insertion sites down to the periosteum. The skin incision should be centered slightly distally for distal physeal fractures, and slightly proximal for proximal fractures, to account for anticipated pin trajectory. Pins are always placed from the epiphyseal or apophyseal segment toward the metaphyseal/diaphyseal segment to maximize

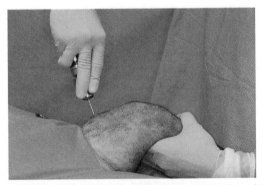

Fig. 2. Closed reduction of a distal femoral physeal fracture can be achieved with manual traction and leverage. For the left hind limb, the surgeon's left palm is placed under the stifle and the distal tibia is firmly grasped. In this case, a temporary half pin is used to assist manipulation of the proximal fragment. Distal traction and cranial leverage is applied to the distal segment with the stifle partially flexed, while the proximal segment is pushed caudally.

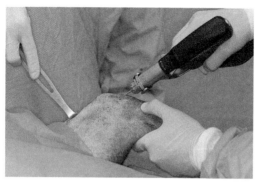

Fig. 3. Pins should always be placed with an air-driven or battery-driven drill. An oscillating function is useful to decrease the risk of entangling surrounding soft-tissue structures.

purchase. This placement is fortuitous, as the epiphysis is often superficial and deep soft-tissue dissection is not typically required. The approaches should be large enough to be able to sufficiently countersink the pins and check that the implants are seated adequately. Good exposure is especially important if the insertion site is intra-articular. Adequate exposure also decreases the incidence of soft-tissue entrapment during pin placement.

Surgical Procedure

Principles of physeal fracture repair must be adhered to with percutaneous pinning. To decrease the risk of premature closure, pins must be placed as perpendicular to the physeal plate as possible. Angulation of pins greater than 45° to the physis predisposes to epiphysiodesis.[10] Threaded pins are not used because of inherent weakness at the thread-shaft interface, risk of hindering longitudinal bone growth, and difficulty with pin removal if required. Trocar-tipped pins enable precise entry to the epiphysis, which is important with percutaneous pinning because the use of pilot holes is not often possible.

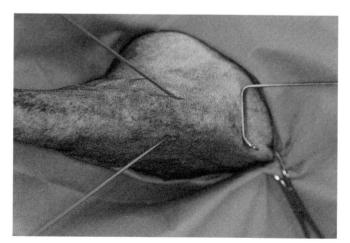

Fig. 4. Percutaneous placement of cross pins before trimming the pins. Note that the precise trajectory of the pins can be difficult because of the very limited approaches; intraoperative fluoroscopy is highly recommended when performing percutaneous pinning.

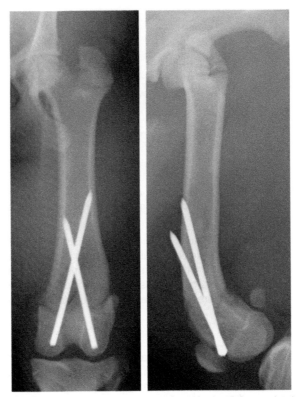

Fig. 5. Orthogonal-view postoperative radiographs of a distal femoral Salter-Harris type I fracture treated with percutaneous pinning. Note that the pins cross proximal to the fracture; pin-entry sites are cranial to the weight-bearing surfaces, and seated to the level of the subchondral bone.

Although immature bone may be soft enough to place pins by hand, battery-driven or air-driven drills should be used for optimal accuracy. An oscillating drill function is useful to prevent soft tissues from entangling around the pin during insertion. Intraoperative fluoroscopy should be used before, during, and after applying the pins to ensure optimal positioning. Without fluoroscopy, it is often extremely difficult to place pins accurately, owing to the limited exposure with percutaneous pinning. It is important to bear in mind that the number of pins and size of pins should be kept to a minimum to decrease iatrogenic physeal damage, yet large enough provide adequate stability. When using cross pins, the implants should cross away from the fracture site to achieve optimal stability. Pins must be seated into the transcortex, carefully measured, backed out, then cut to length accurately such that they can be countersunk to beneath the surface of the bone without protruding into soft tissue. If the pin-insertion site is extra-articular, the pin may be bent to decrease risk of pin migration. Bending the pin also improves the ability to fully seat the pin to the bone through the limited exposure site. Pins should never be bent or left exposed beyond the cartilage surface when they are placed within a joint. Pins may be cut long to be left protruding through the skin, but the sites may be especially prone to draining and infection because they are often periarticular and subject to a high degree of skin motion.

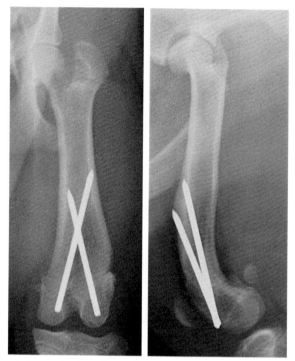

Fig. 6. Orthogonal-view recheck radiographs showing complete healing of a distal femoral Salter-Harris type I fracture treated with percutaneous pinning.

Immediate Postoperative Care

Pin placement and fracture reduction is carefully assessed on postoperative radiographs (**Fig. 13**). For all cases, parenteral analgesia is administered for up to 12 hours to address immediate postoperative pain. Because of the limited soft-tissue trauma induced by surgery, analgesic requirements are expected to be substantially lower than if the procedure was performed with a traditional open approach. There are very few risk factors for infection (clean procedures, young patients, minimal surgical exposure), hence postoperative prophylactic antibiotics are not indicated with routine percutaneous pinning. Local cryotherapy and passive range-of-motion exercises can be instituted in the immediate postoperative period for stabilized fractures at the level of the shoulder, hip, and stifle. Range-of-motion exercises of the stifle for distal femoral physeal fractures are especially important to minimize the risk of quadriceps contracture. Distal tibial and radial physeal fracture repairs must be protected from failure with external coaptation.

Rehabilitation and Recovery

Early return to weight bearing and good limb function is anticipated following percutaneous pinning. Because the minimum size and number of pins that provide adequate stability are used, cage rest should be strictly enforced until complete union of the fracture is documented; these repairs are otherwise at high risk for implant failure and pin migration. With preservation of surrounding soft-tissue structures and tremendous capacity for healing in young animals, clinical union is expected within 3 to 4 weeks. For these reasons, the authors advocate taking radiographs of

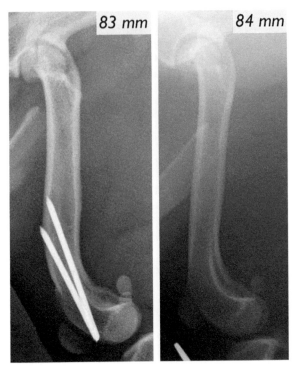

Fig. 7. Lateral view of the operated and the contralateral femurs 12 months after percutaneous pinning of a distal femoral Salter-Harris type I fracture. Notice the absence of length disparity between the operated and nonoperated femurs.

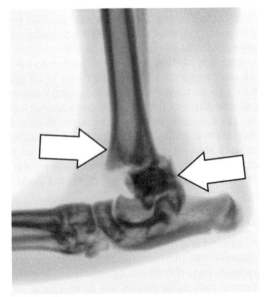

Fig. 8. Lateral-projection intraoperative fluoroscopic image of a Salter-Harris type I distal tibial fracture. *Arrows* indicate direction of force applied on the fracture segments for closed reduction.

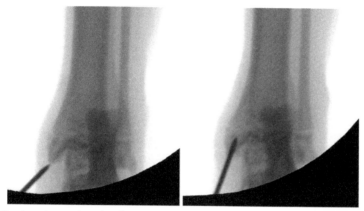

Fig. 9. The location and angle of insertion of the pins is crucial. Pins must engage the malleolus without entering the joint.

the repair every 2 weeks to identify potential complications and assess fracture healing early. For distal tibial and radial physeal fractures, external coaptation should be maintained until clinical union. Bandages should be checked and changed on a weekly basis to minimize the risk of complications such as pressure sores.

As precise application of pins may be more difficult than with a traditional open approach, there may be a higher risk of requiring implant removal for cases of percutaneous pinning. Even very mild protrusion of pins beyond the surface of articular cartilage can cause persistent lameness and pin loosening, and initiate osteoarthritis; long pins extending into surrounding extra-articular soft tissues can predispose to local irritation and seroma formation. Owners should be informed that pin migration could still occur after clinical union, which would also require pin removal.

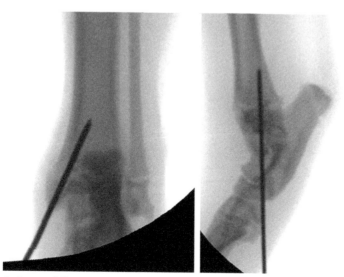

Fig. 10. Orthogonal fluoroscopic views are necessary to accurately assess pin positioning.

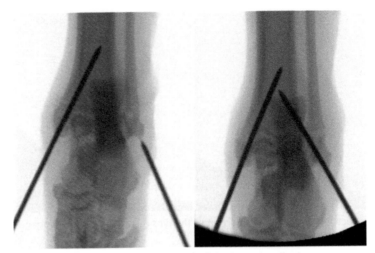

Fig. 11. The second pin is inserted at the level of the lateral malleolus.

CLINICAL RESULTS IN THE LITERATURE

Percutaneous pinning for tibial and femoral fractures was first described in 1989, although it was performed in a "blind" manner without intraoperative fluoroscopy.[11] Osseous union was achieved in 55 of 56 fractures treated in this manner. Age, body weight, fracture type, and time from injury to repair were found to influence overall outcome in these cases. A recent retrospective case series on percutaneous pinning under fluoroscopic guidance has been recently described in abstract format.[12] In this report, 3 dogs were treated for distal femoral fracture (Salter-Harris II) and 2 dogs were

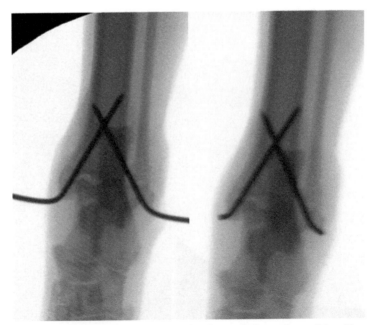

Fig. 12. Pins are carefully bent, then trimmed to beneath the surface of the skin.

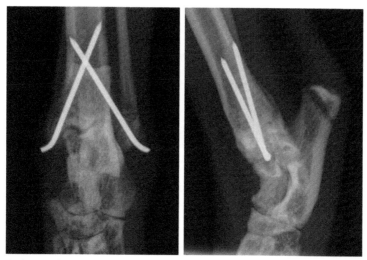

Fig. 13. Orthogonal-view recheck radiographs showing complete healing of a distal tibial Salter-Harris type I fracture treated with percutaneous pinning 3 weeks after fixation.

treated for proximal humeral fracture (Salter-Harris II). The mean age at presentation was 6 months. Breeds included English Springer, Yorkshire Terrier, and mixed breeds. The mean duration from trauma was 2 days. All fractures were closed and mildly to moderately displaced. Mean duration of surgery was 67 minutes. Mean time to radiographic union was 3.5 weeks. No major complications occurred. Mild rotational malalignment occurred in one of the humeral fractures. Good function (subjectively evaluated by the clinician and by the owner) was achieved in all cases.

SUMMARY

Percutaneous pinning is a feasible method for stabilizing Salter-Harris type I and II physeal fractures in dogs and cats. Surgical intervention must be performed soon after the time of trauma, otherwise closed reduction cannot be achieved. The procedure is technically demanding; surgeon experience, intraoperative fluoroscopy, appropriate surgical instrumentation, and strict case selection are all required for a successful outcome. Although clinical comparisons between open and closed pinning have not been described, percutaneous pinning may offer the advantages of decreased postoperative morbidity, earlier return to normal function, and decreased risk of infection. Prospective clinical studies should be performed to better define the role of this minimally invasive method of fracture repair in dogs and cats.

REFERENCES

1. Parker RB, Bloomberg MS. Modified intramedullary pin technique for repair of distal femoral physeal fractures in the dog and cat. J Am Vet Med Assoc 1984; 184(10):1259–65.
2. Presnell KR. Pins versus plates: the orthopedic dilemma. Vet Clin North Am 1978; 8(2):213–7.
3. Campbell JR. The technique of fixation of fractures of the distal femur using rush pins. J Small Anim Pract 1976;17(5):323–9.
4. von Laer L. General observations on treatment. In: von Laer L, editor. Pediatric fractures and dislocations. Stuttgart (Germany): Thieme; 2004. p. 69–77.

5. Cheng JC, Lam TP, Shen WY. Closed reduction and percutaneous pinning for type III displaced supracondylar fractures of the humerus in children. J Orthop Trauma 1995;9(6):511–5.

6. Kaewpornsawan K. Comparison between closed reduction with percutaneous pinning and open reduction with pinning in children with closed totally displaced supracondylar humeral fractures: a randomized controlled trial. J Pediatr Orthop B 2001;10(2):131–7.

7. de Buys Roessingh AS, Reinberg O. Open or closed pinning for distal humerus fractures in children? Swiss Surg 2003;9(2):76–81.

8. Dua A, Eachempati KK, Malhotra R, et al. Closed reduction and percutaneous pinning of displaced supracondylar fractures of humerus in children with delayed presentation. Chin J Traumatol 2011;14(1):14–9.

9. Skaggs DL. Extra-articular injuries of the knee. In: Beaty JH, Kasser JR, editors. Fractures in children. 5th edition. Philadelphia: Lippincott Williams and Wilkins; 2006.

10. Piermattei DL. Fractures in growing animals. In: Piermattei DL, Flo GL, DeCamp CE, editors. Handbook of small animal orthopaedics. St Louis (MO): Saunders; 2006. p. 737–46.

11. Newman ME, Milton JL. Closed reduction and blind pinning of 29 femoral and tibial fractures in 27 dogs and cats. J Am Anim Hosp Assoc 1989;25(1):61–8.

12. Pozzi A, Thieman KM. Percutaneous pinning of growth plate fractures in dogs. Vet Comp Orthop Traumatol 2011;4:A13.

MIPO Techniques for the Humerus in Small Animals

Don Hulse, DVM

KEYWORDS

- Minimally invasive plate osteosynthesis • Humerus • Small animals

KEY POINTS

- Knowledge of regional and topographic anatomy is paramount for success when using minimally invasive plate osteosynthesis (MIPO) for fracture management.
- Preoperative planning is essential for an optimal outcome and reducing stress among the surgical team; factors to consider include biologic assessment, mechanical assessment, clinical assessment, portal placement, and implant selection.
- MIPO is a useful technique for the direct or indirect reduction of humeral diaphyseal fractures.
- Implants should span the length of the bone for ease of implant application and to optimize the mechanical advantage of the implant.
- After surgery, incision care and controlled activity are 2 primary considerations.

REGIONAL ANATOMY

Knowledge of regional and topographic anatomy is paramount for success when using minimally invasive plate osteosynthesis (MIPO) for fracture management.[1–5] The surgeon is working through small incisions (portals) that are 3 to 4 cm in length, and often dissection is carried through muscle fibers rather than between muscles and standard surgical planes. Awareness of the position of nerves and blood vessels relative to the surgical dissection and avenue for plate placement is necessary to prevent the injury of vital structures and serious postoperative morbidity. A visual knowledge of the topographic anatomy is also necessary with MIPO. Working through small portals prevents the surgeon from observing the bone surface proximally to distally as is done with open exposures. Familiarity with the relationship of proximal bony land marks relative to distal bony landmarks as well as the normal curvature and internal torsion of the humerus is necessary to prevent postoperative malalignment. Proper placement of surgical incisions (portals) is essential. Considerations for portal placement include regional anatomy, fracture configuration, and whether direct or indirect reduction is the chosen method of reconstruction.

Department of Small Animal Surgery, College Veterinary Medicine, Texas A&M University, College Station, TX 77843, USA
E-mail address: dhulse@cvm.tamu.edu

Vet Clin Small Anim 42 (2012) 975–982
http://dx.doi.org/10.1016/j.cvsm.2012.07.006
0195-5616/12/$ – see front matter © 2012 Elsevier Inc. All rights reserved.

The application of bone plates or plate/rod constructs with MIPO is best achieved with the implants spanning the length of the bone. In general, this requires a plate that will extend from the region of the proximal metaphysis to the region of the distal metaphysis. A bone plate spanning this length of the bone has a significant mechanical advantage as well as an anatomic advantage for portal placement. The proximal and distal metaphysis of the humerus is more superficial and has less soft tissue overlying the bone surface than the central diaphysis. In general, 2 to 3 small incisions (portals) are used: a proximal portal; a distal portal; and, on occasion, a central observational portal.

INDICATIONS AND CASE SELECTION

MIPO is a useful technique for most humeral fractures. Exceptions are when the fracture configuration is such that there is an articular component or when a reducible comminuted fracture or long oblique fracture is to be stabilized with anatomic reduction (direct reduction) and rigid stabilization. If the fracture is articular, open-exposure direct anatomic reduction and rigid stabilization of the articular surface is paramount for an optimal long-term outcome. With reducible comminuted diaphyseal fractures, (comminuted, long oblique) the length of the fracture site does lend itself to anatomic reduction and rigid stabilization via small incisions (portals). Nonreducible comminuted metaphyseal or diaphyseal fractures are well suited for MIPO; spatial alignment (indirect reduction) with rigid or semirigid stabilization can be readily achieved via small incision (portals). Likewise, anatomic reduction with rigid or semirigid stabilization of transverse fractures or short oblique fractures can be accomplished with the MIPO technique.

PREOPERATIVE PLANNING

Preoperative planning is essential for an optimal outcome and reducing stress among the surgical team. Factors to consider include biologic assessment, mechanical assessment, clinical assessment, portal placement, and implant selection.

Biologic Assessment

The assessment of biologic factors provides the surgeon with an estimate of how rapidly (or slowly) a callus will be formed. This evaluation gives the surgeon an indication of how much she or he can rely on callus formation to provide the stability needed to achieve bone healing. Additionally, this assessment gives the surgeon an indication of how long the stabilization system must remain functional (ie, provide most of the support). Two biologic factors of great importance are the age and general health of the patients. Other biologic factors include the determination of open versus closed fracture and low-energy or high-energy fracture. If the fracture is an open or high-energy fracture (gunshot), the veterinarian can assume a significant degree of soft tissue injury. In terms of bone union, this simply means prolonged healing and that the implant-bone construct must remain rigid during fragile neovascularization. The location of the fracture in terms of the specific bone and site of the fracture within the bone are also important biologic considerations. For example, distal radial and ulnar fractures are recipes for nonunion in the toy canine breeds. If the biologic assessment is very good or excellent (callus formed rapidly), the implant can be less stiff and the implant-bone interface need not remain functional for an extended period. Intermediate biologic assessment warrants moderate strength and stiffness and, at a minimum, a moderate functional life of the implant.

Mechanical Factors

Which reduction technique to use is an important decision the surgeon must make before surgery.[6–8] The surgeon must decide whether to use direct reduction or indirect reduction. The advantage of direct reduction (anatomic reduction) is immediate load sharing between the implant and bone. This concept reduces stress on the implant system and, therefore, results in fewer implant-related complications. However, to apply the technique of direct reduction, several criteria must be fulfilled. First, the fracture configuration must be such that anatomic reduction and interfragmentary stabilization are possible (reducible fracture). Second, the surgeon must be able to achieve anatomic reduction and stabilization without significant injury to the surrounding soft tissue. If the soft tissues are excessively damaged, the biologic response needed for bone union will be delayed. This delay prolongs bone healing and increases the likelihood of complications. Reducible fractures amendable to direct reduction are those with single fracture lines (transverse, oblique) or comminuted fractures having 1 or 2 large fragments. Direct reduction creates fracture planes with small gaps between fragments. For example, transverse fractures have small gap lengths (when reduced) and, therefore, inherently concentrate motion. Because high interfragmentary strain (motion) impedes bone formation, small gap lengths created with the use of direct reduction must be stabilized (rigid or semirigid) to eliminate interfragmentary strain (motion).

If the fracture configuration is such that anatomic reconstruction and stabilization of fracture planes of the bone column are not possible, the surgeon should then use the technique of indirect reduction. Fracture configurations treated with this method are commonly comminuted diaphyseal fractures. The use of the implant in this situation is referred to as a bridging or buttress implant because it is crossing an area of bone fragmentation. The implant must, therefore, be strong enough and stiff enough to withstand all weight-bearing loads until a sufficient callus is formed. Because the goal is to achieve rapid callus (bio-buttress) formation to unload the implant, the surgeon must create an environment where this will occur. Indirect reduction preserves the biology (soft tissue) because there is no attempt to reduce small fragments of bone in the area of comminution. The fracture area length with multiple bone fragments is maintained, which distributes interfragmentary strain (motion) over a larger area. This distribution, therefore, lowers the strain within the fragmented zone, favoring rapid bone formation.

In summary, choose direct reduction when the fracture configuration allows for anatomic reduction and interfragmentary stabilization. The load sharing between the implant-bone construct is a powerful method to avoid implant failures and accelerate early return to function. Choose indirect reduction if the fracture configuration is such that anatomic reduction is not possible or if reduction cannot be accomplished without significant injury to the soft tissue. The implant must be strong and stiff to bridge the fracture area until a callus is formed. Do all that is possible to preserve the soft tissue environment and maintain an environment of low interfragmentary strain to enhance callus formation.

Clinical factors are important in developing a fracture fixation plan. A client who is not observant and does not wish to participate in the postoperative management is not a client to give the responsibility of caring for an external cast or a complex external skeletal fixator. Actually, the same consideration essentially applies for uncooperative *patients*. If the animal is uncontrollable, then external support is not a wise choice. It is vital to consider postoperative limb function. Different kinds of implants allow for varying degrees of comfort. As a general rule, internal devices are more comfortable and allow for greater limb use than external devices. For example, a bone plate with screws is more comfortable for the dog or cat than an external cast or external fixation, depending, of course, on the individual and the area of application. The type of animal is an important consideration. For example, it is difficult to control the activity of cats following fracture repair. Stronger fixation and one that will have an extended functional life (locking plate systems) are best suited for cats.

Implant Selection

The length of the bone plate should be such that the plate spans the length of the bone from the proximal epiphyseal/metaphyseal juncture to the distal epiphyseal/metaphyseal juncture. This length provides superior mechanical advantage by extending the moment arm of the plate/bone construct. Additionally, the soft tissue envelope at the metaphyseal/epiphyseal area of a long bone is less dense and allows for easier access to the surface of the bone. The size of the bone plate depends on the weight and activity level of the dog/cat. Most bone plate systems have a reference chart that provides guidelines for plate size relative to patient size. For many reasons, locking plate systems have become the standard for fracture care.[9] They preserve periosteal vascularity and provide angular stability of the plate/bone construct. The locking plate systems are ideal for most fracture applications. It is important to remember that the strength of a locking plate and resistance to deformation and breakage depends on the size of the plate and not the locking mechanism. Plate/rod constructs are ideal for MIPO application. The rod (Steinman pin) serves to assist in fracture alignment as well as protecting the plate from catastrophic or fatigue failure.

Operating Room Setup, Surgical Approach, Reduction Technique

Patients should be positioned in lateral recumbence with the leg that is to be operated in the uppermost position. Ample clipping and standard surgical asepsis must be used even though small incisions (portals) are to be used for exposure. A hanging limb preparation is used to allow maximal manipulation of the limb during surgery. It is preferable not to apply stockinet covering the surgical site because the surgeon must have full visualization of limb landmarks to facilitate proper spatial alignment of the limb. Standard surgical instrumentation for portal incisions is used. Suction and electrocautery assist with visualization through the small incisions (portals). Special equipment, such as a power drill, hand retractors, gelpi retractors, periosteal elevator, and bone-holding forceps, are indispensable. The type of bone plates and screws that are used is the surgeon's preference. If an alignment pin or plate/rod construct is used, an intramedullary pin set is needed. A surgical fluoroscopy unit is helpful but not essential for conducting MIPO.

Surgical Approach

Proper portal placement is necessary to achieve anatomic alignment (direct reduction) with a transverse or short oblique fracture or spatial alignment (indirect reduction) with nonreducible comminuted fractures. Further, proper portal placement facilitates access to the metaphyseal/epiphyseal bone surface while preserving vital neurovascular structures and unnecessary soft tissue trauma. The proximal portal is 2 to 3 cm in length and made craniolaterally overlying the region of the crest of the greater tubercle of the proximal metaphysis. The axillobrachial vein is caudal to the incision, and the cephalic vein courses beneath the cleidobrachialis muscle. Care is used to isolate and reflect both veins. The cleidobrachialis, acromial head of the deltoid muscle, lateral head of the triceps, and brachialis muscle are partially reflected to expose the craniolateral surface of the proximal metaphysis. The distal portal is made caudolaterally overlying the lateral epicondyloid ridge. Superficial branches of the radial nerve are preserved as they course distally in the subcutaneous tissue. The lateral head of the triceps is reflected caudally, and the origin of the extensor carpi radialis is partially reflected from the epicondyloid ridge. An accessory observational portal may be necessary if the fracture is mid-diaphyseal. The observational portal is used to assure anatomic reduction of the fracture (direct reduction) or to assure intra-medullary placement of the pin as it passes from the proximal parent bone into the medullary cavity of the distal parent bone. The observational portal is positioned over-lying the fracture site. The surgeon must visualize the fracture in the reduced position when planning for the site of the portal. If positioned overlying the bone end of one of the parent bones, the portal is no longer at the fracture site when the fracture is reduced.

Direct Reduction

MIPO can be used with transverse or short oblique humeral fractures. A portal that allows visualization for the fracture site for anatomic (direct) reduction must be established. Bone plate placement is facilitated by creating an avenue along the lateral surface of the bone that enables the surgeon to slide the plate beneath the soft tissue envelop to rest on the surface of the bone. Beginning at the distal portal, an avenue is made in a distal-to-proximal direction with a periosteal elevator deep to the brachialis muscle and radial nerve. The periosteal elevator glides along the surface of the bone to the region of the fracture site. The periosteal elevator is then inserted into the proximal portal and guided distally deep to the brachialis muscle along the surface of the bone in a distal direction to reach the fracture site. Anatomic reduction (direct reduction) is achieved with bone-holding forceps grasping the bone through the proximal and distal portals. A conventional plate is precontoured using a radiograph of the opposite normal humerus as a template and applied as a compression plate. The principles of compression plate application (rigid stabilization) or reduction without compression (semirigid stabilization) are fol-lowed. The plate is slid from the distal portal through the avenue to the proximal portal. With rigid stabilization, plate screws are loaded on either side of the fracture site and the plate is contoured to achieve compression of the fracture. With semirigid stabilization, plate screws are placed in a neutral position 1 to 2 cm on either side of the fracture site. A minimum of 3 screws is placed proximally and 3 screws are placed distally to the fracture site.

Placement of the Alignment Pin with Indirect Reduction

The alignment pin may be retrograded or normograded depending on fracture loca-tion and surgeon preference. If the surgeon has chosen to apply a plate/rod construct, the pin should approximate 40% the diameter of the humeral isthmus. When the frac-ture is supracondylar, the pin is retrograded from the fracture site, entering the marrow cavity at the medial humeral epicondyloid ridge. The pin exits medially to the olecranon and is driven distally until the proximal pinpoint is level with the fracture. Alignment is achieved with bone-holding forceps grasping the bone through the prox-imal and distal portals. The pin is then driven into the marrow cavity of the proximal parent bone to exit at the greater tubercle. The drill is proximally placed on the pin, and the distal point is pulled within the bone surface at the distal exit point at the medial epicondyloid ridge. If the fracture is located midshaft or proximally, the pin is retrograded in a distal-to-proximal direction to exit at the greater tubercle. The frac-ture is aligned, and the pin is driven distally to sit in the medial epicondyloid ridge. Once the fracture is aligned, a conventional or locking plate is applied as described earlier.

CLINICAL CASES
Case 1

A 3-year-old male Labrador that was hit by an automobile sustained a distal third comminuted diaphyseal fracture. The fracture was treated with MIPO (**Fig. 1**).

Case 2

An adult Labrador sustained a gunshot injury resulting in a comminuted midshaft humeral fracture (**Fig. 2**).

Postoperative Management and Rehabilitation

After surgery, incision care and controlled activity are 2 primary considerations. A protective bandage is placed over the portal incisions during the hospitalization period. Once the pet leaves the hospital, the protective dressing can be removed. Daily observation of the incisions is necessary. Although uncommon, the dog/cat may lick or scratch the small portal incisions introducing inflammation and bacteria into the surgical site. It is advisable for the pet to wear a protective device, such as an Elizabethan collar, for 7 to 10 days following surgery. After this period, the incisions are healed and are no longer a source of irritation to the dog.

Controlled activity is important for an optimal outcome. Excessive activity may result in catastrophic or cyclic failure of the implants and necessitate a revision surgery. In general, the pet can function as he or she normally would when inside the house. However, the owner must prevent playful activity with other pets or children and confine the pet when the owner is absent from the home. When outside, the pet must be under leash control. Controlled, purposeful walks are begun immediately following discharge from the hospital. During the first postoperative week, the pet should be taken outside for short walks on a leash (5 minutes, 2–3 times per day or more, if the owner has the time). During these sessions, one should encourage limb use. To encourage limb use, the pace of walking should be very slow; if walking is very slow, the leg is more likely to be used with each step. If walking is too fast, it is easier to skip off the leg and walk on 3 legs. If this occurs, the owner should slow the pace to a level whereby the operated leg is placed down with each step. As comfort increases, frequency, pace, and distance of walking each day may increase. Increase the frequency of exercise sessions up to 3 times daily as the owner's schedule permits. Increase the time of each exercise session by 5 minutes per week; if soreness occurs

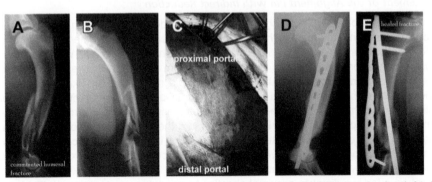

Fig. 1. Three-year-old male Labrador that was hit by an automobile sustained a distal third comminuted diaphyseal fracture: (*A, B*) Preoperative cranial-caudal and lateral radiographs, (*C*) proximal and distal portal placement, and (*D, E*) radiographs taken 7 weeks following surgery showing healed fracture.

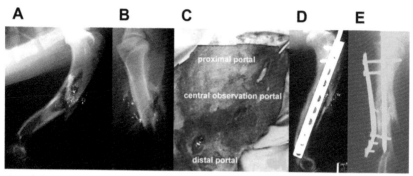

Fig. 2. Adult Labrador sustained a gunshot injury resulting in a comminuted midshaft humeral fracture: (*A, B*) preoperative radiographs, (*C*) position of portals (proximal, central observational, distal), and (*D, E*) radiographs taken 9 weeks following surgery showing bone union.

(less comfortable use of the limb), stop the exercise sessions and rest for 48 hours. Resume exercise sessions at the level used before the soreness occurred. For the initial 2 weeks after surgery, the pet should walk on a flat surface (sidewalk, pavement) with no incline. After 2 weeks, the owner should begin to walk in a higher-cut surface (grass); this results in an increase of active flexion/extension of the shoulder/elbow joints. The height of the surface (higher grass, fields) and, if possible, the degree of the incline is gradually increased. Continue to progress as the owner's time and the comfort of the pet allows.

Cats are more difficult to control postoperatively than dogs. It is best to prepare a site within the home for them to recover from their injuries and surgery. An example would be to prepare a small closet with no items for the cat to jump on and off. The area should have ample room for a litter box, food, and water but should be confined so that harmful activity is not likely.

If available, the owner should seek a veterinary physical therapy/rehabilitation center. The rehabilitation practitioner can perform in-house activities, such as aquatic therapy, physioball, balance board, and floor exercises, to maintain joint motion and muscle strength. The rehabilitation practitioner will also prescribe home activities and work with the pet owner to insure that the in-home activities are performed properly. In-home activities help regain muscle strength, balance, and joint motion.

COMMON ERRORS WITH MIPO
Poor Case Selection: Failure to Convert to OBDT

MIPO is a useful clinical tool, which, when performed properly, will decrease healing time and morbidity. However, MIPO is more demanding than an open exposure. Improper varus/valgus and/or rotational alignment are the most common errors associated with the MIPO technique. The surgeon is working through small incisions (portals) and cannot see anatomic landmarks that are normally used to assure proper bone and limb alignment. The surgeon must understand the relationship of bone and soft tissue landmarks in the proximal epiphysis relative to the distal epiphysis. It is also important for the surgeon to know the normal joint motion angles (internal/external rotation) of the joint above and the joint below the fracture.

Failure to Follow Principles of Implant Application

A second difficulty with the MIPO technique is ensuring that the principles of application for the chosen implant system are followed. Once again, the surgeon is working through small incisions (portals) and is unable to appreciate the proximity of all the fracture planes. The surgeon may inadvertently place screws within or close to a fracture line, which violates the principles of screw insertion; the number of screws securing the implant to the parent bone is, therefore, decreased and may not be sufficient. Another difficulty with MIPO is that the surgeon may not be able to recognize errors until postoperative radiographs are taken. If an error is recognized, correction will necessitate revision.

REFERENCES

1. Guiot LP, Dejardin LM, editors. Minimally invasive percutaneous plate-rod osteosynthesis for treatment of extra-articular humeral fractures in dogs. Abstracts from the American College of Veterinary Surgeons Symposium. Washington, DC: American College of Veterinary Surgeons; 2009.
2. Hudson C, Pozzi A, Lewis D. Minimally invasive plate osteosynthesis: applications and techniques in dogs and cats. Vet Comp Orthop Traumatol 2009;22(3):175–82.
3. Krettek C, Muller M, Miclau T. Evolution of minimally invasive plate osteosynthesis (MIPO) in the femur. Injury 2001;32(Suppl 3):SC14–23.
4. Pozzi A, Lewis D. Surgical approaches for minimally invasive plate osteosynthesis in dogs. Vet Comp Orthop Traumatol 2009;22(4):316–20.
5. Schmokel HG, Hurter K, Schawalder P. Percutaneous plating of tibial fractures in two dogs. Vet Comp Orthop Traumatol 2003;16:191–5.
6. Johnson AL, Smith CW, Schaeffer DJ. Fragment reconstruction and bone plate fixation versus bridging plate fixation for treating highly comminuted femoral fractures in dogs: 35 cases (1987-1997). J Am Vet Med Assoc 1998;213(8):1157–61.
7. Johnson AL, Houlton JEF, Vannini R. AO principles of fracture management in the dog and cat. Davos (Switzerland): AO Publishing; 2005.
8. Perren SM. Evolution of the internal fixation of long bone fractures. The scientific basis of biological internal fixation: choosing a new balance between stability and biology. J Bone Joint Surg Br 2002;84(8):1093–110.
9. Haaland P, Sjostrom L, Devor M, et al. Appendicular fracture repair in dogs using the locking compression plate system: 47 cases. Vet Comp Orthop Traumatol 2009;22(4):309–15.

Minimally Invasive Plate Osteosynthesis in Small Animals
Radius and Ulna Fractures

Caleb C. Hudson, DVM, MS, Daniel D. Lewis, DVM,
Antonio Pozzi, DMV, MS*

KEYWORDS

- Plate osteosynthesis • MIPO • Fracture • Radius • Ulna

KEY POINTS

- Minimally invasive plate osteosynthesis for radius and ulna fractures is performed by reducing the radius in a closed, indirect fashion and applying a dorsal bone plate through two small plate insertion incisions made remote from the fracture site.
- The surgical approach for minimally invasive plate osteosynthesis of the radius preserves the soft tissue structures and vascular supply supporting the fracture site which results in rapid bone healing.
- A simple circular fixator frame is an excellent tool for facilitating closed reduction and alignment of radius and ulna fractures prior to minimally invasive plate stabilization.
- Minimally invasive plate osteosynthesis is most suited for acute, comminuted radius and ulna fractures, but can be applied to chronic fractures or simple fractures in selected cases.
- Open reduction and internal fixation may be a better surgical option than minimally invasive plate osteosynthesis for most simple oblique, open, or chronic mal-aligned radius and ulna fractures.

INTRODUCTION

Radius and ulna fractures are common in dogs and cats with the radius being the third most commonly fractured bone in dogs in one study.[1,2] The most common cause of fractures of the radius is traumatic injury due to a fall.[2] Surgical management of radius and ulna fractures typically consists of the application of a bone plate and screws or an external skeletal fixator to stabilize the radius.[2,3] Bone plates have traditionally been applied to the cranial or, less commonly, the medial surface of the radius using an open surgical approach and direct reduction of the fracture.[4–6] More recently, minimally invasive bone plating techniques have been developed that minimize soft tissue

Department of Small Animal Clinical Sciences, College of Veterinary Medicine, University of Florida, 2015 SW 16th Avenue, Gainesville, FL 32610-0126, USA
* Corresponding author.
E-mail address: pozzia@ufl.edu

Vet Clin Small Anim 42 (2012) 983–996
http://dx.doi.org/10.1016/j.cvsm.2012.06.004
0195-5616/12/$ – see front matter © 2012 Elsevier Inc. All rights reserved.

trauma and preserve the vascular supply to the fracture site to a greater extent than is possible with an open surgical approach.[7–12] The technique of minimally invasive plate osteosynthesis (MIPO) entails the stabilization of a fractured bone with a bone plate and screws that are applied without performing an extensive open surgical approach to directly expose, reduce, and stabilize the fracture. When MIPO is performed, the fracture segments are aligned using indirect reduction techniques in a closed fashion. Small plate insertion incisions are made over the anticipated (intended) locations of the proximal and distal ends of the bone plate. An epiperiosteal tunnel is developed adjacent to the fractured bone, beneath the overlying soft tissues. The epiperiosteal tunnel extends from one plate insertion incision to the other, spanning the fracture site. The plate is inserted through the tunnel and fixed in place with screws inserted through the plate insertion incisions. Small stab incisions can be made over unexposed plate holes to insert additional screws if necessary. MIPO techniques can result in superior preservation of blood supply to the fracture site,[13–15] less disruption of supporting soft tissue structures, and potentially a faster return to function and more rapid bone healing than would be achieved with an open surgical approach to facilitate bone plating.[16]

ANATOMY OF THE RADIUS AND ULNA

The closed reduction techniques and small plate insertion incisions used when performing MIPO do not allow direct observation of the fascial layers and neurovascular structures around the fracture site. A thorough knowledge of the anatomy of the antebrachium is essential for performing MIPO to stabilize radial fractures to prevent complications.

The radius and ulna articulate by means of the proximal radioulnar joint, the distal radioulnar joint, and along their length are bound together by a strong interosseus ligament. The architecture of the joints and supporting ligaments permit minimal translational motion between the radius and the ulna while some rotational motion, known as pronation and supination of the distal limb, is allowed.[17] The caudal interosseus branch of the common interosseus artery, which originates from the median artery, runs in the interosseus space between the radius and ulna and supplies a nutrient artery to both the radius and ulna. The nutrient arteries enter at the level of the proximal third of the radius and the distal third of the ulna.[18]

Under the skin, the antebrachium is surrounded by a delicate superficial antebrachial fascia layer. Underneath and protected by the superficial antebrachial fascia, the cephalic vein, two branches of the cranial superficial antebrachial artery, and two branches of the superficial radial nerve course together on the dorsomedial aspect of the antebrachium. During the surgical approach to the distal aspect of the radius, the superficial fascia is incised lateral to the cephalic neurovascular bundle, after which the neurovascular bundle is gently retracted medially. Under the superficial antebrachial fascia is a deep antebrachial fascia layer that surrounds and protects the antebrachial muscles. The deep antebrachial fascia will also be incised during the surgical approach to the radius to expose the underlying antebrachial muscles.

INDICATIONS AND DECISION-MAKING
Simple Versus Comminuted Fractures

Proper case selection is important to achieve good outcomes with MIPO. MIPO is not the optimal fixation technique for all radius and ulna fractures. When MIPO is performed to stabilize a radial fracture, the bone plate is typically applied in bridging fashion and secondary bone healing with proliferative callus formation is expected.[19]

The ideal radius and ulna fracture configuration for MIPO would be a closed, minimally displaced, mildly comminuted fracture with minimal associated soft tissue trauma. Fractures that fit perfectly into this narrowly defined category are likely to be rare. Simple transverse fractures may benefit from direct, anatomic reduction and application of a bone plate in compression fashion; however, simple fractures that can be easily indirectly reduced into anatomic reduction or that are minimally displaced can be managed using MIPO (**Fig. 1**).

Diaphyseal Versus Metaphyseal Fractures

MIPO is well-suited for diaphyseal fractures of the radius. Distal metaphyseal fractures in toy breed dogs can also be managed successfully with MIPO, but placement of the screws may be more challenging. Fractures that involve the metaphysis or epiphysis of the radius may not allow appropriate screw purchase distally to be suitable for bone plate application. A good rule of thumb is that at least two bicortical screws should be placed in each of the major fracture segments. Metaphyseal or epiphyseal radius fractures that are not suitable for bone plate application may be more appropriately stabilized with the use of a circular or linear-circular hybrid external skeletal fixator.

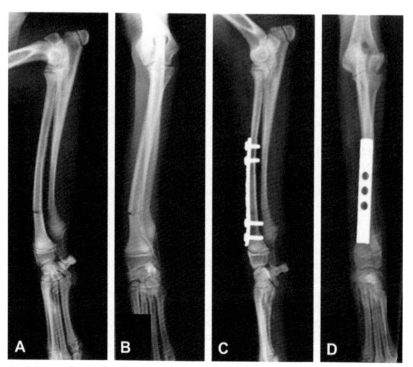

Fig. 1. A 5-month-old female Australian Shepherd that presented after acute trauma. Preoperative lateral (A) and craniocaudal (B) radiographic projections demonstrate a simple transverse fracture of the distal radial diaphysis. The fracture was reduced in an indirect, closed fashion and a 7-hole plate was applied with MIPO technique. Postoperative lateral (C) and craniocaudal (D) radiographic projections demonstrate that near anatomic reduction of the fracture segments has been achieved.

Acute Versus Chronic Fractures

In the authors' experience, MIPO can be effectively applied to most acute fractures but may not be the best option for chronic fractures. Chronic overriding fractures may require direct reduction because the organizing callus may not allow distraction of the fracture segments. Minimally displaced chronic fractures with acceptable alignment may be amenable to MIPO. In these cases, the minimally invasive approach of MIPO may be more efficacious than exposing the fracture site and disrupting the ongoing healing process.

Locking Versus Nonlocking Plates

Implant selection is important to maximize successful outcomes. MIPO can be performed with standard or locking bone plates. The advantage of using nonlocking bone plates for MIPO of radius and ulna fractures is that the plate can be used to reduce and align the fracture in the sagittal plane. The flat cranial surface of the radius allows precise reduction of the proximal and distal fracture segments as long as the plate has been appropriately contoured. Precise plate contouring can be performed preoperatively using radiographs of the contralateral normal limb. Locking bone plates provide the advantage of not requiring precise contouring as the screws lock into the bone plate and the fracture segments are not displaced as the screws are tightened, even when the plate is not in contact with the bone. Owing to the angular stability achieved by the screws locking into the plate, locking constructs function as internal fixators.[20] The major disadvantages of using locking implants are the inability to vary the angle of screw insertion through the bone plate and the increased cost of locking implants compared with standard plates and screws. The authors routinely use non-locking dynamic compression plates and limited contact dynamic compression plating systems, as well as locking compression plates and Fixin plates (TraumaVet S.l.r., Rivoli, Italy) for MIPO of radial fractures. Specially designed Y-plates or T-plates have proven very useful for MIPO stabilization of distal diaphyseal or metaphyseal fractures of the radius that would normally be difficult to stabilize using straight plates.

PREOPERATIVE PLANNING

Careful preoperative planning is critical to facilitate any MIPO procedure. Well-positioned craniocaudal and mediolateral projection radiographs of the fractured and the contralateral antebrachium should be obtained. The radiographs should be scaled to actual size. Information regarding the diameter and length of the fractured radius obtained from the preoperative radiographs is used in combination with the weight, age, breed, and activity level of the animal to select the appropriate implant type and size. Plate selection is important as undersizing implants increases the risk of implant failure, whereas applying overly stiff implants can result in stress protection and delayed healing. Screw diameter should not exceed 40% of the diameter of the fractured radial diaphysis as measured on the craniocaudal projection radiograph.[21] When performing MIPO, the bone plate is applied in buttress fashion in most cases. Long plates that span the length of the radius are preferable to shorter plates because longer plates provide mechanical advantages. Long plates also allow the plate insertion incisions to be made remote to the fracture site. Preoperative planning should include the position and order of insertion of all of the screws that will be placed. In most cases, we prefer to insert the first screw distally to center the plate over the distal segment. The most proximal screw is then placed in the proximal fracture segment to align and stabilize the fracture. Additional screws are inserted and used to reduce the radius to the plate. When using a locking plate, we recommend first inserting a single nonlocking screw in both the distal and proximal bone segments to reduce the distance between the plate and the bone. After stabilizing the fracture with the two nonlocking screws, locking screws are sequentially placed.

Availability of intraoperative fluoroscopy is invaluable when performing MIPO. Fluoroscopy allows fracture reduction, accuracy of plate contouring, and location of screws relative to the fracture site to be assessed. If MIPO is performed without intraoperative fluoroscopy there is a high risk of obtaining suboptimal fracture reduction, less than ideal plate contouring and application, as well as a risk of inserting screws too close to the fracture site. We routinely use intraoperative fluoroscopy when performing MIPO of radial fractures and believe that its use results in shorter procedure times and more appropriate fracture reduction and implant application than is achieved without the use of fluoroscopy during the procedure. Intraoperative fluoroscopy should be used judiciously during MIPO procedures to avoid exposure of the animal and operating room personnel to unnecessary amounts of radiation.

PREPARATION AND POSITIONING

In preparation for surgery, the fractured forelimb should be clipped from digits to dorsal midline and a dirty scrub should be performed in routine fashion. In the operating room, the animal should be positioned in dorsal recumbency with a foam pad under the shoulder of the fractured limb. The fractured limb should be sterilely scrubbed using a hanging limb technique. The limb should be draped so that both the brachium and antebrachium are in the surgical field to allow intraoperative manipulation of the limb and facilitate positioning of the limb in the fluoroscopy unit. The entire paw on the affected limb should be scrubbed in sterile fashion or the paw can be wrapped with a barrier drape so that it can remain in the surgical field. If a barrier drape is used to cover the paw, the drape should not extend proximal to the carpometacarpal joint to allow manipulation of the carpus intraoperatively and to allow the distal plate insertion incision to be made without interference. Both the elbow and the carpus need to be included in the surgical field so both joints can be flexed and extended simultaneously to assess limb alignment after fracture reduction.

INDIRECT REDUCTION TECHNIQUES

Indirect reduction refers to the reduction of a fracture by application of distraction forces to fracture segments applied distant from the fracture site. Indirect reduction techniques allow for fracture segment alignment without direct exposure of the fracture.[22,23] Indirect reduction techniques are used when performing MIPO because the fracture site is never exposed. The goals of indirect reduction are to restore the fractured radius to normal length and to properly align the elbow and carpal joints. In general we do not attempt to anatomically reduce radial fractures before performing MIPO, nor do we attempt to manipulate any small, comminuted fracture fragments. Reduction efforts are focused on the major fracture segments and any smaller fragments are left to be incorporated in the fracture callus and remodeled over time. The exceptions to this rule are the cases in which MIPO is used in simple transverse radial fractures. Simple transverse fractures can, in some animals, be reduced nearly anatomically using indirect reduction techniques.

Several techniques may be used to assist in the closed, indirect reduction of radius and ulna fractures. These techniques include suspending the limb, placement of an ulnar intramedullary pin, and using a circular fixator to distract the fracture. The hanging limb technique involves suspending the fractured forelimb from the paw.

The animal's body weight provides the distraction force to stretch out contracted muscles and return the fractured limb segment to normal length.[23,24]

If the hanging limb technique does not adequately distract the fractured radius to allow closed reduction to be performed, we recommend the application of a simple two-ring circular fixator to facilitate radial distraction and limb alignment. Rings should be selected that allow at least 1 cm of space (more space is optimal) between the inner circumference of the ring and the soft tissues of the antebrachium. Rings that are oversized relative to the diameter of the animal's limb make the surgical approach and plate application easier to perform. A single Kirschner wire is inserted from medial-to-lateral through the distal radial epiphysis, perpendicular to the longitudinal axis of the radius and parallel to the radiocarpal articulation. A second Kirschner wire is inserted in the proximal radial diaphysis, perpendicular to the longitudinal axis of the radius and parallel with the articular surface of the radial head (**Fig. 2**). Each Kirschner wire is attached to its respective ring using a pair of fixation bolts and the radius is centered in the rings. The rings are articulated using two segments of threaded rod that are secured to each ring using a pair of nuts. The rods are placed medial and lateral to the radius. Initially the threaded rod should be inserted through the same holes in both the proximal and distal rings, relative to the position of the fixation bolts securing the Kirschner wires (**Fig. 3**). The nuts on the segments of threaded rod on the interior of the construct are serially tightened to distract the fractured antebrachium to the desired length (**Fig. 4**). Once the desired length is achieved, the nuts on the threaded rod on the exterior of the construct are tightened to maintain the position of the rings and secured limb segment. With the limb distracted, the fracture is indirectly reduced using closed digital manipulation of the two major radial fracture segments. If necessary, the fracture segments can be translated along the Kirschner wires using digital pressure to improve fracture reduction.[25] The elbow and carpus should be flexed to assess rotation as well as limb alignment. Rotational alignment can be adjusted by altering the position of the Kirschner wire about the circumference of the ring. The fixation bolts holding the distal Kirschner wire in place on the distal ring are removed and the distal limb segment is rotated inside the ring until appropriate alignment is achieved. The fixation bolts are reinserted to maintain the position of the distal limb segment. The fixator is left in place to maintain reduction and alignment while the surgical approach is developed and the bone plate is applied.

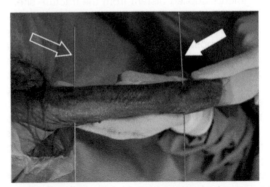

Fig. 2. Antebrachium with the elbow to the left and the paw to the right demonstrating proper positioning of two Kirschner wires inserted parallel to the radiocarpal joint (*solid white arrow*) and the proximal radial articular surface (*white outline arrow*).

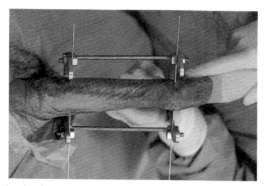

Fig. 3. A two-ring circular fixator frame using incomplete 5/8 rings and two connecting rods has been applied to the antebrachium. The Kirschner wires are fixed to the rings using cannulated-slotted fixation bolts. The circular frame facilitates closed, indirect fracture distraction and reduction as well as limb alignment.

SURGICAL APPROACH

The authors recommend a craniomedial surgical approach (see previous discussion) for MIPO of the radius.[26] The limb is extended caudally alongside the thorax for the surgical approach. The surgical approach should begin by making the distal plate insertion incision. Digital palpation combined with flexion of the carpal joint and, if necessary, insertion of a 25-gauge hypodermic needle is used to locate the antebra-chiocarpal joint. A 2 to 4 cm long skin incision is made, starting at the antebrachiocarpal joint and extending proximally. The incision should be centered over the cranial aspect of the radius. The skin edges are retracted laterally and medially using Senn retractors (Sontec Instruments, Inc. Centennial, CO) or a small Gelpi retractor (Sontec Instruments, Inc. Centennial, CO). The incision is continued through the superficial and then the deep antebrachial fascia between the tendon of the extensor carpi radialis and the tendon of the common digital extensor muscles (**Fig. 5**). The cephalic neuro-vascular bundle should be gently retracted medially if necessary. The tendon of the abductor pollicis longus muscle can be transected where the tendon crosses the radius in the surgical field, which will increase the ease of positioning the bone plate.

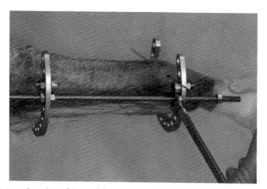

Fig. 4. Fracture distraction is achieved by sequentially tightening the connecting rod nuts on the inside of the circular rings. Once sufficient distraction has been achieved, the nuts on the outside of the circular rings are tightened down to secure the fixator frame.

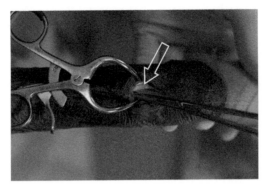

Fig. 5. The distal plate insertion incision is 2 to 4 cm in length extending proximally from the antebrachiocarpal joint. The incision extends through skin, superficial antebrachial fascia, and deep antebrachial fascia. Gelpi retractors can be used to provide better exposure. Metzenbaum scissors are used to separate between the extensor carpi radialis tendon (*white outline arrow*) and the common digital extensor tendon and to create an epiperiosteal soft tissue tunnel for plate insertion. The paw is to the right in this image.

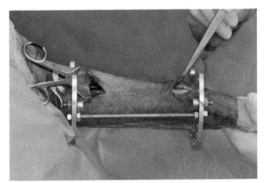

Fig. 6. A Gelpi retractor exposes the proximal shaft of the radius through the proximal plate insertion incision while the distal end of the radius is exposed with a baby Hohman retractor through the distal plate insertion incision. The circular fixator maintains the antebrachial alignment and fracture reduction during the surgical approach.

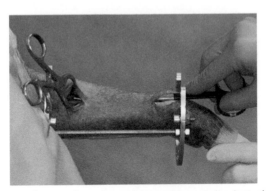

Fig. 7. A pair of Metzenbaum scissors is used to create an epiperiosteal soft tissue tunnel starting at the distal plate insertion incision and extending to the proximal plate insertion incision. The tip of the Metzenbaum scissors is visible in the proximal incision.

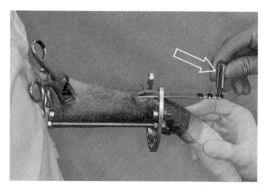

Fig. 8. Plate insertion starts at the distal insertion incision. The plate will then be slid proximally through the epiperiosteal soft tissue tunnel. The handle of the locking drill guide (*white outline arrow*) can be used to direct and slide the plate.

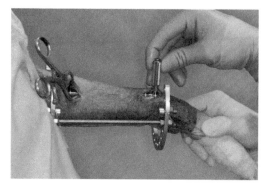

Fig. 9. A locking plate has been slid through the epiperiosteal soft tissue tunnel into final position. The proximal end of the plate is visible in the proximal insertion incision.

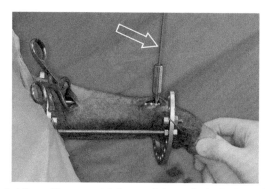

Fig. 10. A drill bit (*white outline arrow*) is inserted through the locking drill guide and used to drill the first hole in the distal segment of the radius.

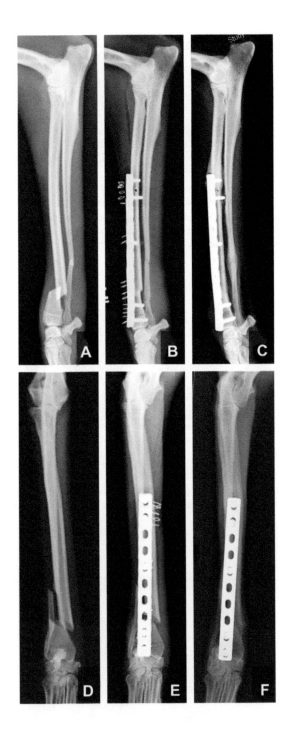

The anticipated location of the proximal portion of the plate over the radius can be marked on the skin on the craniomedial aspect of the antebrachium. A 2 to 4 cm skin incision is created at the previously marked location. The skin edges are retracted, similarly to the distal incision, and the incision is continued through the deep antebrachial fascia between the extensor carpi radialis and the pronator teres muscles. The extensor carpi radialis muscle belly is retracted laterally to expose the shaft of the radius (**Fig. 6**). An epiperiosteal soft tissue tunnel is developed, typically from distal-to-proximal, along the cranial surface of the radius using Metzenbaum scissors (Sontec Instruments, Inc. Centennial, CO) or a Freer Periosteal Elevator (Sontec Instruments, Inc. Centennial, CO) (**Fig. 7**). It may be necessary to insert the instrument from proximal to distal, particularly if the fracture is not yet fully reduced to completely develop the epiperiosteal tunnel.

APPLICATION OF IMPLANTS

Limb alignment and fracture reduction should be assessed immediately before plate insertion. Limb alignment is assessed by flexing the elbow and carpus simultaneously. Fracture reduction is assessed with intraoperative fluoroscopy, if available, or by digital palpation over the fracture site. Adjustments to alignment and reduction are made, if necessary, using the previously described techniques. The precontoured bone plate is inserted through one of the insertion incisions and advanced along the cranial surface of the radius through the epiperiosteal tunnel that was previously created until the end of the plate is appropriately positioned in the second insertion incision (**Fig. 8**). We have found that it is easiest to insert the plate through the distal insertion incision and advance the plate toward the proximal insertion incision. The plate can also be inserted from the proximal incision toward the distal incision if the distal segment of the radius is caudally displaced at the fracture site.[26] If a locking implant is used, it is useful to use the drill guide inserted in the end plate hole as a handle to insert and position the bone plate on the radius (**Fig. 9**). Proper positioning of the bone plate on the radius can be assessed with fluoroscopy. Once the position of the plate is deemed appropriate, a screw is inserted through the distalmost hole in the bone plate into the distal radial segment (**Fig. 10**). Care should be taken to ensure that the screw is centered in the radius. The screw should be marginally, but not fully, tightened so that the plate position on the proximal radial segment can still be adjusted. Limb alignment and fracture reduction is again assessed. The bone plate is adjusted so that the proximal end of the plate is centered over the radius. A screw is then inserted into the proximal radial segment through the most proximal hole in the bone plate. The proximal screw is tightened securely and then the first screw that was placed in the distal end of the plate is also tightened securely. Limb alignment and fracture reduction is again assessed. One or two additional screws are then

◄───

Fig. 11. A 20-month-old female, spayed, mixed-breed dog presented for a non–weight-bearing right forelimb lameness. Preoperative mediolateral (*A*) and craniocaudal (*D*) radiographic projections revealed a short oblique fracture of the distal diaphysis of the radius and ulna. The fracture was reduced in an indirect, closed fashion and a 10-hole plate was placed using MIPO technique. Immediate postoperative radiographs revealed good alignment in the craniocaudal plane on the mediolateral projection (*B*) and the presence of a 3 mm translational malalignment in the mediolateral plane on the craniocaudal projection (*E*). Six-week postoperative recheck radiographs demonstrated bridging osseous callus formation at both the radial and ulnar fracture sites on both the mediolateral projection (*C*) and the craniocaudal projection (*F*). The fracture was pronounced healed at the six-week recheck examination.

sequentially inserted into both the proximalmost and the distalmost holes in the bone plate. Typically, we insert three screws in the proximal segment and either two or three (length of the segment permitting) screws in the distal segment of the radius. All screws should obtain bicortical bone purchase if possible. Typically, the two insertion incisions are sufficient for placing all the necessary screws because a Senn retractor can be used to shift the commissure of the incision either proximally or distally, as necessary, to expose additional holes in the bone plate. If a screw needs to be placed in a plate hole that cannot be accessed through the insertion incisions, a stab incision can be created over the desired plate hole using fluoroscopic guidance. Once the fracture has been adequately stabilized with the plate, both insertion incisions and any additional stab incisions are closed in routine fashion using a three-layer closure (deep fascia, subcutaneous tissue, and skin). Tenorrhaphy of the previously transected abductor pollicis longus tendon is not necessary. The closure should be performed meticulously to prevent postoperative incision dehiscence that could result in exposure of the bone plate and surgical site infection.

IMMEDIATE POSTOPERATIVE CARE

Postoperative radiographs should be obtained with the animal still anesthetized so that revision surgery can be performed immediately if necessary. The alignment of the elbow and carpal joints, as well as apposition at the fracture site and the presence of iatrogenic limb angulation, should be assessed on orthogonal radiographs of the antebrachium. Bone plate positioning on the radius should be assessed and verification that screws have not been placed in the carpal or elbow joints should be obtained. If any significant problems are noted the animal should be returned to the operating room so the problem can be corrected.

Once satisfactory radiographs have been obtained and assessed, the animal can be recovered from anesthesia. A soft padded bandage can be placed for the first night after surgery. Alternately, the limb can be left without a bandage so that cold compresses can be applied over the surgical sites. We typically administer an injectable opioid and a nonsteroidal antiinflammatory agent as analgesia for the first 12 to18 hours following surgery.

MANAGEMENT DURING THE POSTOPERATIVE CONVALESCENT PERIOD

We usually discharge animals that have had radius and ulna fractures stabilized with MIPO the day following surgery. Typically, animals are discharged with a seven-day to ten-day supply of oral tramadol and dogs are given a seven-day to ten-day course of an oral nonsteroidal antiinflammatory agent. Some animals are discharged with a 3-week course of oral cephalexin, depending on surgeon preference.

We do not splint animals with radial fractures treated with MIPO unless we think that there has been significant undersizing of the implants relative to the size of the animal. We have seen problems, particularly in toy breeds, with stress shielding and delayed union when splints are used as additional stabilization for a plated radius fracture. We typically do not discharge patients with any bandage except for a light, adhesive, sterile dressing to cover the incisions.

Animals should be confined to a crate following surgery until clinical and radiographic documentation of bone healing has been obtained. Owners should be instructed to restrict their dog's activity to short walks on a leash mainly for the purposes of urinating and defecating. We advise owners to initially support their dog's weight with a sling placed under the thorax when walking their pet.

ASSESSMENT OF REPAIR AND OUTCOME

Recheck orthopedic examinations and radiographs should be performed at 3 weeks after surgery and at subsequent 3-week intervals until radiographic evidence of osseous union is obtained. We recommend repeat radiographs every 3 weeks because, in our experience, some radial fractures treated with MIPO obtain radiographic union by 3 weeks and many fractures obtain radiographic union by 6 weeks (**Fig. 11**).[27] Radiographs should consist of orthogonal views of the antebrachium. Additional oblique views of the antebrachium may be desirable in small or toy breeds if the plate obscures assessment of radial fracture healing on the craniocaudal projection radiograph. Because many MIPO-treated fractures of the radius have not been anatomically reduced, and most are plated in buttress fashion, most heal with bridging, secondary callus formation. Once confluent bridging bone is noted on mediolateral and craniocaudal projections of the radius and the animal is clinically bearing weight on the stabilized limb without lameness, the fracture is pronounced healed, and the animal is allowed to return to normal activity over a period of several weeks.

SUMMARY

MIPO is a biologically friendly approach to fracture reduction and stabilization that is applicable to many radius and ulna fractures. An appropriate knowledge of the anatomy of the antebrachium and careful preoperative planning is a prerequisite for achieving a successful outcome. The initial technical difficulty associated with the inability to directly observe the fracture segments during surgery tends to decrease as experience and familiarity with the procedure is attained. Based on the authors' experience, good outcomes, including rapid return of function and time to union, can be expected when MIPO is applied to radius and ulna fractures.

REFERENCES

1. Harasen G. Common long bone fractures in small animal practice–part 1. Can Vet J 2003;44:333–4.
2. Harasen G. Common long bone fracture in small animal practice–part 2. Can Vet J 2003;44:503–4.
3. Boudrieau RJ. Fractures of the radius and ulna. In: Slatter D, editor. Textbook of small animal surgery, vol. 2, 3rd edition. Philadelphia: Saunders; 2003. p. 1953–73.
4. Harrison JW. Fractures of the radius and ulna in the dog. In: Brinker WO, Hohn RB, Prieur WD, editors. Manual of internal fixation in small animals. New York: Springer-Verlag; 1984. p. 144–51.
5. Sardinas JC, Montavon PM. Use of a medial bone plate for repair of radius and ulna fractures in dogs and cats: a report of 22 cases. Vet Surg 1997;26: 108–13.
6. Piermattei DL, Flo GL, DeCamp CE. Handbook of small animal orthopedics and fracture repair. 4th edition. St. Louis (MO): Saunders Elsevier; 2006. p. 359–381.
7. Garofolo SQ, Pozzi A. The effect of minimally invasive plating osteosynthesis and open plating techniques on the extraosseous blood supply of the canine radius. Proceedings of the Annual Conference of the Veterinary Orthopedic Society; March 5-12, 2011; Snowmass, CO. Vet Comp Orthop Traumatol 2011;24:A10.
8. Miclau T, Martin RE. The evolution of modern plate osteosynthesis. Injury 1997; 28:A3–6.
9. Tong G, Bavonratanavech S. AO Manual of Fracture Management Minimally Invasive Plate Osteosynthesis (MIPO). Clavadelerstrasse (Switzerland): AO Publishing; 2007.

10. Krettek C, Muller M, Miclau T. Evolution of minimally invasive plate osteosynthesis (MIPO) in the femur. Injury 2001;32:SC14–23.
11. Schmokel HG, Hurter K, Schawalder P. Percutaneous plating of tibial fractures in two dogs. Vet Comp Orthop Traumatol 2003;16:191–5.
12. Schmokel HG, Stein S, Radke H, et al. Treatment of tibial fractures with plates using minimally invasive percutaneous osteosynthesis in dogs and cats. J Small Anim Pract 2007;48:157–60.
13. Farouk O, Krettek C, Miclau T, et al. Effects of percutaneous and conventional plating techniques on the blood supply to the femur. Arch Orthop Trauma Surg 1998;117:438–41.
14. Farouk O, Krettek C, Miclau T, et al. Minimally invasive plate osteosynthesis: does percutaneous plating disrupt femoral blood supply less than the traditional technique? J Orthop Trauma 1999;13:401–6.
15. Borrelli J Jr, Prickett W, Song E, et al. Extraosseous blood supply of the tibia and the effects of different plating techniques: a human cadaveric study. J Orthop Trauma 2002;16:691–5.
16. Baumgaertel F, Buhl M, Rahn BA. Fracture healing in biological plate osteosynthesis. Injury 1998;29:C3–6.
17. Evans HE. Arthrology. In: Evans HE, editor. Miller's anatomy of the dog. 3rd edition. Philadelphia: W. B. Saunders; 1993. p. 219–57.
18. Evans HE. The heart and arteries. In: Evans HE, editor. Miller's anatomy of the dog. 3rd edition. Philadelphia: W. B. Saunders; 1993. p. 586–681.
19. Pozzi A, Risselada M, Winter MD. Ultrasonographic and radiographic assessment of fracture healing after minimally invasive plate osteosynthesis and open reduction and internal fixation of radius-ulna fractures in dogs. J Am Vet Med Assoc, in press.
20. Schutz M, Sudkamp NP. Revolution in plate osteosynthesis: new internal fixator systems. J Orthop Sci 2003;8:252–8.
21. Johnson AL, Houlton JE, Vannini R. AO principles of fracture management in the dog and cat. Davos (Switzerland): AO Publishing; 2005.
22. Palmer RH. Biological osteosynthesis. Vet Clin North Am Small Anim Pract 1999;29:1171–85.
23. Johnson AL. Current concepts in fracture reduction. Vet Comp Orthop Traumatol 2003;16:59–66.
24. Aron DN, Palmer RH, Johnson AL. Biologic strategies and a balanced concept for repair of highly comminuted long bone fractures. Comp Cont Ed (Sm Anim) 1995;17:35–47.
25. Anderson GM, Lewis DD, Radasch RM, et al. Circular external skeletal fixation stabilization of antebrachial and crural fractures in 25 dogs. J Am Anim Hosp Assoc 2003;39:479–98.
26. Pozzi A, Lewis DD. Surgical approaches for minimally invasive plate osteosynthesis in dogs. Vet Comp Orthop Traumatol 2009;22:316–20.
27. Pozzi A, Hudson CC, Gauthier C, et al. A retrospective comparison of minimally invasive plate osteosynthesis and open reduction and internal fixation for radius-ulna fractures in dogs. Vet Surg, in press.

Minimally Invasive Osteosynthesis Techniques of the Femur

Michael P. Kowaleski, DVM

KEYWORDS

- Femur • Fracture • Minimally invasive osteosynthesis

KEY POINTS

- A thorough working knowledge of the anatomic landmarks of the femur facilitates anatomic alignment during minimally invasive osteosynthesis (MIO).
- A variety of fixation techniques, including plate, plate-rod, and interlocking nail, are well suited for the stabilization of femoral shaft fractures with MIO techniques.
- Axis and torsional alignment can be assessed with several intraoperative techniques to ensure that anatomic alignment is obtained.

CLINICAL ANATOMY OF THE FEMUR

The proximal end of the femur is comprised of the nearly hemispherical femoral head, which caps the dorsocaudal and medial aspects of the femoral neck. The neck is about as long as the diameter of the femoral head and is slightly compressed from a cranial-to-caudal direction.[1] Femoral neck anteversion describes the cranial (anterior) projection of the femoral head and neck relative to the anatomic axis of the femur. The anteversion angle in normal dogs has been reported to be 12° to 40°, with a mean value of 27° (**Fig. 1**).[2] The femoral inclination angle is the angle formed between the anatomic axis of the femur and the long axis of the femoral head and neck (**Fig. 2A**). The range of motion of the hip joint in healthy Labrador retrievers, as determined by goniometry, was 50° ± 2° of flexion to 162° ± 3° of extension. The hip joint angle was measured at the intersection of the longitudinal axis of the femur and a line that joined the tuber sacrale and ischiadicum.[3] The normal range of motion of the hip in rotation is approximately 45° of internal rotation and 90° of external rotation. These

Financial disclosure and conflict of interest: Dr Kowaleski has acted indirectly through the AO Foundation as a consultant on product development for Synthes Vet as a member of the Veterinary Expert Group of the AO Technical Commission (AOTK).
Department of Clinical Sciences, Cummings School of Veterinary Medicine, Tufts University, 200 Westboro Road, North Grafton, MA 01536, USA
E-mail address: mike.kowaleski@tufts.edu

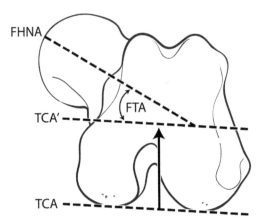

Fig. 1. The anteversion angle is the angle formed by the cranially projecting femoral head and neck and the femoral shaft. In an axial view of the femur, femoral anteversion and femoral torsion are quantified together as the femoral torsion angle (FTA) at the intersection of the femoral head and neck axis (FHNA) and the transcondylar axis (TCA). Note that the TCA is translated vertically (TCA') to highlight the intersection of the axes within the image.

values are important in assessing correct femoral torsional alignment intraoperatively. For instance, if the range of motion in the internal rotation is less than 45° and the range of motion in the external rotation is more than 90° following the femoral diaphyseal fracture reduction, then it is likely that external femoral torsion (decreased angle of anteversion) has been induced and the assessment of alignment using local land-marks or image intensification is warranted.

The greater trochanter is positioned directly lateral to the femoral head and neck; it is connected to the femoral head medially by a ridge of bone referred to as the trochanto-capital ridge (see **Fig. 2**). The trochanteric fossa is caudal to the trochanto-capital ridge. A dorsally arched ridge of the bone, known as the transverse

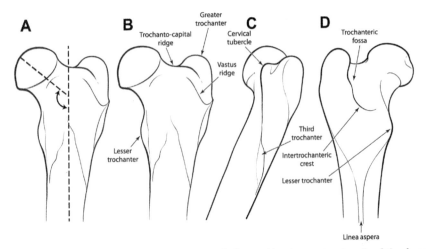

Fig. 2. The femoral inclination angle is the angle formed by the anatomic axis of the femur and the long axis of the femoral head and neck (*curved arrow, A*). The anatomic landmarks of the femur are illustrated in the cranial (*B*), lateral (*C*), and caudal views (*D*).

line, runs across the cranial surface of the trochanto-capital ridge, reinforcing the femoral neck and connecting the femoral head to the laterally placed greater trochanter (see **Fig. 2**). The lesser trochanter is a distinct pyramidal eminence that projects from the caudomedial surface of the femoral metaphysis, near the junction with the proximal diaphysis. It is connected to the greater trochanter by a low but wide arciform crest, known as the intertrochanteric crest (see **Fig. 2**). The most cranio-lateral eminence of the greater trochanter is known as the cervical tubercle. A crest of bone, known as the vastus ridge, arches distocaudally from the cervical tubercle and terminates at the third trochanter.[1]

The femoral shaft is nearly circular in cross section and is straight proximally and curved from cranial to caudal distally, yielding the normal procurvatum of the femur. The medial, cranial, and lateral surfaces cannot be identified from each other, but the caudal surface is somewhat flatter than the others. The caudal surface is marked by a finely roughened surface, the linea (facies) aspera, which is narrow in the middle and wider at both ends. This slightly roughened face is bounded by the medial and lateral lips, which diverge proximally, running into the lesser and greater trochan-ters, respectively (see **Fig. 2**).[1] This anatomic feature is useful in confirming the correct torsional alignment of the femoral shaft following the reduction of shaft fractures.

The quadrangular distal end of the femur protrudes caudally and contains 3 major articular areas, one each on the medial and lateral femoral condyles and the third within the femoral trochlea on the cranial surface. The medial and lateral femoral condyles are thick, rollerlike surfaces that are convex in both the sagittal and trans-verse planes and are separated by the intercondyloid fossa. The femoral trochlea is the smooth, wide articular groove on the cranial surface of the distal femur, which is continuous with the condyles distally.[1]

FEMORAL CAPITAL PHYSEAL AND FEMORAL NECK FRACTURE
Patient Positioning and Surgical Approach

Patients are positioned on a radiolucent operating table in dorsal or dorsolateral recumbence, with the affected leg uppermost. A modified approach to the greater trochanter and subtrochanteric region of the femur is performed to access the region of the third trochanter of the femur (**Fig. 3**A, B).[4–8] A 1- to 2-cm incision is made begin-ning 3 to 4 cm distal to the greater trochanter. The skin and subcutaneous tissue are retracted and the superficial leaf of the fascia lata is incised along the cranial border of the biceps femoris muscle. The biceps muscle is retracted caudally and the fascia lata is retracted cranially with a sharp Volkmann rake or Senn retractor; care should be taken during caudal retraction of the biceps muscle to avoid damage to the sciatic nerve. The deep fascia lata is incised cranial to its insertion on the third trochanter and caudal to the vastus lateralis, leaving enough fascia for closure. The origin of the vastus lateralis is partially incised and elevated from the vastus ridge. The vastus lateralis is retracted cranially with a Hohmann retractor to expose the third trochanter and lateral aspect of the femur.

Reduction

Pointed reduction forceps are placed on the greater trochanter through the surgical approach or skin. The fracture is reduced with a combination of distal and lateral trac-tion, internal rotation, and abduction of the femur. The preoperative and intraoperative position of the bone segments can be used to predict what manipulations will be necessary. Once reduced, medial pressure on the greater trochanter is used to

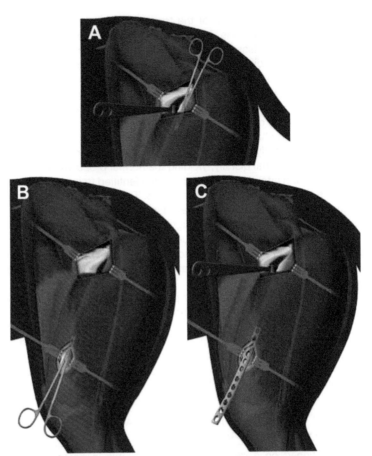

Fig. 3. Modified approach to the greater trochanter and subtrochanteric region of the femur (*A–C*) and modified approach to the distal femur through a lateral incision (*B, C*). (*From* Pozzi A, Lewis DD. Surgical approaches for minimally invasive plate osteosynthesis in dogs. Vet Comp Orthop Traumatol 2009;22:316–20; with permission.)

maintain reduction. Anatomic reduction is confirmed with image intensification or radiographic images in both the craniocaudal and lateral views.

Implants and Fixation

A Kirschner wire is positioned at the distal end of the third trochanter and directed through the lateral femoral cortex parallel to the calcar of the femur, through the femoral neck, and into the femoral head, ensuring that both the inclination and anteversion of the femoral neck are accounted for during the Kirschner-wire insertion. Image intensification is used to assess the alignment of the Kirschner wire during insertion as well as the depth of insertion. Two more Kirschner wires are placed parallel to the first and seated in the femoral head.

Alternatively, a bone screw placed in lag fashion and antirotational Kirschner wire can be used to stabilize the fracture. Once the fracture is reduced, a Kirschner wire is placed as described earlier to maintain reduction. A second Kirschner wire is placed parallel to the first in the proximal aspect of the femoral neck. A cannulated bone screw is placed over the first Kirschner wire to achieve compression of the fracture.

The Kirschner wires are bent over and cut at the lateral femoral cortex, the hip joint range of motion is assessed to ensure that there is no crepitus from inadvertent joint penetration with implants, and the reduction is confirmed with image intensification or orthogonal radiographic images. The biceps fascia, subcutaneous tissues, and skin are closed routinely (**Fig. 4**).

FEMORAL DIAPHYSEAL, PROXIMAL, AND DISTAL METAPHYSEAL FRACTURES
Patient Positioning and Surgical Approach

Patients are positioned on a radiolucent operating table in dorsal or dorsolateral recumbence, with the affected leg uppermost. A foam pad or vacuum bag should

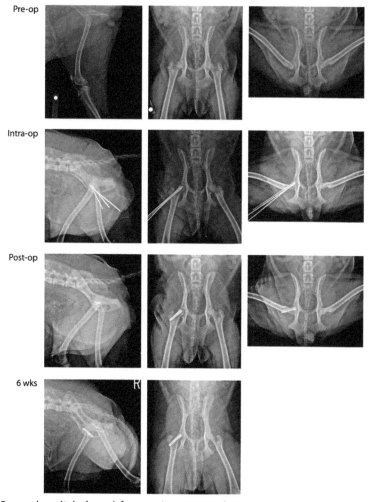

Fig. 4. Femoral capital physeal fracture in a young dog. Note that the proximal femoral epiphysis is minimally displaced in the ventrodorsal view and much more noticeably displaced in the mediolateral and frog leg views. Intraoperative images demonstrate Kirschner wire placement. Postoperative views were obtained after confirming appropriate Kirschner wire placement and cutting the Kirschner wires. Radiographic union is evident in the 6-week follow-up radiographic images. (*Courtesy of* Dr Brian S. Beale.)

be placed under the hip on the affected side to elevate the surgical site from the surface of the table. A modified approach to the greater trochanter and subtrochanteric region of the femur[4,8] is combined with a modified approach to the distal femur and stifle joint through a lateral incision (see **Fig. 3**).[5,8]

To create the proximal portal, a 2- to 4-cm long incision is made starting 1 to 2 cm distal to the greater trochanter. The skin and subcutaneous tissue are retracted, and the superficial leaf of the fascia lata is incised along the cranial border of the biceps femoris muscle. The biceps muscle is retracted caudally and the fascia lata is retracted cranially with a sharp Volkmann rake or Senn retractor; care should be taken during caudal retraction of the biceps muscle to avoid damage to the sciatic nerve. The deep fascia lata is incised cranial to its insertion on the third trochanter and caudal to the vastus lateralis, leaving enough fascia for closure. The origin of the vastus lateralis is partially incised and elevated from the vastus ridge. The vastus lateralis is retracted cranially with a Hohmann retractor to expose the third trochanter and lateral aspect of the femur.

To create the distal portal, a 2- to 4-cm long incision is made extending from just proximal and 1 cm lateral to the base of the patella. The biceps fascia is incised along the same line, just cranial to the cranial border of the biceps femoris muscle. The biceps muscle is retracted caudally, and the fascia lata is retracted cranially with a sharp Volkmann rake or Senn retractor. The aponeurotic septum of the fascia lata is incised, and the vastus lateralis muscle is retracted cranially with a Hohmann retractor to expose the femur.

Alternatively, an approach to the shaft of the femur[6] can be used with an open-but-do-not-touch technique (**Fig. 5**). A skin incision is made along the craniolateral border of the shaft of the femur, extending from the greater trochanter to 1 cm lateral to the base of the patella. The skin and subcutaneous tissue are retracted, and the superficial leaf of the fascia lata is incised along the cranial border of the biceps femoris muscle. The biceps muscle is retracted caudally and the fascia lata is retracted cranially with a sharp Volkmann rake or Senn retractor; care should be taken during caudal retraction of the biceps muscle to avoid damage to the sciatic nerve. The skin and/or fascial incisions can be made as discrete portals as described earlier (see **Fig. 5**). The aponeurotic septum of the fascia lata is incised and the vastus lateralis muscle is retracted cranially with Hohmann retractors to expose the femoral shaft, ensuring that the soft tissue attachments of the fracture fragments and the fracture hematoma are not disturbed.

Methods of Reduction

In multi-fragmentary metaphyseal and diaphyseal fractures, it is only essential to achieve functional reduction, which consists of restoration of length, mechanical, and/or anatomic axis, and torsional alignment of the major bone segments that are attached to the joint surfaces. Precise anatomic reduction of each bone fragment is not necessary and, in fact, doing so may jeopardize the blood supply to these fragments and/or the main bone segments. The stabilization of the 2 major bone segments with relative stability, without disturbing the multi-fragmentary zone and its vascularity, promotes indirect bone healing within 4 to 8 weeks.[9]

In contrast, simple metaphyseal or diaphyseal fractures, such as transverse, oblique, or spiral fractures, should be treated with absolute stability achieved by anatomic reduction and compression fixation. Absolute stability with anatomic reduction and compression reduces the risk of implant failure from stress concentration.

In MIO, the goals are to achieve fracture reduction and fixation without exposure of the fracture site or, at a minimum, without disturbance of the vascularity and fracture hematoma within the zone of comminution (see **Fig. 5**). Thus, whenever possible, indirect reduction techniques should be used. However, the quality of reduction should never be sacrificed simply for the sake of minimally invasive techniques. If adequate reduction cannot be achieved by indirect techniques, then it is necessary to resort to direct reduction to achieve the desired accuracy of reduction. Even if direct reduction techniques are used, small incisions with minimal soft tissue dissection will still achieve the goals of MIO.

Ideally, the choice of reduction technique should be made during preoperative planning. If adequate reduction cannot be achieved with a closed technique and indirect reduction, conversion to direct reduction can be performed. Even with direct methods, there are a variety of techniques, instruments, and implants that can be used to minimize intraoperative trauma to the soft tissues surrounding the fracture. The key to MIO is to leave a small footprint or the least possible damage at the fracture zone.[9]

Indirect reduction

The primary indications for indirect reduction are multi-fragmentary metaphyseal and diaphyseal fractures, although some long oblique and spiral fractures and some minimally displaced simple articular fractures are also amenable to these techniques. An image intensifier is essential to assess the quality of reduction, although arthroscopy can be used in selected articular fractures.

Using indirect reduction techniques, the fracture site is not exposed, thus, it remains covered by the surrounding soft tissues and fracture hematoma, resulting in maximal preservation of the biology intrinsic to the fracture site and bone fragments. Indirect reduction is accomplished using instruments or implants introduced distant to the fracture zone. Reduction is achieved by applying traction along the long axis of the limb as well as rotation, angulation, and translation as necessary. Bone fragments in the zone of comminution are indirectly reduced by ligamentotaxis, which is the application of longitudinal force to bring fracture fragments into reduction. In order for ligamentotaxis to be successful, soft tissue attachments must be present on the bone fragments to pull and guide the fragments into reduction. Because there is no direct visualization or fixation of these fragments, their reduction is usually not anatomic, and healing occurs by callus formation.

Direct reduction

The primary indications for direct reduction are simple transverse and oblique fractures, most long oblique and spiral fractures, and most articular fractures. Absolute stability is achieved with anatomic reduction and interfragmentary compression, resulting in direct bony healing. Using direct reduction, the fracture site is exposed and the fracture fragments are directly manipulated. Because all maneuvers are directly visualized, image intensification is not necessary, although it can still be quite useful. With direct reduction techniques, fracture reduction is typically more precise and easier than when indirect reduction techniques are used. However, the surgical approach and application of reduction instrumentation may damage soft tissues and/or their attachments to bone, affecting the vascularity of the bone fragments. Thus, when using direct reduction techniques, the surgical exposure should be adequate for direct reduction to be used, with minimal stripping of the periosteum or soft tissue attachments. The remainder of the fixation can be done percutaneously to achieve the goals of MIO.

Techniques of Indirect Reduction for Diaphyseal Fractures of the Femur

Indirect reduction of diaphyseal fractures is a demanding technique because the fracture fragments are neither directly visualized nor manipulated. A clear understanding

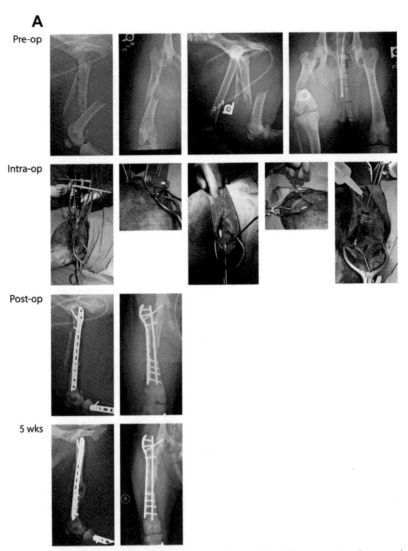

Fig. 5. (A) Plate rod stabilization of a comminuted femoral shaft fracture using the open-but-do-not touch approach. The intraoperative photographs demonstrate anatomic alignment of the femoral shaft using Kern bone-holding forceps and normograde, proximal-to-distal intramedullary pin placement. The tip of the pin is exposed at the fracture site and cut off to mitigate inadvertent penetration into the stifle joint. An epi-periosteal tunnel is created, the plate is slid along the bone within the tunnel, and locking screws are inserted into the plate; the locking drill guide is used to align the drill bit within the plate hole. Clinical union has been obtained at 5 weeks postoperatively.

of normal anatomy is necessary for the surgeon to accurately restore limb length, axis, and rotation. Various methods must be used to assess the accuracy of reduction. Preoperative, intraoperative, and/or postoperative comparison with the intact opposite limb is useful to establish the normal anatomic shape of the limb and relationship of the joints, particularly considering the variety of patient sizes and shapes that are

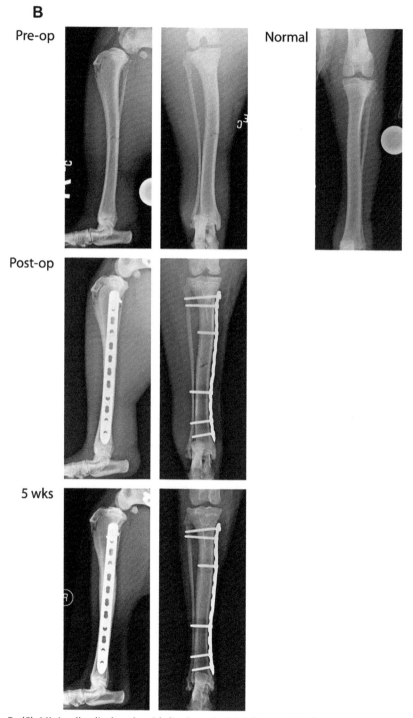

Fig. 5. (*B*) Minimally displaced, mid-diaphyseal tibial fracture in the same patient as in Fig. 5(A) stabilized in a minimally invasive plate osteosynthesis fashion with a Locking Compression Plate (LCP, DePuy Synthes, West Chester, PA). Clinical union has been obtained at 5 weeks postoperatively.

common in small animal practice. Radiographs of the intact opposite limb can be used to determine the correct length of the bone plate, the size of the intramedullary pin, and can be used as a guide to precontour the bone plate; alternatively, a similarly sized plastic or cadaveric bone can used to precontour the bone plate.

Traction

The application of traction is essential to achieve indirect reduction because it restores limb length and can be used to correct torsional and angular malalignment. Traction is the basis for ligamentotaxis; in order for ligamentotaxis to be successful, the soft tissue attachments to the fracture fragments must be intact and preserved. In addition, the fracture must be relatively acute, otherwise soft tissue contracture may prevent effective indirect reduction.

Traction can be applied with a variety of methods. A traction table or external traction device can be used (see article by Peirone and colleagues elsewhere in this issue). This device is particularly useful when surgical assistance is limited. The disadvantages include difficulty in fine adjustments of the reduction, difficulty in assessing adjacent joint orientation because the joint cannot be flexed and extended while traction is applied, and difficulty comparing with the opposite limb.

In many cases, manual traction is adequate to achieve reduction. A fracture distractor or temporary external skeletal fixator can be used to apply and maintain traction and reduction. Once reduction is achieved, the bolts on the distractor or fixator are tightened, locking the fracture fragments in position, and the definitive fixation is applied.

Supports and pads

Muscular forces usually determine the displacement of fracture segments. Although traction is useful to correct limb length, it may exacerbate torsional or axial malalignment. A supporting pad may be used to correct angular or torsional alignment. For instance, because the distal aspect of the pelvic limb is thinner than the proximal aspect, external femoral torsion is commonplace if the limb is laid flat on the surgical table. Elevation of the tarsus off the table with a pad or support corrects the torsional deformity.

External fixators and fracture distractors

External fixators and fracture distractors can be used to achieve and maintain fracture reduction and, therefore, they are indispensible tools for MIO of multi-fragmentary fractures of the diaphysis. These devices can be used to apply longitudinal traction to the bone segments, manipulate the segments into reduction, correct axial and torsional malalignment, and maintain reduction. The primary difference between the two is that the fracture distractor can be used to both distract and compress fractures using the integral threaded rod and nuts. Manual traction must be applied to an external skeletal fixator unless a threaded rod is used as a connecting bar.

Once the limb is prepped and draped, threaded fixation pins are inserted into the bone ends opposite the fracture site through stab incisions. Placing both pins in the same anatomic plane, perpendicular to the axis of the bone, facilitates reduction because the alignment of the pins parallel to each other essentially aligns the bone segments. Manipulation of the fracture is performed, and reduction is assessed with image intensification and/or local landmarks. Once satisfactory reduction is obtained, the clamps on the external fixator or distractor are tightened to maintain reduction.

Push-pull technique

The push-pull technique is used to adjust length and reduction once one bone segment has been secured to an implant, typically a bone plate. A tension device, bone spreader, or bone clamp is applied to the non-secured end of the bone plate.

The bone plate and attached bone segment is pushed away from the opposite segment to achieve reduction. Pulling on the bone plate can be used to achieve compression. An independent screw can be placed as an anchor point for the tensioner, bone spreader, or bone clamp.

Reduction by implants

Anatomically shaped implants can be used to achieve reduction. Although there is a paucity of precontoured, anatomically shaped implants available to the veterinary surgeon, precontouring available implants yields an anatomic shape. This shape can be easily achieved using a radiograph of the unaffected opposite limb or a bone model or cadaver bone. The appropriate plate length and position on the bone can be determined, and the plate can be accurately contoured and sterilized, saving time and facilitating intraoperative reduction. The bone plate is secured in the correct position to one bone segment. Often standard cortex screws are placed first to pull the bone segment to the bone plate. Once the plate is positioned accurately on the first bone segment, an additional standard or locking head screw is placed to stabilize the bone segment to the bone plate. Next, the bone-plate construct is reduced to the other bone segment. A standard cortex screw can be used to pull the bone plate to the bone; this is known as a reduction screw (**Fig. 6**, demonstrates reduction screws in the distal segment). Alternatively, a push-pull reduction device can be used for this purpose. Minor degrees of angulation and translation can be corrected at this time because only a single point of fixation has been applied; however, torsional malalignment cannot be corrected, thus, it is imperative to achieve correct torsional alignment before applying fixation to the second bone segment. If adequate alignment cannot be achieved, the screw or push-pull reduction device can be removed, and reduction can be improved. Once proper reduction is achieved, the fixation can be completed by the placement of additional standard or locking head screws in each bone segment. When locking head screws are used, it is imperative to ensure that accurate reduction has been obtained before placing the locking screws. A poorly reduced fracture will be maintained in position once the locking head screws are placed.

Cerclage wires

Cerclage wiring is a useful technique for the reduction of large butterfly (wedge) fragments (and displaced long oblique or spiral fractures, particularly when the degree of displacement is large enough to delay bone healing) as well as the neutralization of fissure lines (**Fig. 7**). Cerclage wires should be carefully placed using a wire passer, ensuring that there is minimal denuding of the bone segments. Cerclage may be used as temporary reduction aids or can remain as part of the definitive fixation.

Implants and Fixation

Bone plates with compression or neutralization function

Standard and locking bone plates can be placed with a neutralization function, and many of these implants can be placed with a compression function; these methods are typically indicated for the stabilization of transverse or short oblique fractures. The bone plate is precontoured using a bone model, cadaveric bone, and/or radiograph of the unaffected opposite limb; the bone plate is then sterilized before surgery. Because of the normal procurvatum of the femur (**Fig. 8A**), a straight bone plate cannot be applied along the length of the lateral aspect of the bone (see **Fig. 8B**). Doing so would create a recurvatum deformity in the bone (see **Fig. 8C**). To place a bone plate along the length of the femur, the plate must be twisted to match the local anatomy and applied in a helical fashion (so-called helical plating) (see **Fig. 8D**). For instance, in the case of a distal diaphyseal fracture, the plate can be applied relatively caudal

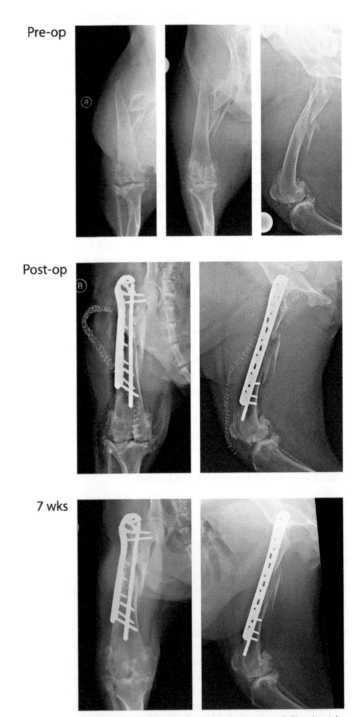

Pre-op

Post-op

7 wks

Fig. 6. A comminuted proximal diaphyseal femoral fracture stabilized with a plate-rod construct. Note that the plate is contoured to the proximal extent of the greater trochanter to obtain multiple converging screw fixation of the proximal segment. Standard cortex screws were used distally to draw the bone plate to the bone; screws used in this fashion are referred to as reduction screws. After reduction, additional locking screws were added. Stable implants and clinical union is evident at 7 weeks postoperatively.

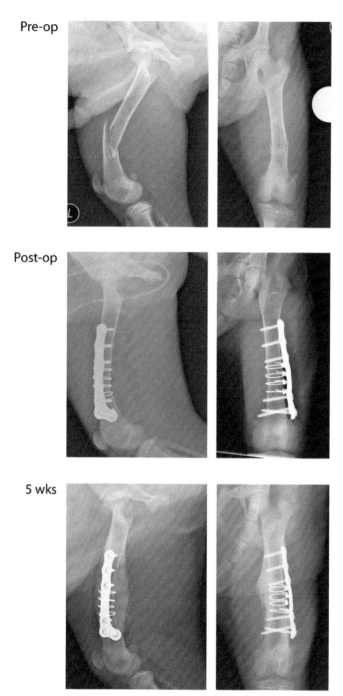

Fig. 7. Distal diaphyseal fracture in an immature dog. Following an open-but-do-not-touch approach, reduction was obtained and maintained with loop cerclage wires. A Fixin locking plate (TraumaVet, Rivoli, Turin, Italy) in a neutralization function was used to stabilize the fracture. Abundant bridging periosteal callus, stable implants, and considerable longitudinal bone growth are radiographically evident at 5 weeks postoperatively.

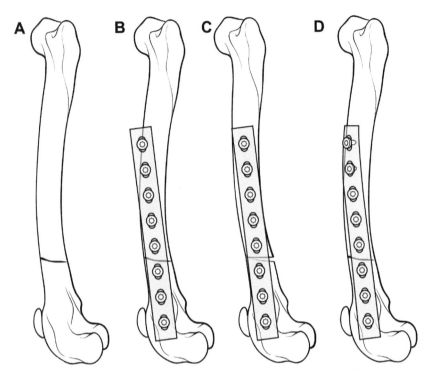

Fig. 8. Procurvatum is normally present in the canine femur (*A*). Because of the normal pro-curvatum of the femur, a straight bone plate cannot be applied along the length of the lateral aspect of the femur because this will cause the plate to be malaligned proximally, which may result in the inability to direct the bone screws into the bone at the proximal extent of the bone plate (*B*). Alignment of the femur along the straight bone plate can result in a recurvatum deformity (*C*). Application of the distal end of the plate on the caudal aspect of the femoral condyle prevents interference with the para-patellar fibrocartilage. The proximal extent of the plate can be twisted to lie on the craniolateral aspect of the femur; this technique is known as helical plating (*D*). Using the helical plating technique, a straight bone plate can be applied along the length of the lateral aspect of the femur while maintaining anatomic alignment.

on the lateral femoral condyle to avoid interference with the patella and para-patellar fibrocartilage and contoured such that it extends to the craniolateral aspect of the proximal femur (see **Fig. 8**D).

Following development of proximal and distal portals, a pathway for the introduction of the bone plate is prepared in a submuscular, epi-periosteal plane using a periosteal elevator, a blunt pair of scissors, a tunneler, or the bone plate itself. A locking bone plate can be attached to a plate holder, which is used as a handle to hold the plate for percutaneous insertion. Usually the screw at the proximal end of the plate is place first. The fracture is reduced, if it has not been reduced already, the accuracy of the plate contouring is confirmed, and the screw at the distal end of the plate is placed. The quality of reduction is assessed using image intensification and/or local land-marks, and minor adjustments in angular and translational alignment are made as needed. The remainder of the bone screws are placed in the plate holes accessible through the proximal or distal portals or through separate stab incisions, based on the preoperative plan.

The sequence of screw insertion can be altered as needed. If both standard and locking head screws are to be placed, it is recommended that the standard screws are placed first. These screws should be placed in plate holes in which the plate is well contoured and lying directly on the bone or they can be used as reduction screws to pull the bone to a well-contoured bone plate as long as adequate plate-bone contact occurs with screw tightening. If a standard screw must be placed after a locking screw has been placed, it is recommended that all the locking screws in that bone segment are loosened before placing the standard screw; the locking head screws are then retightened. The portals are closed routinely.

Screws placed in lag fashion
Independent lag screws, or lag screws placed through the bone plate, can be used to produce and/or maintain reduction and generate interfragmentary compression. Although the placement of a lag screw requires exposure of the fracture site, such screws can be placed with minimally invasive techniques. Lag screws are used to create absolute stability in articular or reconstructible fractures of the metaphysis or diaphysis.

Bone plates with bridging function
Bridging plates are used to span nonreconstructible fractures. Initially, indirect reduction is achieved with manual traction, an alignment pin, and/or the aid of a distractor or external skeletal fixator. The pin, distractor, or external skeletal fixator can be used to maintain reduction once it has been achieved. Alternatively, the plate itself can be used as an additional or the sole indirect reduction tool. To use the plate as a reduction tool, it must be well contoured to the intact proximal and distal bone segments. Contouring the plate anatomically to the nonreconstructible portion of the fracture also aids in the fitment of the device to the local anatomy, particularly within the soft tissue envelope. The placement of standard cortex screws should be done only in areas in which the bone plate is well contoured and lying directly on the bone; these screws should be place before the placement of locking bone screws. If locking screws are used, the plate contour does not need to be as precise; however, the closer the bone plate is applied to the bone, the greater the construct strength. Standard bone screws can be used as reduction screws to pull the bone to a well-contoured bone plate as long as adequate plate-bone contact occurs with screw tightening. If a standard screw must be place after a locking screw has been placed, it is recommended that all of the locking screws in that bone segment are loosened before placing the standard screw; the locking head screws are then retightened.

Appropriate proximal and distal portals are developed, a submuscular, epiperiosteal tunnel is created, and the plate is inserted as described earlier. The bone plate is generally secured to the proximal bone segment first because it is usually easier to adjust the reduction of the distal limb if adjustments are necessary. The adequacy of reduction is assessed, and temporary fixation of the distal segment with a monocortical or bicortical bone screw or bone clamp placed over the plate is applied. The accuracy of the reduction is confirmed using image intensification and/or local landmarks, such as axis alignment and range of motion of the adjacent joints; reduction is adjusted as necessary by removing and replacing the bone screw or bone clamp; and the remaining bone screws are placed through the portals or additional stab incisions. If conventional bone screws are placed, they should be placed in the buttress position using the neutral end of the appropriate load/neutral drill guide or a universal drill guide. The placement of the bone screws in the buttress position eliminates the potential for screw migration toward the fracture site during limb loading, by placing the screw head adjacent to the edge of the bone plate hole near to the fracture site. If an alignment pin is used, it is generally withdrawn slightly, cut, and seated back to its original depth with a mallet and pin punch or similar device after 2 to 3 bone screws are placed in each major bone segment (**Fig. 9**). As a greater number of bone screws are place, the interference of the screws with the pin may make

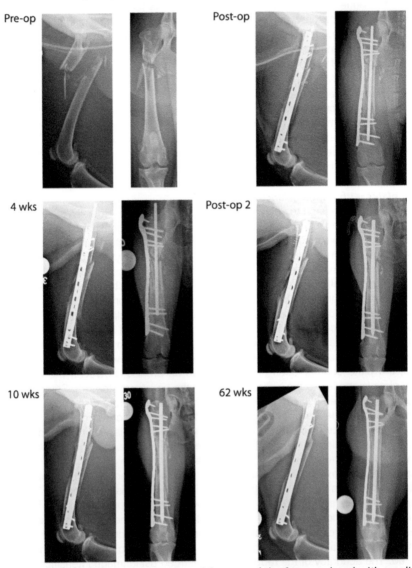

Fig. 9. A comminuted proximal metaphyseal fracture of the femur reduced with an alignment pin that was cut short and countersunk below the greater trochanter; the alignment pin remains as part of the plate-rod fixation. At 4 weeks, the pin has migrated, indicating motion at the fracture site. Inadequate bone healing is present for the pin to be safely removed at this time. The pin was removed and a larger pin was placed to improve stability at the fracture site. In addition, the larger pin will have greater contact with the bone screws, mitigating the risk of pin migration. The new pin has been cut short and countersunk below the greater trochanter. Clinical union is evident at 10 weeks, and fracture site remodeling and stable implants are evident at 62 weeks.

withdrawing the pin for cutting difficult or impossible. Withdrawing the pin enables it to be cut to the desired length without interference from anatomic structures adjacent to the pin entry site. The portals and stab incisions are closed routinely.

Interlocking nail

The interlocking nail is ideally suited to minimally invasive, percutaneous osteosynthesis, since it can be placed through small stab incisions. In addition, the large diameter fills a considerable amount of the medullary cavity, thus, the placement of the nail from the medullary cavity of one major segment to the other achieves good reduction. A nail can be placed normograde in a proximal-to-distal direction or normograde in a distal-to-proximal direction. The latter requires an approach to the stifle joint and placement of the nail through the articular surface in the non–weight-bearing distal portion of the trochlear groove. The nail is countersunk below the cartilage surface and secured with locking bolts. This technique is particularly well suited to fractures of the distal femoral diaphysis or distal metaphysis in which anatomic axis alignment precludes adequate depth of the nail placement in the distal segment (**Fig. 10**). Slight over-reduction of the distal segment (intentional creation of slight recurvatum) is performed such that the medullary canal of the distal segment is axially aligned with that of the proximal segment to facilitate nail placement (see **Fig. 10; Fig. 11**).

The diameter, length, hole pattern, depth of insertion, and bolt position of the interlocking nail are determined by preoperative planning (see **Fig. 11**). A radiograph of the opposite intact femur is invaluable for planning purposes (see **Fig. 11**). A small approach to the greater trochanter and trochanteric fossa is performed, which is a modification of the approach to the craniodorsal and caudodorsal aspects of the hip joint by osteotomy of the greater trochanter.[7] A 1- to 2-cm incision is made in a proximal-to-distal direction, centered over the greater trochanter. The subcutaneous tissue is retracted with the skin, and the superficial leaf of the biceps fascia is incised along the cranial border of the biceps femoris muscle. An incision in the deep leaf of the biceps fascia is made caudal to or through the superficial gluteal muscle with a muscle-splitting technique. The nail is introduced medial to the medial border of the greater trochanter, is aligned along the anatomic axis of the femur, and is inserted into the medullary canal of the proximal segment. The nail is directed into the distal segment using fluoroscopic guidance, closed palpation, or an open-but-do-not-touch approach to the fracture site as described earlier. The accuracy of the reduction is confirmed using image intensification and/or local landmarks, such as axis alignment and range of motion of the adjacent joints; reduction is adjusted as necessary. When using an interlocking nail, the axis alignment in the coronal and sagittal planes is usually good because of the intramedullary location and canal fill of the device; torsional alignment must be carefully assessed to prevent torsional deformity. Once adequate reduction is confirmed, the locking bolts are placed in a proximal-to-distal direction through stab incisions as described in the article by Déjardin and colleagues elsewhere in this issue, and the incisions are closed routinely.

External skeletal fixation

External skeletal fixation is well suited to provide distraction and temporary stabilization during implant (typically bone plate) placement. Because of the overlying muscle mass of the femur and the associated morbidity with long-term application of fixation pins, external skeletal fixation is not typically the first choice of definitive fixation for most femoral fractures. In select cases, particularly metaphyseal or diaphyseal fractures in feline or small canine patients, an alignment pin can be used in a tie-in configuration with a laterally applied type I external skeletal fixator for definitive stabilization.

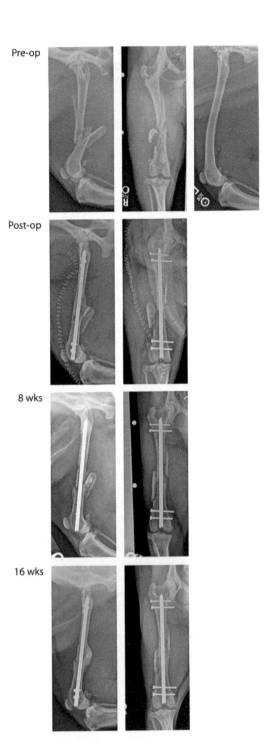

Elastic plate osteosynthesis

Several factors must be considered when stabilizing femoral shaft fractures in growing animals. The growth plates must be preserved for normal growth to occur; ideally, the periosteum should not be damaged during the surgical approach or application of fixation; and the cortices are thin and, therefore, the purchase of bone screws is poor. In a review of 8 cases of femoral diaphyseal fracture in young, growing dogs treated by intramedullary pin fixation, 7 out of 8 puppies developed subluxation of the hip joint and/or malformations of the proximal femoral epiphysis following the procedure.[10] These abnormalities were likely caused by the disruption of proximal femoral physis during pin insertion; thus, intramedullary pin fixation of such fractures should be performed with caution or avoided. The application of bone plates in the standard manner may result in fixation failure because of screw pullout caused by the high stress imposed on bone screws by rigid implants and the poor screw holding power of the thin cortices in young dogs. To overcome the limitations of standard plate fixation. Cabassu[11] described the application of a relatively elastic implant, the veterinary cuttable plate, with 2 screws in the proximal and distal segments, as far from the fracture site as possible, known as elastic plate osteosynthesis. Using this technique, 21 puppies aged 6 to 20 weeks were successfully treated.[11] In another report, 17 cases of femoral and tibial fractures in puppies were successfully managed.[12] The elasticity of the implant coupled with the young age of the patient leads to the rapid formation of a large periosteal callus in these cases. The most common complication seems to be plate bending,[12] thus, this technique is best applied to young puppies in which cortical bone thinness creates concern for the adequacy of bone-screw holding power. In addition, patient factors, such as body weight, age, activity level, and presence of other injuries in other limbs, must be considered when considering this technique.[12] In older, larger puppies with adequate cortical thickness and, thus, bone-screw holding power, a conventional rigid fixation bone plate may be more safely used than elastic fixation (see **Fig. 7**).

Assessment of Axis and Torsion with Local Landmarks

Intraoperative image intensification is the ideal method to assess limb alignment and the adequacy of reduction. However, this modality is not available to every veterinary surgeon. Therefore, the surgeon must be well versed in several intraoperative methods to assess the alignment of the limb using local landmarks and anatomic features.

Hip rotation test

The hip rotation test is a clinical method that compares the hip range of motion with the unaffected normal side or normal range-of-motion values. The technique is easy to perform and does not require fluoroscopy. However, the estimation of the range of motion may be incorrect and depends on the position of the pelvis on the surgical table. Ideally, the range of motion of the unaffected normal hip is assessed preoperatively in

◀───

Fig. 10. A comminuted, distal diaphyseal fracture of the femur stabilized with an interlocking nail. A radiograph of the intact opposite femur was obtained to facilitate preoperative planning. Note the normal procurvatum of the intact femur and the slight recurvatum of the affected femur following repair with a straight interlocking nail. Because of the distal location of the fracture, the interlocking nail was inserted normograde in a distal-to-proximal direction through a non–weight-bearing portion of the femoral articular surface, just proximal to the intercondylar notch. Slight over-reduction (recurvatum deformity) is introduced, and then the nail is passed into the proximal bone segment. Clinical union has been obtained at 16 weeks postoperatively.

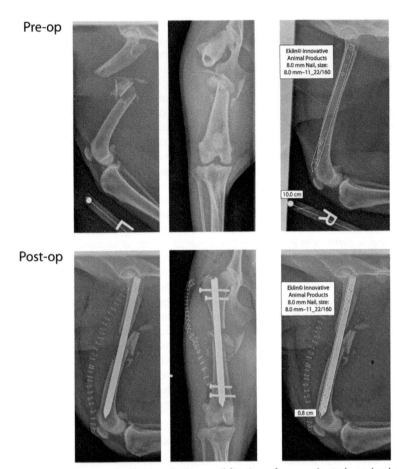

Fig. 11. Preoperative planning for interlocking nail fixation of a comminuted proximal diaphyseal femoral fracture. A radiograph of the intact, opposite femur was obtained to facilitate preoperative planning. Note that the straight interlocking nail template does not fit into the medullary canal of the intact, curved femur because of the normal procurvatum of the femur. Slight over-reduction (recurvatum deformity) of the femur is necessary to insert the interlocking nail, and this is evident in the postoperative lateral view. A digital template (Sound-Eklin, Carlsbad, CA, USA) applied to the postoperative lateral view reveals an exact match of the digital template and the actual interlocking nail (Innovative Animal Products, Rochester, MN, USA).

both internal and external rotation. To perform this test, the hip is flexed to a normal standing angle of 120°[13,14] and the stifle is extended to a normal standing angle of 135°[13]; the hip range of motion in both internal and external rotation is assessed. The normal range of motion of the hip of the dog is approximately 45° of internal rotation and 90° of external rotation. Increased internal rotation and diminished external rotation indicates an internal femoral torsion malalignment, whereas increased external rotation and diminished internal femoral rotation indicates an external femoral torsion malalignment.

Lesser trochanter shape sign
The lesser trochanter shape sign is an intraoperative radiologic or palpation assessment in which the shape of the lesser trochanter is compared with that of the

contralateral femur. Obtain a true cranio-caudal view of the contralateral femur using a horizontal beam, angled beam, or elevated torso view[15]; alternatively, an image can be taken and stored in the image intensifier. Before fixing the distal main fracture segment to the proximal main segment, the patella is oriented cranially, and the proximal segment is rotated until the shape of the lesser trochanter on the ipsilateral side matches the shape of the contralateral lesser trochanter.

In cases of external torsion of the distal segment, the lesser trochanter is smaller and partially hidden behind the proximal femoral shaft. In cases of internal torsion of the distal segment, the lesser trochanter seems enlarged. If intraoperative fluoroscopy or radiography is not available, this assessment can be made clinically by palpation or radiologically on the immediate postoperative radiographs.

Greater trochanter position sign

The position of the greater trochanter can be used in a fashion similar to that of the shape of the lesser trochanter to assess the rotational alignment of the 2 main bone segments. With the distal femur positioned such that the patella faces cranially, the greater trochanter is typically in a true lateral position. This position can be confirmed by preoperative palpation of the unaffected contralateral limb and/or by the assessment of the mediolateral radiograph of the unaffected contralateral limb.

In cases of external torsion of the distal segment, the greater trochanter is positioned cranial to the proximal femoral shaft. In cases of internal torsion of the distal segment, the greater trochanter is positioned caudal to the proximal femoral shaft. If intraoperative fluoroscopy or radiography is not available, this assessment can be made clinically by palpation or radiologically on the immediate postoperative radiographs.

Cortical step sign

The correct rotation of simple transverse or oblique fractures may be assessed by the thickness of the cortices of the proximal and distal segments. This assessment is accurate when considerable torsional deformity is present in human patients[16] but is not likely as accurate in dogs and cats because the femoral cortices are quite thin.

Diameter difference sign

The assessment of the similarity in the periosteal (clinical) or endosteal (radiological) diameter of the proximal and distal main bone segments is useful to diagnose rotational alignment and malalignment in reducible simple transverse or oblique fractures. This test is only relevant in areas in which the cross section of the bone is oval rather than round; this is known as the diameter difference sign. The diameter difference sign is positive in the presence of rotational malalignment, since the diameters of the apposed bone segments are different.

Femoral head and neck version sign

In a normal femur, approximately one-half of the femoral head projects cranial to the greater trochanter in a true mediolateral view. This position can be confirmed preoperatively by the assessment of the mediolateral view of the unaffected contralateral femur. With the distal femur positioned such that the patella faces cranially, palpation of the femoral head and neck through the proximal portal can be used to clinically evaluate the version of the femoral head and neck. In addition, intraoperative fluoroscopy, if available, can be used to assess the version.

In cases of external torsion of the distal segment, the less than half of the femoral head projects cranial to the greater trochanter. In cases of internal torsion of the distal segment, more than half of the femoral head projects cranial to the greater trochanter. The findings of palpation and/or intraoperative fluoroscopy are confirmed radiologically on the immediate postoperative radiographs.

Radiographs of Intact Opposite Limb

A mediolateral view and a true cranio-caudal view of the contralateral femur using a horizontal beam, angled beam, or elevated torso view[15] are invaluable for preoperative planning and intraoperative reference (**Fig. 12**). The mediolateral view is more useful for assessing limb length than the cranio-caudal view because it is more likely that the femur is parallel to the radiographic cassette or detector in this view, mitigating the likelihood of foreshortening caused by malposition. In addition, the mediolateral view is useful to assess the greater trochanter position and femoral head and neck version. The cranio-caudal view is useful to assess the lesser trochanter shape and can be used as a guide for precontouring a bone plate.

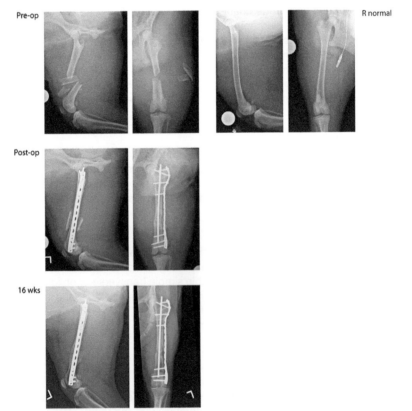

Fig. 12. A comminuted distal diaphyseal fracture of the femur with mediolateral and cranio-caudal views of the intact opposite femur for preoperative planning. The metallic sphere in the image is a 30-mm diameter magnification marker situated at the same distance from the digital detector as the femur; this marker is used to quantify magnification and calibrate the digital image. The fracture has been stabilized with a plate-rod construct in a minimally invasive plate osteosynthesis fashion. Clinical union is evident at the 16-week follow-up radiographic examination.

Prevention of Femoral Malrotation

- Keep in mind that this complication can occur, is a common pitfall, and aim to prevent it.[16]
- Be familiar with the various methods to detect this complication intraoperatively so it may be addressed before the application of the final fixation.
- If possible, use a radiolucent operating table and intraoperative fluoroscopy to assess alignment rather than a traction table. Although a traction table can be used to maintain the length of the limb, the torsional alignment cannot be assessed clinically while traction is applied. If a traction table is used, radiological methods of torsional assessment, such as the lesser trochanter sign, must be relied on to assess alignment.
- If a radiolucent table is used, torsional alignment should be assessed with the hip rotation test following preliminary fixation of the proximal and distal segments and adjusted as needed.
- Drape both lower limbs into the surgical field if possible to compare the hip rotation and to measure the length. Alternatively, obtain a lateral radiographic projection of the unaffected opposite femur to measure the length, and measure and record the hip range of motion of the opposite limb before surgery for intraoperative reference.

Intraoperative correction or early revision of any torsional deformity is essential. It is much easier, less time consuming, and preferable to correct a malreduced fracture than a malunion. In addition, patients can return to normal function earlier.

Coronal Plane: Varus-Valgus Malalignment

Coronal plane malalignment occurs more commonly in metaphyseal fractures than diaphyseal fractures because the metaphyseal cortex is not as straight as that in the diaphysis. Therefore, the bone plate must be accurately precontoured and positioned on the bone in the same location as during the precontouring process. An intraoperative technique to assess coronal plane alignment of the pelvic limb is the cable technique.[16] In this technique, image intensification and a sterile marking pen are used to identify and mark the center of the femoral head and the distal intermediate ridge of the tibia. A cautery cable is spanned between the center of the femoral head and the distal intermediate ridge of the tibia, and a radiographic image of the stifle is obtained. The position of the cautery cable relative to the center of the stifle joint indicates the axial deviation in the coronal plane. Although this is a reliable method, it is radiation dependent.

Sagittal Plane: Procurvatum-Recurvatum Malalignment

In proximal femoral fractures with the lesser trochanter attached to the proximal segment, the proximal segment has a tendency to be positioned in flexion, abduction, and external rotation because of the strong pull of the gluteals and external rotators. Counteracting these forces is necessary for accurate anatomic reduction of this segment. This counteraction can be achieved with bone-holding forceps and manual reduction; an external skeletal fixator or fracture distractor; or a joystick, which is a pin placed in the proximal segment that is manipulated to counteract the muscle pull.

Sagittal plane alignment of femoral diaphyseal fractures can be assessed clinically by visual inspection or radiologically with intraoperative lateromedial radiographs or fluoroscopy. Because of the normal procurvatum of the femur, fixation of a simple fracture with a bone plate that is centered on the lateral cortex tends to create a recurvatum deformity (see **Fig. 8C**). To avoid this, the ends of the bone plate should be positioned roughly centered on the lateral cortex, and the plate could be positioned closer to the caudal cortex near the fracture; however, this may not result in adequate alignment of the bone plate and femur if a long bone plate is chosen or the normal pro-curvatum of the femur is profound. Another strategy to accommodate for the normal procurvatum of the femur is to contour the bone plate in the coronal plane to create a cranial-to-caudal curvature. Alternatively, the plate must be twisted to match the local anatomy and applied in a helical fashion (so-called helical plating). Twisting the plate such that it begins on the cranio-lateral cortex proximally and ends on the lateral cortex distally (see **Fig. 8**D) will achieve an anatomic contour; this is known as helical plating.

Limb-Length Discrepancy

The femur is more commonly affected with limb-length discrepancy than the tibia or radius/ulna because of the difficulty in evaluation caused by the overlying muscle mass. The most common form of limb-length discrepancy is shortening, whereas

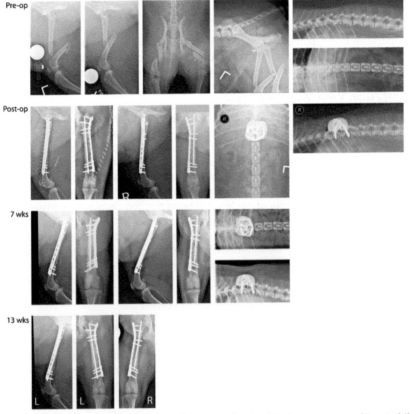

Fig. 13. Case study: A young mixed-breed dog sustained vehicular trauma resulting in bilateral comminuted femoral fractures and a T12-T13 vertebral fracture luxation. The femoral fractures were stabilized with plate-rod constructs using minimally invasive plate osteosynthesis techniques, and the vertebral fracture was stabilized with direct reduction, pins, and polymethyl methacrylate. Progressive bony union is evident at 7 weeks and clinical union is apparent at 13 weeks.

lengthening rarely occurs. Clinical or radiologic comparison with the unaffected contralateral limb is an accurate and reproducible method to determine limb length. The overall length of the femur from the greater trochanter to the femoral condyle is measured on the mediolateral view of the contralateral femur and compared with a clinical measurement of the ipsilateral femur made with a sterilized ruler. The meter-stick technique involves the measurement of the femoral length from the top of the femoral head to the distal margin of the lateral femoral condyle using a radiographic ruler or meter stick and fluoroscopic guidance.

SUMMARY

Indirect reduction techniques (**Fig. 13**, case study) and carefully planned and executed direct reduction techniques (see **Fig. 13**, case study) result in the maximal preservation of the biology of the fracture site and bone fragments. These techniques, coupled with the use of small soft tissue windows for the insertion of instruments and implants, result in minimal additional trauma to the soft tissues and fracture fragments. Without direct visualization, MIO techniques are more demanding than open reduction and internal fixation; however, the biologic advantages are vast. As such, MIO techniques represent a fascinating new armamentarium in fracture fixation.

REFERENCES

1. Evans HE. The skeleton, arthrology, the muscular system. In: Evans HE, editor. Millers anatomy of the dog. 3rd edition. Philadelphia: WB Saunders; 1993. p. 122–384.
2. Nunamaker DM, Beiry DN, Newton CD. Femoral neck anteversion in the dog: its radiographic measurement. Am J Vet Radiol Soc 1973;14:45–8.
3. Jaegger G, Marcellin-Little DJ, Levine D. Reliability of goniometry in Labrador retrievers. Am J Vet Res 2002;63:979–86.
4. Piermattei DL, Johnson KA. Approach to the greater trochanter and subtrochanteric region of the femur. In: Piermattei DL, Johnson KA, editors. An atlas of surgical approaches to the bones and joints of the dog and cat. 4th edition. Philadelphia: Saunders; 2004. p. 332.
5. Piermattei DL, Johnson KA. Approach to the distal femur and stifle joint through a lateral incision. In: Piermattei DL, Johnson KA, editors. An atlas of surgical approaches to the bones and joints of the dog and cat. 4th edition. Philadelphia: Saunders; 2004. p. 338.
6. Piermattei DL, Johnson KA. Approach to the shaft of the femur. In: Piermattei DL, Johnson KA, editors. An atlas of surgical approaches to the bones and joints of the dog and cat. 4th edition. Philadelphia: Saunders; 2004. p. 336.
7. Piermattei DL, Johnson KA. Approach to the craniodorsal and caudodorsal aspects of the hip joint by osteotomy of the greater trochanter. In: Piermattei DL, Johnson KA, editors. An atlas of surgical approaches to the bones and joints of the dog and cat. 4th edition. Philadelphia: Saunders; 2004. p. 336.
8. Pozzi A, Lewis DD. Surgical approaches for minimally invasive plate osteosynthesis in dogs. Vet Comp Orthop Traumatol 2009;22:316–20.
9. Leung FK, Chow SP. Reduction techniques. In: Tong GO, Bavonratanavech S, editors. Minimally invasive plate osteosynthesis (MIPO). Stuttgart (Germany), New York: Georg Thieme Verlag; 2007. p. 67–77.
10. Black AP, Withrow SJ. Changes in the proximal femur and coxofemoral joint following intramedullary pinning of diaphyseal fractures in young dogs. Vet Surg 1979;8:19–24.

11. Cabassu JP. Elastic plate osteosynthesis of femoral shaft fractures in young dogs. Vet Comp Orthop Traumatol 2001;14:40–5.

12. Sarrau S, Meige F, Autefage A. Treatment of femoral and tibial fractures in puppies by elastic plate osteosynthesis. Vet Comp Orthop Traumatol 2007;20: 51–8.

13. Hottinger HA, DeCamp CE, Olivier B, et al. Noninvasive kinematic analysis of the walk in healthy large breed dogs. Am J Vet Res 1996;57:381–8.

14. Hudson CC, Pozzi A, Lewis DD. Minimally invasive plate osteosynthesis: applications and techniques in dogs and cats. Vet Comp Orthop Traumatol 2009;22: 175–82.

15. Kowaleski MP, Boudrieau RJ, Pozzi A. Stifle joint. In: Tobias KM, Johnston SA, editors. Veterinary surgery: small animal. St Louis (MO): Elsevier; 2012. p. 906–98.

16. Apivatthakakul T. Complications and solutions. In: Tong GO, Bavonratanavech S, editors. Minimally invasive plate osteosynthesis (MIPO). Stuttgart (Germany), New York: Georg Thieme Verlag; 2007. p. 67–77.

Minimally Invasive Plate Osteosynthesis: Tibia and Fibula

Brian S. Beale, DVM*, Ryan McCally, DVM

KEYWORDS

- Tibia • Fracture • Minimally invasive plate osteosynthesis • Dog • Cat

KEY POINTS

- Tibial fractures are often times amenable to repair using the minimally invasive plate osteosynthesis (MIPO) technique.
- The rationale for MIPO is preservation of blood supply to encourage more rapid healing, lower patient morbidity, and provide a more rapid return to function.
- Locking bone plates are often used with MIPO because of the lack of a need for anatomic contouring of the plate, preservation of periosteal blood supply below the plate, greater screw security, and an enhanced ability to prevent collapse of the fracture gap.
- MIPO repair of tibial fractures uses indirect reduction to return the limb to normal length and establish proper limb alignment.

INTRODUCTION

Fracture of the tibia and fibula is common in dogs and cats.[1–4] Tibial fractures occur most commonly as a result of substantial trauma. Common causes include vehicular trauma, rough play, sports-related injury, and gunshot.[3,4] Fractures may be closed or open, but tibial fractures have a higher incidence of open fractures compared with other bones owing to the sparse soft tissue covering medially. Fracture treatment is determined after careful consideration of mechanical, biologic, and patient compliance factors.[5] Nonsurgical treatment of tibial fractures may be possible with minimally displaced fractures, particularly in immature patients.[3,4] Nonsurgical stabilization includes casting or splinting. Surgical stabilization of tibial and fibular fractures is more commonly required.[3,4] The goal of repair is stabilization of the tibia only. The fibular fracture is rarely repaired. Minimally invasive techniques have become popular for repair of most types of tibial fractures in recent years.[6,7] The rationale for using minimally invasive fracture repair is preservation of blood supply to encourage more rapid healing, lower patient morbidity, and provide a more rapid return to function.[6–11] Surgical trauma is minimized during the stabilization procedure in an effort to preserve

Gulf Coast Veterinary Specialists, 1111 West Loop South, Suite 160, Houston, TX 77027, USA
* Corresponding author.
E-mail address: drbeale@gcvs.com

Vet Clin Small Anim 42 (2012) 1023–1044
http://dx.doi.org/10.1016/j.cvsm.2012.08.001
0195-5616/12/$ – see front matter © 2012 Elsevier Inc. All rights reserved.

vetsmall.theclinics.com

blood supply to the fracture fragments.[11–19] Less invasive surgical approaches include a closed approach, the "open but don't touch approach (OBDT) and the minimally-invasive surgical (MIS) approach.[6–11,19] Use of a bone plate with the MIS approach is referred to as minimally invasive plate osteosynthesis (MIPO).[11,13,19] MIPO has been associated with decreased surgical times and this can lead to a lower risk of infection.[11]

Surgical stabilization using the MIS technique can be achieved using a variety of implant systems, including external fixator, interlocking nail, plate-rod construct, clamp-rod internal fixator, and bone plate and screws.[3,4,10,12,13] Two types of bone-plating systems are commonly used for MIPO. Traditional bone plates, such as the veterinary cuttable plate (VCP), dynamic compression plate (DCP), and limited contact dynamic compression plate (LCDCP), can be placed using cortical screws in compression, neutralization and buttress modes as previously described.[4,10] Locking plates, also known as internal fixators, can be applied using locking or cortical screws.[4] Locking screws provide fixed angle stabilization.[4] Locking bone plates have certain advantages, including the lack of a need for anatomic contouring of the plate, preservation of periosteal blood supply below the plate, greater screw security, and an enhanced ability to prevent collapse of the fracture gap.[18,20,21] Bone plates are traditionally applied to the medial surface of the tibia using direct or indirect reduction of the fracture.[3,4,19] Occasionally, a second plate is applied to the cranial surface of the tibia to supplement the fixation.

Certain tibial fractures are amenable to repair using closed technique and application of an external fixator. External fixators commonly used to stabilize tibial fractures include linear, circular, and hybrid fixators. Closed reduction and fracture stabilization results in the least amount of iatrogenic surgical trauma to the tibia and regional soft tissues. When using closed or MIS techniques, it is imperative to restore proper length and alignment to the limb.

ANATOMY OF THE TIBIA AND FIBULA

The proximal aspect of the tibia is triangular with its apex facing cranially (**Figs. 1 and 2**). The proximal articular surface lies on the medial and lateral condyles. A sagittal, nonarticular region and 2 eminences called the intercondyloid eminence separate the condyles (see **Figs. 1 and 3**).[22] This nonarticular region is not covered with hyaline cartilage. The eminences are called the medial and lateral intercondylar eminences.[22] The meniscal ligaments attach just cranial and caudal to the intercondyloid eminence.[22] The medial condyle is oval in shape, and the lateral condyle is circular.[22] The extensor groove (or muscular groove) of the tibia is a small notch in the cranial aspect of the lateral condyle, through which the tendon of the extensor digitorum longus courses.[22] The popliteal notch is found on the caudal aspect of the proximal tibia between the condyles.[22] The head of the fibula attaches to a flat area at the caudolateral aspect of the proximal tibia. The tibial tuberosity is a large, quadrangular process found at the proximal and cranial aspect of the tibia. The patellar tendon and portions of the biceps femoris (lateral) and sartorius (medial) muscles insert on the tibial tuberosity.[22] The extension of the tibial tuberosity distally along the cranial edge of the tibia is called the cranial border (formerly known as the tibial crest).[22] Portions of the gracilis, semitendinosus, sartorius (medial), and biceps femoris (lateral) muscles insert on the tibial crest.[22]

The tibia shaft is triangular in the proximal half and cylindrical in the distal half. The medial surface of the tibia is relatively flat along it entire length and is an ideal location for placement of a bone plate. The medial surface of the bone is easily accessed because of the sparse soft tissue covering in this region. The popliteus muscle lies along the caudal surface of the tibia and attaches to the caudomedial edge at the intersection

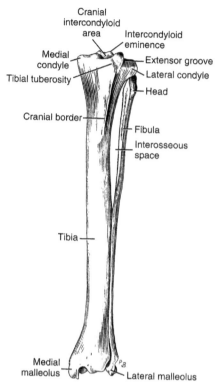

Fig. 1. Cranial aspect of tibia and fibula. (*From* Evans HE and Christensen GC, editors. Miller's Anatomy of the Dog. 2nd edition. Philadelphia: WB Saunders; 1979. p. 210–5; with permission.)

of the proximal and middle thirds.[22] The medial collateral ligament of the stifle inserts on the caudomedial aspect of the proximal tibia just cranial to the insertion of the popliteus muscle. The flexor hallucis longus, tibialis posterior, and flexor digitorum longus muscles lie lateral to the popliteus on the caudal aspect of the tibia and course the length of the bone.[22] The tibialis cranialis arises from the craniolateral aspect of the tibia and courses along the lateral surface of the tibia along its entire length.[22] The distal third of the tibial shaft has a slight degree of torsion. A slight caudal twist in the distal end of the bone plate may be needed if the plate extends the entire length of the tibia.

The distal end of the tibia is quadrilateral and larger than the adjacent shaft.[22] The distal articular surface is formed by 2, nearly sagittal arciform groves called the tibial cochlea tibiae.[22] The grooves are separated by an intermediate ridge. The medial aspect of the tibia extends more distal than the lateral end and is called the medial malleolus. The medial collateral ligament complex of the tarsus originates from the medial malleolus. A large sulcus for the tendon of the flexor hallucis longus muscle lies on the caudal aspect of the distal tibia. No muscles attach to the distal half of the tibia.[22]

The fibula is long and thin and attaches to the proximal and distal aspects of the tibia laterally. The head of the fibula is flattened and broader than the shaft. The head of the fibula serves as the insertion of the lateral collateral ligament of the stifle and a portion of the origin of the flexor digitorum longus, tibialis caudalis, peroneus brevis, and peroneus longus muscles.[22] The shaft of the fibula is slender and irregular and is the site of attachment of a portion of the origin of the flexor hallucis longus muscle.[22] The distal

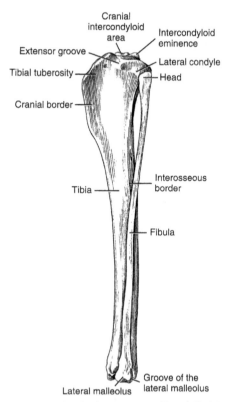

Cranial intercondyloid area

Intercondyloid eminence

Extensor groove

Lateral condyle

Tibial tuberosity

Head

Cranial border

Interosseous border

Tibia

Fibula

Lateral malleolus

Groove of the lateral malleolus

Fig. 2. Lateral aspect of tibia and fibula. (*From* Evans HE and Christensen GC, editors. Miller's Anatomy of the Dog. 2nd edition. Philadelphia: WB Saunders; 1979. p. 210–5; with permission.)

end of the fibula is known as the lateral malleolus, which is the origin for the lateral collateral ligament complex of the tarsus.

The saphenous artery and vein courses along the medial aspect of the tibia and has a cranial and caudal branch. The cranial branch courses over the medial surface of the tibia in a distocranial direction near the mid to distal third of the diaphysis. The caudal saphenous artery is the direct continuation of the saphenous artery and it lies between the tibia and the medial head of the gastrocnemius muscle.[22] The popliteal artery is a continuation of the femoral artery.[22] It courses caudal to the stifle and divides into the cranial tibial and caudal tibial arteries.[22] The cranial tibial artery runs between the tibia and fibula distally.[22] Many muscular branches arise from the cranial tibial artery supplying the extensor hallucis longus and tibialis cranialis muscles.[22] The caudal tibial artery runs adjacent to the flexor hallucis longus and supplies a branch that forms the nutrient artery of the tibia.[22]

The sciatic nerve branches into the tibial and common peroneal nerves.[22] The tibial nerve runs caudal to the tibia between the semimembranosus and the biceps femoris muscles.[22] The common peroneal nerve lies below the terminal part of the deep portion of the biceps femoris muscle and it courses over the lateral head of the gastrocnemius muscle.[22] It continues to run distally between the flexor hallucis longus and extensor digitorum lateralis muscles caudally and the peroneus longus cranially.[22] The common peroneal nerve divides into a superficial and deep branch slightly distal to the stifle.[22] The superficial peroneal nerve courses toward the cranial aspect of the crus.[22] The tibial nerve courses toward the plantar aspect of the crus.[22]

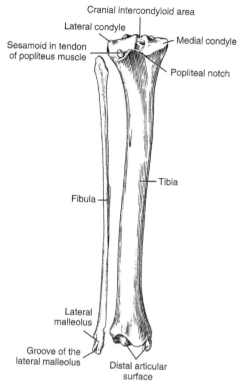

Fig. 3. Caudal aspect of tibia and fibula. (*From* Evans HE and Christensen GC, editors. Miller's Anatomy of the Dog. 2nd edition. Philadelphia: WB Saunders; 1979. p. 210–5; with permission.)

INDICATIONS

Most tibial fractures requiring surgical fixation are amenable to MIPO (**Fig. 4**). An exception would be articular fractures of the tibia, which may require an open approach to ensure accurate anatomic reduction of the joint surface to reduce the risk of future osteoarthritis. Even in this instance, MIPO can be used under fluoroscopic guidance. MIPO is particularly advantages in comminuted, open, and highly traumatic fractures associated with extensive soft tissue trauma.[10,11] The preservation of blood supply to the comminuted fragments not only speeds formation of bone callus, but also reduces the chance of infection. There are no specific contraindications to MIPO repair of tibial fractures. A recent study of 36 tibial fractures treated with MIPO found a very high rate of success regardless of size, species, or breed of patients.[8,10]

DECISION MAKING
Simple versus Comminuted

Patients should be evaluated for the potential use of MIPO technique versus a traditional open technique when treating tibial and fibular fractures. The contralateral leg should be radiographed preoperatively to assist in contouring of the plate and assessment of normal limb length.[10] MIPO is an excellent choice for minimally displaced fractures in which little fracture reduction is needed (**Fig. 5**). MIPO can also be used in

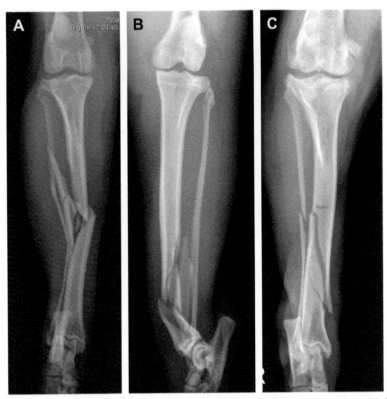

Fig. 4. Examples of common fractures that are good candidates for MIPO. Dogs with highly comminuted diaphyseal fractures (*A*) can be treated with MIPO technique reasonably easily because of minimal soft tissue covering over the medial surface of the tibia and ample healthy bone proximally and distally for screw placement. MIPO can also be used effectively for comminuted fractures in cats (*B*). Less comminuted fractures can also be treated effectively using MIPO technique (*C*).

highly comminuted fractures when there is no chance of reconstructing the bone column (**Fig. 6**). Traditional open reduction and rigid stabilization using fundamental AO principles can lead to successful healing with minimum morbidity. Simple transverse, long oblique, and spiral fractures are examples of fractures that could be handled well with a traditional open approach. These simple types of fractures can also be handled using minimally invasive technique with direct reduction if desired. Because MIPO of comminuted fractures relies heavily on biologic osteosynthesis, plates are often applied in a bridging fashion and secondary bone healing and large callus formation are expected (see **Fig. 6**).[10,11,23] External fixation is also an excellent option for bridging osteosynthesis of the tibia because of the minimal soft tissue coverage over the tibia (**Fig. 7**).[5]

With comminuted fractures, it is recommended to choose a bone plate that is at least 2-3 times the length of the fracture gap.[10,11] Longer plates with fewer screws are stronger than shorter plates with more screws.[11] A longer plate, with screws only at the ends, has increased compliance.[10,11] This relative stability can stimulate secondary bone healing and result in profound callus formation. Simple, transverse fractures have a small fracture gap, and consequently high interfragmentary strain.[24] If MIPO is used

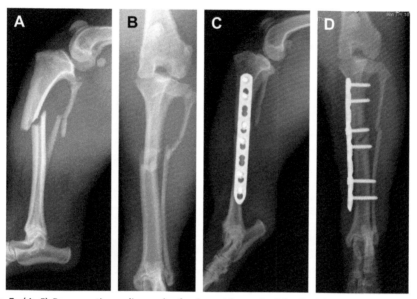

Fig. 5. (*A, B*) Preoperative radiograph of a dog with a reducible tibial fracture that could be repaired using a traditional open reduction technique. This type of fracture is also a good candidate for MIPO in an effort to reduce patient morbidity and preserve blood supply to the fracture zone. (*C, D*) Postoperative radiograph showing use of a locking plate with MIPO technique. The goals of stabilization are to apply a long plate along the shaft of the tibia. Screws are typically inserted at the proximal and distal aspect of the plate. Additional screws are inserted near the fracture when the fracture is simple and when using direct reduction.

for these fractures, it is necessary to place additional screws near the fracture site (see **Fig. 5**).[10,11] This adds stiffness to the construct, reducing motion and interfragmentary strain. Regardless of the application of the bone plate, it is recommended to span as much of the bone as possible with the plate.[10,11]

Immature versus Mature

External coaptation may be considered in young puppies and kittens having minimally displaced tibia fractures. External coaptation provides less stability, but preserves the soft tissue envelope of the bone. A splint or cast can provide adequate stability because of the minimal displacement and robust healing in the immature puppy or kitten (**Fig. 8**). MIPO can be used effectively in immature and mature dogs. Elastic osteosynthesis is a technique to reduce the chance of screw pull-out in thin, soft bone found in puppies when using cortical screws.[25] Typically, VCP plates are used to span the entire tibia and are attached with 2 to 3 screws at the end of the plate on the proximal and distal aspect of the bone (**Fig. 9**). A very thin plate is used to allow elasticity and decrease the tendency for screw pull-out.[25] This technique had a favorable outcome in all but 1 patient in a recent study.[25] Healing was typically seen as bridging callus in approximately 5 weeks.[25] Mature dogs are expected to require slightly heavier plates, but healing with bridging callus also occurs quickly, usually in 4 to 6 weeks.[7,10] These types of fracture can also be repaired using locking plates and screws to prevent the chance of screws pulling out of the soft bone of a puppy.

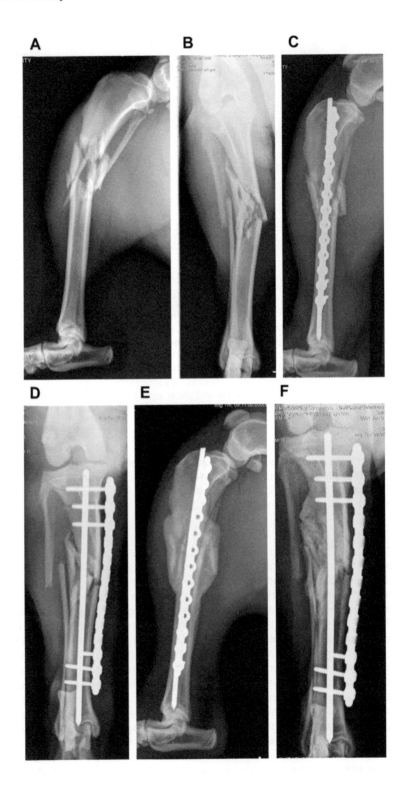

Diaphyseal versus Metaphyseal

Metaphyseal fractures are seen less commonly than diaphyseal fractures. Metaphyseal fractures may be simple or comminuted and may extend to the articular surface. Fractures having an articular component require anatomic reduction for that component. This portion of the reduction can be accomplished using an open or minimally invasive technique. If an open approach is used to reduce and stabilize the articular portion of the fracture, the remaining portion of the fracture can be repaired using the MIPO technique. Diaphyseal fractures of the tibia and fibula are particularly well suited for MIPO techniques because the medial surface of the bone is readily accessible and has little soft tissue covering. Fracture stabilization can be accomplished with minimal disturbance of the fracture site. Distal metaphyseal fractures may provide for little room distal to the fracture site to gain screw purchase. Care must be taken not to interfere with the stifle joint when placing screws proximally or the talocrural joint when placing screws distally. The risk of placing a screw in the joint when stabilizing metaphyseal fractures is increased when using locking screws because it is necessary to place the screws perpendicular to the plate. Typically the most proximal or distal screw is at greatest risk. Two options exist to avoid placement of the screw into the joint. A cortical screw can be angled away from the joint surface or a short locking screw can be used (**Fig. 10**). It is generally recommended to have at least 2 bicortical screws in each of the major fracture segments, although 3 screws are preferred if allowed by the fracture configuration. MIPO technique has been found to be an equally effective method of treating metaphyseal and diaphyseal fractures of the tibia in dogs and cats.[8,10]

Acute versus Chronic

MIPO is best applied to acute fractures that have a fresh hematoma. MIPO can be used very successfully in fractures of duration less than 2 weeks. With chronic fractures that require significant reduction to regain length and alignment, muscle contracture and preexisting callus formation may not allow for adequate indirect reduction. In these cases, it may be necessary to open the fracture site to help achieve appropriate length and acceptable alignment. The exception may be chronic fractures with minimal displacement and little need for reduction. These fractures respond well to MIPO technique. Many of these cases may heal appropriately with external cooptation as well. Chronic fractures treated with MIPO may benefit from percutaneous injection of biologic catalysts of healing, such as platelet-rich plasma or stem cells. Adjunctive techniques, such as shock-wave therapy or magnetic therapy, may also help to stimulate the biologic status of fracture healing.

Locking versus Nonlocking Plates

Locking plates have several advantages over nonlocking plates when stabilizing tibia and fibular fractures using MIPO, particularly in the metaphyseal regions.[11] Although the authors prefer locking plates for many fractures of the tibia and fibula, it should be emphasized that conventional plating systems can and have been used for

◀───

Fig. 6. (*A, B*) An open comminuted mid diaphyseal fracture in a 42-kg mixed breed dog was evaluated for surgical repair. MIPO was selected over an external fixator because of patient management concerns postoperatively. (*C, D*) The fracture was repaired using a plate-rod technique in MIPO fashion. The intramedullary pin was placed first to establish partial stability and regain limb length and alignment. A locking plate was placed next, increasing axial, bending, and rotational stability. (*E, F*) Good healing is seen 7 weeks after surgical stabilization using MIPO technique. The dog was gradually returned to normal activity over a 4-week period.

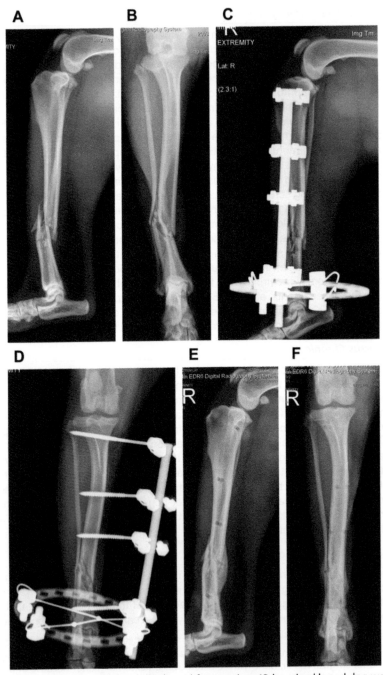

Fig. 7. (*A, B*) A comminuted distal diaphyseal fracture in a 13-kg mixed breed dog was evaluated for surgical repair. (*C, D*) A hybrid external fixator was applied using minimally invasive technique. External fixators are a good option for stabilizing comminuted fractures of the tibia because of the ability to place fixator pins easily without disruption of soft tissues overlying the tibia. (*E, F*) Good healing is seen 6.5 weeks after surgery at the time of removal of the external fixator. The dog was gradually returned to normal activity over a 4-week period.

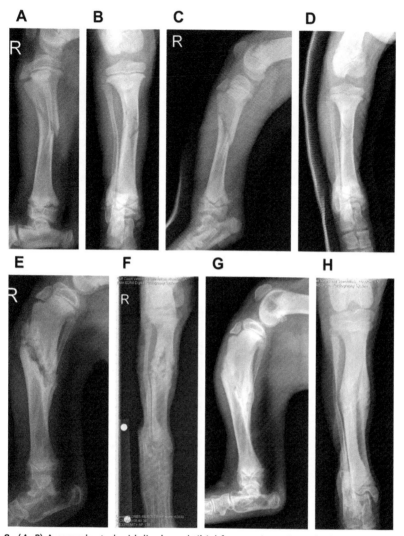

Fig. 8. (A, B) A comminuted mid diaphyseal tibial fracture in a 12-week old, 13.5-kg English Mastiff was evaluated for fracture stabilization. (C, D) A lateral fiberglass splint was used to stabilize the fracture owing to the minimally displaced nature of the fracture and the young age of the puppy. Activity was prevented for 3 weeks after applying the splint. The splint was changed weekly. (E, F) Good bridging callus is seen 3 weeks after stabilization of this fracture using a lateral fiberglass splint. Good stability of the tibia could be appreciated on palpation. The fracture appears healed on the anteroposterior view, but healing is incomplete on the lateral view. The splint was removed at this time and the dog was gradually returned to normal activity over a 4-week period. (G, H) Good healing and remodeling of the callus is seen 6 months after fracture stabilization with a lateral splint. Good alignment and continued growth of the bone was achieved.

many years to successfully treat simple and comminuted fractures of these bones. A recent study showed no difference in outcome when treating tibial fractures in dogs and cats with MIPO technique using VCP, LCP, or LCDCP plates.[10] The density of bone in the proximal metaphyseal region of some large and giant breed dogs, such

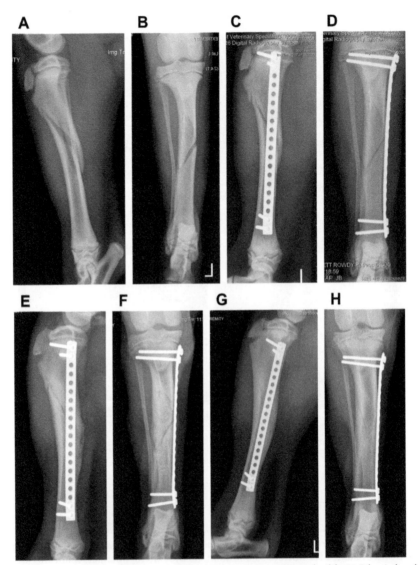

Fig. 9. (A, B) A spiral mid diaphyseal tibial fracture in a 13-week-old, 14.5-kg Labrador retriever puppy was evaluated for fracture stabilization. (C, D) An elastic plating technique was used to stabilize the fracture because of the minimally displaced nature of the fracture and the young age of the puppy. A plate is applied along the entire length of the medial tibia and 2 screws are placed proximally and distally in MIPO fashion. Activity was limited to leash walk for 2 weeks postoperatively. (E, F) Good bridging callus is seen 2 weeks after stabilization of this fracture. Good stability of the tibia could be appreciated on palpation. The dog was allowed increased walking exercise for 2 additional weeks then a gradual return to normal activity over a 2-week period. (G, H) Good healing and remodeling of the callus is seen 6 weeks after fracture stabilization. Good alignment and continued growth of the bone was achieved.

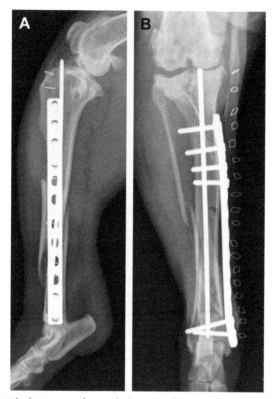

Fig. 10. (*A, B*) A cortical screw can be angled proximally away from the distal tibial articular surface to avoid penetrating the tibiotarsal joint. The medial malleolus can be used as a landmark to help estimate the needed angle for the screw. This fracture was stabilized using indirect reduction and an "open but don't touch" surgical approach.

as the German Shepherd, Mastiff, and Great Dane, can be suboptimal. Locking screws provide increased protection against backing out of screws in soft bone. Very proximal and distal metaphyseal fractures of the tibia may not be amenable to placement of 3 screws. Use of 2 locking screws in these fractures improves stability and the risk of implant failure. Locking screws provide fixed-angle stability and are unlikely to loosen. Cortical screws are more likely to loosen, particularly when using only 2 screws in a bone segment. Instability may ensue, increasing the possibility of delayed bone healing or loss of limb alignment. Nonlocking or locking bone plates can be used successfully for diaphyseal fractures of the tibia and fibula. Anatomic plate contouring of the bone plate is required at sites where nonlocking screws are placed. The plate contour can be approximated preoperatively using radiographs of the contralateral normal limb. If the plate is not contoured properly in the regions where cortical screws are placed, loss of alignment will occur as the bone is drawn toward the plate during screw tightening (**Fig. 11**). The need to anatomically contour the plate adds surgical time and increases the technical difficulty. Precise contouring of locking plates is not needed because the head of the screws lock into the plate, preventing the lag effect on the bone as the screw is tightened (**Fig. 12**). Fracture alignment is thus maintained despite the presence of small gaps between the plate and

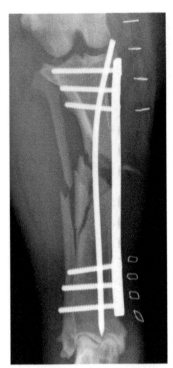

Fig. 11. If the plate is not contoured properly in the regions where cortical screws are placed, loss of alignment will occur as the bone is drawn toward the plate during screw tightening. The proximal tibial fragment was drawn up to an inadequately contoured bone plate causing valgus deformity.

the bone. It is recommended that the gaps between the plate and the bone be kept to 2 mm or less to prevent significant loss of construct stability.[26] The lack of need for precise contouring of the plate with MIPO is a tremendous advantage because of the lack of accessibility to the surface of the bone owing to the minimally-invasive nature of the technique. The disadvantages of using locking screws are an inability to angle the screws and the increased cost. The surgeon must be careful to avoid placing screws into the stifle or tarsus when inserting locking screws proximally or distally if the plate is contoured to match the flared surface of the bone. The contouring of the plate proximally or distally directs the holes of the plate toward the joint. Locking screws are presently placed perpendicular to the plate with most of the present systems available, and thus accidental placement of the screw into the joint can occur if this possibility is not anticipated. The surgeon typically can use a short screw in this situation to avoid penetration into the joint. The cost of locking screws is greater than nonlocking screws; however, it is minimal especially when considering the time savings from not having to precisely contour the plate and cost savings should a revision surgery be needed. In addition, surgeons typically use fewer screws when using locking systems. Another advantage of using locking screws is the increased stability achieved when using screws in a monocortical fashion. The use of a plate in combination with an intramedullary pin for fixation (plate-rod construct) of tibial fractures has become common owing to the ease of application and increased resistance to bending forces.[8,10,24] The intramedullary pin may interfere with placement of some of the screws, requiring use of a monocortical rather than a bicortical screw. It is also possible to use a combination of nonlocking and locking screws. Use of both types of screws reduces the cost, while still gaining additional screw stability from the locking screws. When using a combination of locking and nonlocking screws, it is important to place the cortical screws first to created the desired compression between the plate and the bone to increase the frictional forces that supply the stability. If a locking screw is placed before the cortical screw, the plate is unable to be pulled against the bone creating this frictional force. It should be emphasized that nonlocking screws should be placed in areas where good plate-bone contact is present to avoid undesirable displacement of bone fragments when the screw is tightened. Many different locking plate systems are available. Because of the lack of soft tissue covering over the medial aspect of the tibia, a low-profile plate is preferred by many surgeons. If a thin plate is used, supplemental stability can be provided if needed using an intramedullary pin or a second plate on the cranial surface (**Fig. 13**). Bone plates are typically applied to the medial surface of the tibia where most tensile forces occur during weight bearing. The cranial surface of the bone is also an acceptable site when applying a second plate to the distal two-thirds of the bone.

Patient positioning
The leg is clipped and prepped in routine fashion from the mid femur to the metatarso-phalangeal joints. It is helpful to have the stifle and the tarsus in the surgical field to facilitate evaluation of limb alignment and to give access for placement of an intrame-dullary pin if needed. The patient is usually positioned in dorsal recumbence. This allows good access for fracture repair using the MIPO technique as well as an optimal view to assess limb alignment. A hanging limb preparation should be used. It is helpful to hang the leg under tension to fatigue the muscles to aid reduction. An effective means of providing tension is to hang the leg, placing tension while securing to an anchor point above the table. Lowering the table a short distance while leaving the leg suspended increases the amount of tension on the limb, thus adding reduction by distracting the fracture further. The leg can be left suspended during closed reduc-tion and fixation using external fixation. The leg is typically lowered from its suspended position when using MIPO technique.

Indirect reduction for MIPO
Fracture reduction is attained indirectly in most comminuted tibial fractures repaired with MIPO. Sustained distractive forces are applied across the fracture to fatigue muscles causing overriding of the fragments to regain limb length. Distraction can be applied manually, by suspending the leg from above, using a distraction table, using a fracture distractor or a temporary external fixator with linear motors.[10,11,19,27] As limb length is regained, the fracture fragments are drawn more closely toward their original position because of the preservation of muscle attachments. Limb length was restored to 99% of normal length following indirect reduction in tibial fractures treated with MIPO.[10] Indirect fracture reduction can lead to very good reduction if the fracture is treated early. Reduction of fragments can be assisted using bone-holding forceps through the proximal and distal incisions (**Fig. 14**).[10] Guiot and Dejardin[10] achieved good or adequate reduction in all patients after MIPO repair of tibial fractures in 36 dogs. Once the limb length is restored to as normal as possible, axial and rotational alignment must be restored. Axial alignment is assessed by evaluating the limb along the sagittal and frontal planes. It is important for the joint surfaces of the stifle and tarsus to be aligned properly. The alignment of the joint surfaces can be evaluated by flexing and extending the stifle and the tarsus and ensuring that the plane of motion

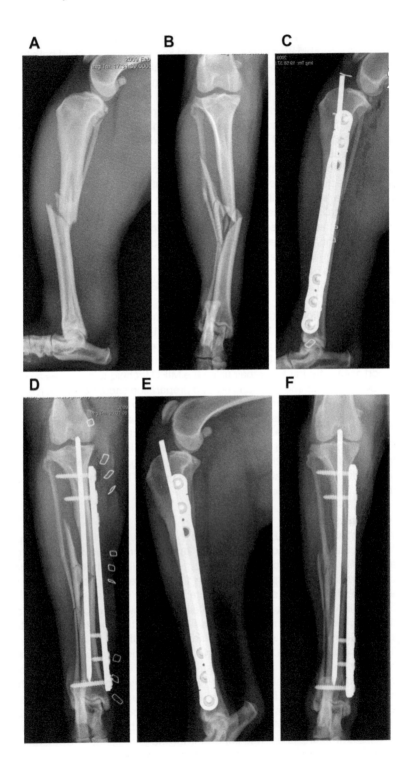

of both joints are in the same direction The alignment of the joint surfaces can be evaluated by flexing and extending the stifle and the tarsus. Rotational or varus/valgus malalignment can lead to suboptimal function and increase the risk of osteoarthritis. It is often helpful to place an intramedullary pin in normograde fashion to assist in restoring length to the limb and to help attain proper axial alignment. The pin provides temporary stabilization and facilitates application of the plate in MIPO. Any rotational malalignment can be easily resolved by rotating the fracture fragments around the pin. The pin can be either left in place when using a plate-rod construct or it can be removed after the plate is partially secured to the bone. The intramedullary pin is typically placed normograde from the medial aspect of the tibial plateau, midway between the medial collateral ligament and patellar tendon. The pin should be carefully directed down the medullary canal to avoid accidental penetration of the lateral cortex. Fracture reduction can be assessed by palpation, using fluoroscopy, or through a small incision over the fracture (observation portal).[8,10,11,19]

SURGICAL APPROACH

A medial surgical approach has been previously described for MIPO of the tibia.[8,10,19] The location of the proximal and distal incisions is based on the plate selected for MIPO.[19] Typically the incisions will be near the proximal and distal extent of the bone because most comminuted fractures treated with MIPO use a plate that spans the entire bone (**Fig. 15**). The authors prefer to make the proximal incision first when using a plate-rod technique or an intramedullary pin for alignment purposes. The distal incision is made second at the site of the intended position of the distal end of the plate. Occasionally a third incision is made over the fracture to confirm accurate placement of the intramedullary pin or to assess fracture alignment (see **Fig. 15**). This incision, if used, is termed the observation portal. It should be emphasized that this portal should not be used to excessively manipulate the fragments and risk disturbing blood supply. The incisions are typically 2 to 4 cm in length. This is usually ample length for placement of 2 to 3 screws proximally and distally. There is little risk of disturbing muscular or neurovascular structures when using MIPO for tibial fracture repair. An epiperiosteal soft tissue tunnel is developed below the subcutaneous tissues by passing Metzenbaum scissors or a periosteal elevator from the distal to proximal incision. Elevation of the periosteum is not necessary or desired.

SURGICAL PROCEDURE

The intramedullary pin is inserted initially if a plate-rod construct is planned (**Fig. 16**). If using a pin, it is important that the diameter of the pin be 40% of the diameter of the isthmus of the medullary cavity of the tibia.[8,10,24] This will allow ample room for placement of bicortical plate screws without interference by the pin. After fracture reduction

---

Fig. 12. (*A, B*) Preoperative views of a 4-year-old Spitz with an open comminuted mid diaphyseal tibial fracture. (*C, D*) The fracture was repaired with a plate-rod implant using MIPO technique. Precise contouring of locking plates is not needed because the head of the screws lock into the plate, preventing the lag effect on the bone as the screw is tightened. The advantages of not anatomically contouring the plate distally are decreased surgical time and ability to place the most distal locking screw in bicortical fashion without being directed toward the joint. (*E, F*) Good bridging callus is seen 7 weeks after stabilization of this fracture. Monocortical screws were needed because of the intramedullary pin present. Locking screws are less likely to loosen and back out compared with traditional cortical screws.

A   B

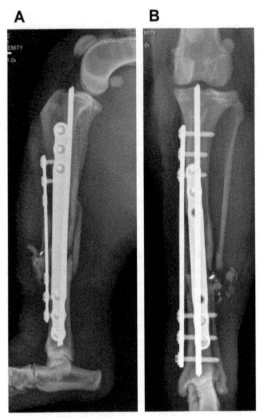

Fig. 13. (*A, B*) A second plate was added to the cranial surface of the tibia in this dog after stabilizing this comminuted tibial fracture with a plate-rod MIPO technique. Adding a second plate to the cranial surface of the tibia added additional bending and rotational stability to this very excitable dog with a very unstable fracture. The open screw holes in the cranial plate pose very low risk due to the presence of the IM pin and medial bone plate that counteract the bending forces that could result in plate breakage.

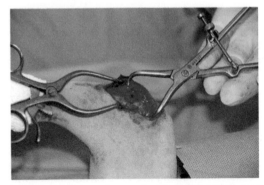

Fig. 14. Pointed reduction forceps can be used with MIPO technique to manipulate fragments when using indirect reduction or to temporarily stabilize the fracture with direct reduction.

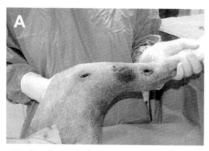
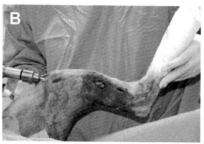

Fig. 15. (*A, B*) Typically the incisions for placement of screws will be near the proximal and distal extent of the bone because most comminuted fractures treated with MIPO use a plate that spans the entire bone (*A*). A third incision can be made over the fracture zone to allow a view of the medullary canal of the distal fragment to aid placement of the intramedullary pin when using a MIPO plate-rod technique (*B*).

is confirmed, the plate is applied. The plate is contoured as needed. Contouring can be facilitated using a radiograph of the opposite normal limb. Limb alignment and fracture reduction should be assessed immediately before plate insertion. The stifle and tarsus should be flexed and extended, making sure the sagittal plane of motion is the same for both joints. Fracture reduction is assessed by palpation, by direct visualization through an observation portal, or with fluoroscopy. The precontoured bone plate is inserted through one of the insertion incisions and advanced along the medial surface of the tibia through the epiperiosteal tunnel that was previously created until the end of the plate is appropriately positioned in the second incision. It is often easiest to insert the plate through the distal incision and slide the plate toward the proximal incision. If a locking implant is used, it is useful to use the drill guide inserted in the end plate hole as a handle to insert and position the bone plate on the tibia. The position of the bone plate on the tibia can be checked with direct observation and digital palpation. A screw is inserted through the most distal hole in the bone plate into the distal tibial segment. The screw is centered in the distal tibia unless a plate rod construct is being used. In this case, it may be necessary to adjust the position of the plate slightly more cranial or caudal to allow screw insertion past the intramedullary pin. The screw should be tightened enough to hold the position of the plate on the

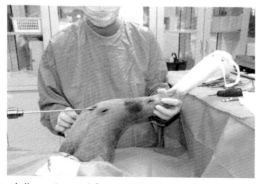

Fig. 16. The intramedullary pin used for a MIPO plate-rod technique is placed initially to help align the fracture and provide bending stability. The pin is placed in normograde fashion through a stab incision over the medial aspect of the tibial plateau midway between the patellar tendon and the medial collateral ligament.

distal tibia, but still allow adjustment of the plate on the proximal tibia. Proper limb alignment and fracture reduction should be confirmed and adjusted as needed before insertion of the first proximal screw. The bone plate is adjusted so that the proximal end of the plate is positioned slightly caudal to the center of the proximal tibia. The caudal half of the proximal tibia is wider, therefore provides optimal bone purchase by the screw. The position of the plate should be adjusted as needed to avoid screw interference with an intramedullary pin if used. The first screw is then inserted into the proximal tibial segment through the most proximal hole in the bone plate. The proximal screw is tightened securely and then the first screw that was placed in the distal end of the plate is also tightened securely. Limb alignment and fracture reduction is again assessed. One or 2 additional screws are then sequentially inserted into both the most proximal and the most distal holes in the bone plate. Typically the authors insert 3 screws in the proximal segment and either 2 or 3 (length of the segment permitting) screws in the distal segment of the tibia. All screws should obtain bicortical bone purchase if possible. If a combination of screws is used, nonlocking screws should be placed first in each bone segment, followed by locking screws. Typically the 2 incisions are sufficient for placing all the necessary screws as a Senn retractor can be used to shift the end of the incision either proximally or distally as necessary to expose additional holes in the bone plate. If a screw needs to be placed in a plate hole that cannot be accessed through the insertion incisions, then a stab incision can be created over the desired plate hole using digital palpation or fluoroscopic guidance. The incisions are closed in routine fashion after the plate is applied.

IMMEDIATE POSTOPERATIVE CARE

Immediate postoperative radiographs should be obtained in the anesthetized patient. Fracture apposition and limb alignment should be assessed. The proper alignment of the stifle and tarsal joints is confirmed by checking for proper angulation and rotational orientation. Excessive varus/valgus or rotational deformity should be revised immediately if the patient is stable under anesthesia. The position of the bone plate and screws, as well as the intramedullary pin if used, should be assessed. If screw purchase is inadequate, the screws should be replaced by opening the appropriate incision. If screws have inadvertently penetrated the stifle or tarsal joints, the offending screws should be redirected, removed or replaced with a shorter screw. The position of the intramedullary pin should be adjusted as needed to obtain optimal position. The pin is then bent over at its proximal end and cut or it is cut short and countersunk based on surgeon preference. A soft-padded bandage is applied as the patient is recovered from anesthesia. Pain management is used as needed to keep the patient calm and pain-free.

MANAGEMENT DURING THE POSTOPERATIVE CONVALESCENT PERIOD

The soft-padded bandage is typically replaced with a nonadherent bandage applied over the incision the morning following surgery. Most patients undergoing tibial fracture repair with MIPO are sent home the day following surgery. The patients are treated with postoperative analgesics as needed for 5 to 10 days. Postoperative antibiotic treatment is determined on a case-by-case basis. Activity should be restricted to a short leash walk to urinate and defecate for the initial 2 weeks following surgery. Walks can be increased to 3 to 4 walks of 5-minutes each after suture removal 10 to 14 days following surgery. Running and jumping are strictly prohibited. Patients will benefit from rehabilitation exercises provided by a trained physiotherapist. Patients can typically walk up and down stairs beginning 6 weeks postoperatively. Swimming can begin 6 weeks after surgery in most patients, depending on the status of the individual patient. Animals should be confined to a crate following surgery if needed to achieve the activity goals. Owners may assist walking using a sling as needed. Activity is restricted as described until clinical and radiographic documentation of bone healing has been obtained.

ASSESSMENT OF REPAIR AND OUTCOME

Recheck orthopedic examinations should be performed at 2, 4, 6, and 8 weeks. Follow-up radiographs should be obtained at 4 and at subsequent 3-week to 4-week intervals until radiographic evidence of bone union is obtained. Radiographs should consist of orthogonal views of the tibia. Limb alignment, fracture apposition, and integrity of the implants should be assessed and compared with the immediate postoperative radiographs. Fractures are considered healed when bony bridging is evident across the fracture zone on the medial-lateral and cranio-caudal views. Bridging callus is expected in 3 to 5 weeks in immature patients and 4 to 6 weeks in mature patients.[8,10,11] The animal is allowed to return to normal activity gradually over a period of several weeks.

SUMMARY

Tibial fractures can be repaired successfully using MIPO technique with low risk of complication in dogs and cats. Use of MIPO technique in cats can be very rewarding due to their susceptibility to postoperative stress. Cats typically tolerate MIPO extremely well due to the lower morbidity, quick recovery and lack of need of postoperative bandaging. The authors believe tibial fractures are the least complicated to repair using MIPO technique and thus is an ideal starting point for novice MIPO surgeons. The ability to readily palpate the medial surface of the tibia, because of the lack of soft tissue covering, greatly aids indirect reduction of the fracture and placement of implants. The success of MIPO for repair of tibial fractures is dependent on adequate indirect fracture reduction, appropriate selection of an implant that will provide adequate stability until bridging callus has developed, proper contouring of the plate, preservation of soft tissues and blood supply, and appropriate postoperative management of the patient.

REFERENCES

1. Harasen G. Common long bone fractures in small animal practice–part 1. Can Vet J 2003;44:333–4.
2. Harasen G. Common long bone fracture in small animal practice–part 2. Can Vet J 2003;44:503–4.
3. Piermattei DL, Flo GL, DeCamp CE. Handbook of small animal orthopedics and fracture repair. 4th edition. St Louis (MO): Saunders Elsevier; 2006. p. 359–81.
4. Schwarz G. Fractures of the tibial diaphysis. In: Johnson AL, Houlton JEF, Vannini R, editors. AO principles of fracture management in the dog and cat. Davos (Switzerland): AO Publishing; 2005. p. 319–31.
5. Palmer RH. Biological osteosynthesis. Vet Clin North Am Small Anim Pract 1999; 29:1171–85.
6. Schmokel HG, Hurter K, Schawalder P. Percutaneous plating of tibial fractures in two dogs. Vet Comp Orthop Traumatol 2003;16:191–5.
7. Schmokel HG, Stein S, Radke H, et al. Treatment of tibial fractures with plates using minimally invasive percutaneous osteosynthesis in dogs and cats. J Small Anim Pract 2007;48:157–60.

8. Reems MR, Beale BS, Hulse DA. Use of a plate-rod construct and principles of biological osteosynthesis for repair of diaphyseal fractures in dogs and cats: 47 cases (1994-2001). J Am Vet Med Assoc 2003;223:330–5.

9. Hortsman CL, Beale BS, Conzemius MG, et al. Biological osteosynthesis versus traditional anatomic reconstruction of 20 long bone fractures using an interlocking nail: 1994-2001. Vet Surg 2004;33:232–7.

10. Guiot LP, Dejardin LM. Prospective evaluation of minimally invasive plate osteosynthesis in 36 nonarticular tibial fractures in dogs and cats. Vet Surg 2011;40: 171–82.

11. Hudson CC, Pozzi A, Lewis DD. Minimally invasive plate osteosynthesis: applications and techniques in dogs and cats. Vet Comp Orthop Traumatol 2009;22: 175–82.

12. Johnson AL, Smith CW, Scheffer DJ. Fragment reconstruction and bone plate fixation versus bridging plate fixation for treating highly comminuted femoral fractures in dogs: 35 cases (1987-1997). J Am Vet Med Assoc 1998;213:1157–61.

13. Tong G, Bavonratanavech S. AO manual of fracture management minimally invasive plate osteosynthesis (MIPO). Clavadelerstrasse (Switzerland): AO Publishing; 2007.

14. Krettek C, Muller M, Miclau T. Evolution of minimally invasive plate osteosynthesis (MIPO) in the femur. Injury 2001;32:SC14–23.

15. Farouk O, Krettek C, Miclau T, et al. Effects of percutaneous and conventional plating techniques on the blood supply to the femur. Arch Orthop Trauma Surg 1998;117:438–41.

16. Farouk O, Krettek C, Miclau T, et al. Minimally invasive plate osteosynthesis: does percutaneous plating disrupt femoral blood supply less than the traditional technique? J Orthop Trauma 1999;13:401–6.

17. Borrelli J Jr, Prickett W, Song E, et al. Extraosseous blood supply of the tibia and the effects of different plating techniques: a human cadaveric study. J Orthop Trauma 2002;16:691–5.

18. Johnson AL, Houlton JE, Vannini R. AO principles of fracture management in the dog and cat. Davos (Switzerland): AO Publishing; 2005.

19. Pozzi A, Lewis D. Surgical approaches for minimally invasive plate osteosynthesis in dogs. Vet Comp Orthop Traumatol 2009;22:316–20.

20. Schutz M, Sudkamp NP. Revolution in plate osteosynthesis: new internal fixator systems. J Orthop Sci 2003;8:252–8.

21. Baumgaertel F, Buhl M, Rahn BA. Fracture healing in biological plate osteosynthesis. Injury 1998;29:C3–6.

22. Evans HE, de Lahunta A, editors. Miller's anatomy of the dog. 4th edition. St Louis: Elsevier; 2013. p. 148–51.

23. Pozzi A, Hudson CC. A retrospective comparison of minimally invasive plate osteosynthesis and open reduction and internal fixation for radius-ulna fractures in dogs. Veterinary Surgery, in press.

24. Hulse D, Hyman W, Nori M, et al. Reduction in plate strain by addition of an intramedullary pin. Vet Surg 1997;26:451–9.

25. Sarrau S, Meige F, Autefage A. Treatment of femoral and tibial fractures in puppies by elastic plate osteosynthesis. A review of 17 cases. Vet Comp Orthop Traumatol 2007;20:51–8.

26. Stoffel K, Dieter U, Stachowiak A, et al. Biomechanical testing of the LCP—how can stability in locked internal fixators be controlled. Injury 2003;34(Suppl 2):11–9.

27. Rovesti GL, Margini A, Cappellari F, et al. Clinical application of intraoperative skeletal traction in the dog. Vet Comp Orthop Traumatol 2006;19:14–9.

Minimally Invasive Repair of Meta-bones

Alessandro Piras, DVM, MRCVS[a],*, Tomás G. Guerrero, Dr med vet, DECVS[b]

KEYWORDS

- Metacarpal • Metatarsal • Meta-bones • Fractures • Biologic

KEY POINTS

- A minimally invasive approach to the repair of meta-bone fractures represents a viable option with several benefits related to the preservation of the local biology.
- Fractures of the body of meta-bones III and IV can be approached by creating 1 or 2 small skin incisions proximally and distally to the fractured area.
- The 4 bones are parallel to each other and diverge distally.

INTRODUCTION

Metacarpal and metatarsal fractures are common injuries in small animals and usually result from direct trauma, such as a road traffic accident or collision with a stationary object.[1–3] Fractures of the metacarpal/tarsal bones are classified according to their anatomic location as fractures of the base, fractures of the shaft, and fractures of the head.[2,4] Depending on the location in the bone, number of fractured bones, displacement, type of activity of the patients, and other factors, meta-bone fractures can be treated in a conservative or surgical manner.[2,5] Surgical treatment is recommended for active and working dogs in which a fast and full recovery is desired.[2,4] Surgical treatment should also prevent healing disturbances, like misalignment or nonunions.[2,4]

A minimally invasive approach to the repair of meta-bone fractures represents a viable option with several benefits related to the preservation of the local biology. Fractures of the base and of the head may be treated via stab incisions above the fractured fragment and lag screw insertion. Fractures of the body of meta-bones III and IV can be approached by creating 1 or 2 small skin incisions proximally and distally to the fractured area. Implants can be slid through an epi-periosteal tunnel; both bones can be plated dorsally by a single portal centered between the two bones. Meta-bones II

[a] University College Dublin, Belfield, Dublin 4, Ireland; [b] Small Animal Medicine and Academic Program, St. George's University, School of Veterinary Medicine, True Blue, Grenada, West Indies
* Corresponding author.
E-mail address: alexpvet@mac.com

Vet Clin Small Anim 42 (2012) 1045–1050
http://dx.doi.org/10.1016/j.cvsm.2012.07.003
0195-5616/12/$ – see front matter © 2012 Elsevier Inc. All rights reserved.

and V are plated medially and laterally, respectively, by individual portals and in a similar fashion to meta-bones III and IV. The small skin incisions reduce the risk of suture dehiscence and protect the local biology, which enhances the healing potential of the fractured bones.

META-BONES ANATOMY

Of the 5 meta-bones, the ones that are amenable to surgical repair are II, III, IV, and V. These 4 bones are parallel to each other and diverge distally. This divergence is more evident in the II and V meta-bones and starts at the distal third of the bone. The II and IV meta-bones are the weight-bearing meta-bones and they tend to be straight along all their length.

The proximal portion of each bone, named the base, articulates with the numbered carpal or tarsal bones and has a close anatomic relationship with the adjacent meta-bones. The body, or shaft, runs distally, losing contact with the adjacent meta-bones to end in the articular portion known as the head.

The shape and cross section of the different meta-bones affect either the position or the direction of the implants and should be kept in mind during the surgical planning. The soft tissue structures of surgical interest differ slightly between metacarpal and metatarsal regions. The 3 tendinous groups of the common digital extensor, the lateral digital extensor, and the extensor of the first and second digits (medially) glide along the dorsal aspect of the metacarpal bones. The dorsal common digital artery and vein enter the dorsal aspect of the metacarpal region between the bases of the II and III meta-bones to divide into 3 distinct branches that run between the II and III, III and IV, and IV and V meta-bones.

The tendon of the long digital extensor runs over the dorsal aspect of the metatarsal region. The vascular arrangements of the metatarsal bone are slightly more complex in comparison with the metacarpal region as the dorsal common vv. and its numerous branches cover quite extensively the dorsal aspect of every single metatarsal bone.

PREOPERATIVE PATIENT ASSESSMENT AND DECISION MAKING

Preoperative dorso-palmar/plantar (DP) and mediolateral (ML) views are usually sufficient to assess the type and location of the injuries (**Fig. 1**A). In addition, DP 15° oblique views and ML 45° oblique views may be necessary to evaluate the extension of fissures or the degree of comminution of complex and multiple fractures.

The application of a well-padded Robert Jones bandage supported by a meta splint for 24 to 48 hours before surgery helps to decrease the swelling, which will in turn facilitate fracture reduction.

Preoperative planning consists of the precise measurement of the length and diameter of the intact contralateral meta-bones to size the implants and precontour the plate when requested.

ORTHOPEDIC EQUIPMENT, IMPLANTS, AND ANCILLARY EQUIPMENT

Minimally invasive surgical repair of fractures of the meta-bones do not usually require the use of intraoperative fluoroscopy (C-arm). The scarcity of soft tissues around the meta-bones facilitates the palpation of the bony structures and fracture reduction.

The orthopedic equipment used for the reduction of fractures of meta-bones includes small-point reduction forceps, periosteal elevators, and internal fixation implants and set. The implants commonly used vary according to surgeon preferences from traditional plating to locking systems.

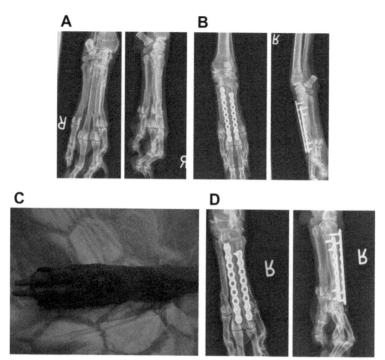

Fig. 1. (*A*) DP and ML radiographs of the right carpus and metacarpus of a 13-year-old Borzoi showing diaphyseal fractures of metacarpal bones II to IV. The carpal joint was partially fused because of a previous trauma unrelated to the actual fractures. (*B*) DP and ML postoperative radiographs after reduction and stabilization of Mc III and IV with 2 ALPS 8-mm plates positioned via dorsally performed tunnels. Good alignment and reduction are observed. Plates were not precontoured, and the most distal screws were applied mono-cortically to avoid interference with the sesamoid bones. (*C*) Picture taken immediately post-operative showing the sutures where the skin incisions were performed between Mc III and IV to position the plates. Skin incisions were displaced medially and laterally to fix both metacarpal bones. (*D*) DP and ML radiographic follow-up 6 weeks after surgery. Clinical bone union is documented. The implants were not removed because they did not affect performance of the dog.

The Veterinary Cuttable Plate (Synthes; 1.5 mm/2.0 mm and 2.0 mm/2.7 mm) is an excellent traditional implant for the repair of metacarpal/tarsal fractures. Other commonly used implants are locking plates of appropriate size, such as LCP (Locking Compression Plates) (Synthes), Fixin (Traumavet), and Pax (Securos), or cuttable to length, like ALPS (Advanced Locking Plates) (Kyon).

PREOPERATIVE PREPARATION

A standard orthopedic aseptic preparation for surgery is performed. Patients are positioned in dorsal recumbence with the affected limb extended and hanging from a ceiling hook or a drip stand.

SURGICAL TECHNIQUE

Bone segments could be reduced using indirect reduction techniques. If severely dislocated, hanging patients from the affected leg until enough relaxation is obtained facilitates reduction. Alignment is restored with the help of pointed bone-holding forceps applied percutaneously or through the proximal and distal incisions. The assessment of reduction is evaluated by palpation of the bone fragments.

The plate's length is measured in radiographs, and, as rule of thumb, the longest possible plates are selected (**Fig. 1**B). Minimal contouring is needed for plates applied to meta-bones III and IV, whereas contouring is needed for meta-bones II and V.

Meta-bones III and IV are approached via 2 small skin incisions performed in the area between the proximal and distal ends of both bones (**Fig. 1**C). The incisions should be large enough to accommodate the passage of the instruments and implants. By displacing the incisions medially and laterally, epi-periosteal tunnels above meta-bones III and IV are prepared. Tunnels are made by carefully elevating the soft tissues from the dorsal aspect of the bones until the proximal and distal incisions are connected. Hypodermic needles can be used to landmark the proximal and distal joints. The extensor tendons are gently retracted medially or laterally to facilitate the insertion of the implants through the tunnels. The most proximal screw is usually inserted first, and reduction and alignment are achieved by traction and manipulations applied to the distal end of the meta-bones. A small, pointed reduction forceps applied on the condyle of the head of the bone is used for this purpose. In patients less than 15 kg, the application of a pointed reduction forceps as described earlier could be cumbersome because of the size of the bones and the lack of space. In this case, the pointed reduction forceps can be applied on the body of the first phalanx, and the fracture can be reduced indirectly.

When acceptable, reduction and alignment are achieved, and the other end of the plate is secured to the bone. Depending on the type of implants used, 2 or 3 screws per segment are applied. If using locking plates, 2 screws per fragment are generally considered sufficient.

Meta-bones II and V can be stabilized using plates applied medially and laterally, respectively, using the same technique. The approach to these bones is simplified by the scarcity of soft tissue structures, but the reduction and alignment are more demanding because of the curved shape of the bones. Perfect plate contouring is essential, particularly when using nonlocking implants; rigorous alignment is necessary to avoid torsional deformities caused by malreduction.

The postoperative care of patients is similar to treatment using an open approach. The amount of postoperative support of the repair will depend on the number of fractured bones, the location of the fractures, and the number of bones repaired. Generally for fixations of weight-bearing meta-bones, a combination of a well-padded bandage and a palmar/plantar protective splint is recommended for the first 2 to 3 weeks postoperatively. For repairs of non–weight-bearing meta-bones, a padded bandage for the first 2 weeks is generally sufficient. Strict confinement and controlled activity should be imposed until there are signs of radiographic healing, usually around the third to fourth week (**Fig. 1**D).

Follow-up radiographs are taken between 3 and 4 weeks postoperatively because bone healing is expected to occur at this time. In sporting dogs, plates are generally removed as soon as bone healing has occurred. The implants can be removed via small incisions in the same place as the first approach.

DISCUSSION

Minimally invasive stabilization of meta-bone fractures is a very effective method of treatment of injuries affecting this anatomic location. The main advantages are related to the relatively simple local anatomy and less demanding surgical technique.

Expected outcomes are fast healing of the fracture because of adequate stabilization and respect of the local biology at the fracture site.

Meta-bones have some anatomic particularities that make these bones ideal to be treated by minimally invasive techniques. The minimal amount of soft tissues covering the meta-bones allows for easy reduction of the fractures and assessment of reduction by palpation, making the use of intraoperative diagnostic imaging unnecessary. The possible presence of intact meta-bones adjacent to the repaired ones enhances stability by natural splinting, which decreases the need of heavy fixation.

Despite the relative simplicity of the surgical techniques, there are a few important considerations that should be kept in mind to avoid complications. The III and IV meta-bones are straight but with a tendency to diverge from each other in their distal third. The minimally invasive approach does not allow proper visualization of the centering of the plate over the bone and, for this reason, there is a tendency to place the implant off-line in its distal portion. If this happens with a traditional implant, it is sufficient to orient the screws in the plate accordingly, but it represents a major limitation when dealing with angle stable implants. This problem can be avoided by inserting guide needles perpendicular to the medial and lateral margin of the bone in the space between them. The needles placed in such a fashion will prevent the plate from slipping sideways, keeping it centered over the dorsal aspect of the bone. Another consideration regards the cross section of the III and IV meta-bones. Proximally, it is triangular with the dorsal aspect flat and evened to the other adjacent bones; distally, the section is round as the bone loses contact with the next one. A common pitfall is to start securing the plate to the bone by inserting the distal screws. This practice will constrain the plate in such a way that when it is applied over the dorsal surface of the proximal portion, as the plate is tightened against the bone, the distal portion can rotate and generate a torsional malalignment. This problem can be avoided by simply starting to secure the proximal portion of the plate to the bone, then the distal portion is reduced; the alignment is checked; and when screws are inserted, the plate can still adapt to the bone surface.

Fixation of the II and V meta-bones offers some challenge relative to the curved and twisted shape of the bones. A typical error here consists of poor contouring of the implant that could result in straightening the bone and possibly creating a rotational defect. The immediate consequence will be that the full digit will enter in conflict with the adjacent toe with an obvious impediment to normal function. This problem is avoided by meticulous precontouring of the implant, even when dealing with locking plates.

The use of a tourniquet is described mostly in human surgery but is not required with our patients. As stated earlier, the need of a postoperative support associated with a padded bandage depends on the type and strength of the fixation and is left as the surgeon's decision.

REFERENCES

1. De La Puerta B, Emmerson T, Moores AP, et al. Epoxy putty external skeletal fixation for fractures of the four main metacarpal and metatarsal bones in cats and dogs. Vet Comp Orthop Traumatol 2008;21:451–6.
2. Wernham B, Roush J. Metacarpal and metatarsal fractures in dogs. Compend Contin Educ Vet 2010;32:E1–8.
3. Muir P, Norris JL. Metacarpal and metatarsal fractures in dogs. J Small Anim Pract 1997;38:344–8.

4. Brinker WO, Piermattei DL, Flo GL. Fractures and other orthopedic conditions of the carpus, metacarpus and phalanges. 4th edition. Philadelphia: Saunders; 2006.
5. Seibert RL, Lewis DD, Coomer AR, et al. Stabilisation of metacarpal or metatarsal fractures in three dogs, using circular external skeletal fixation. N Z Vet J 2011;59: 96–103.

Minimally Invasive Osteosynthesis Technique for Articular Fractures

Brian S. Beale, DVM*, Grayson Cole, DVM

KEYWORDS

- Minimally invasive osteosynthesis • Articular • Fracture • Dog • Cat

KEY POINTS

- The repair of articular fractures requires anatomic reduction, rigid fixation, and early return to joint mobility.
- Minimally invasive approaches decrease morbidity and allow earlier return to function.
- Minimally invasive approaches include mini-arthrotomy and arthroscopic-assisted and percutaneous techniques.
- Minimally invasive osteosynthesis articular fracture repair is performed using implant systems and stabilization methods that are similar to those used in traditional open reduction and internal fixation.

INTRODUCTION

Articular fractures occur commonly in dogs and cats. Articular fractures can occur in any diarthrodial joint, but the most commonly affected joints are the elbow and hip. Repair of articular fractures requires anatomic reduction and rigid fixation to reduce the chance of osteoarthritis and joint dysfunction. Traditional arthrotomy can be used to accomplish these goals, but anatomic reduction can be difficult with certain fractures because of an inability to adequately view the joint surfaces. Minimally invasive osteosynthesis (MIO) using a minimally invasive or mini-arthrotomy approach, arthroscope-assisted approach, or percutaneous techniques have been used to treat articular fractures in humans and in dogs and cats.[1–11] Arthroscope-assisted surgery has the advantages of superior visualization and less invasiveness, improved outcome, and accurate reduction, in addition to the diagnosis and repair of related injuries.[1–3,10] Disadvantages of arthroscopic repair of articular fractures include a learning curve and initial expense of the needed equipment.

Dr Grayson Cole is now with the University of Tennessee Veterinary Medical Center, 2407 River Dr Knoxville, TN 37912
Gulf Coast Veterinary Specialists, 1111 West Loop South #160, Houston, TX 77027, USA
* Corresponding author.
E-mail address: dogscoper@aol.com

Vet Clin Small Anim 42 (2012) 1051–1068
http://dx.doi.org/10.1016/j.cvsm.2012.07.008
0195-5616/12/$ – see front matter © 2012 Elsevier Inc. All rights reserved.

GOALS OF REPAIR OF ARTICULAR FRACTURES

The goal of surgical repair of articular fractures is a return to pain-free motion and absence of osteoarthritis. The principles of articular fracture repair include:

1. Anatomic reduction of the articular surface
2. Rigid stabilization
3. Early surgical repair
4. Early mobilization of the joint

Adherence to these important principles is critical to giving the patient the greatest opportunity of maintaining a healthy articular surface, viable hyaline cartilage, normal periarticular supporting connective tissues, and less muscle atrophy and fibrosis. Deviation from the principles will likely lead to poor outcome characterized by osteo-arthritis, joint fibrosis, muscle atrophy, and chronic pain.

FRACTURE ASSESSMENT

Articular fractures involve disruption of the articular surface of the joint within the syno-vial cavity. Articular fractures are most common in the elbow and hip, but they can also occur in the shoulder, carpus, stifle, and tarsus. Fractures of the joint surface have a greater likelihood of the development of osteoarthritis. Many of these fractures also occur in growing dogs and cats. The physis is a common site for fracture because of the relatively weak zone of hypertrophied chondrocytes. Fractures through the physis have been classified by Salter and Harris into 6 types.[12] The severity of physeal fractures increases with the increasing numerical type of Salter-Harris fracture. Some Salter-Harris fractures occur within the joint but do not involve the articular surface. Salter III and IV fractures invade the joint surface and result in an articular fracture. Increased severity of physeal fracture is associated with increased chance of growth disturbance of the physis, potentially leading to limb shortening or angular limb defor-mity. Identification of an articular component, presence of preexisting orthopedic conditions, presence of physeal involvement, fracture classification, duration of injury, and expected patient and owner compliance are important to consider in the decision-making process for the treatment plan for articular fractures.

INDICATIONS FOR MIO

The type of surgical approach for articular fractures should be considered carefully before the start of surgery. Traditional surgical approaches to the joints of the dog and cat have been previously reported and can be used to treat all articular frac-tures.[13] A minimally invasive surgical approach using an MIO technique is optimal for repair of certain articular fractures, particularly fractures that are minimally dis-placed, simple (2 pieces), and acute. This may be accomplished using arthroscopy and percutaneous placement of implants or using an arthroscope through a mini-arthrotomy to better view the articular fracture.[1–3,10] The use of an arthroscope within an arthrotomy incision is known as arthroscopic-assisted arthrotomy.[14] The mini-arthrotomy incision is much shorter than the arthrotomy incision used to treat articular fractures using traditional open reduction and stabilization techniques. The mini-arthrotomy incision can be extended as needed to apply implants to stabilize the frac-ture. A MIO technique can be used for articular fractures of the glenoid, humeral head, humeral condyle, anconeal process, carpus, acetabulum, femoral head, femoral condyle, and tarsus. A MIO technique improves the surgeon's view of the articular surface and results in a more precise repair as a result of the magnification provided by the arthroscope.[2,3] Fluoroscopy also can be used to improve the surgeon's spatial orientation and for assessment of fragment alignment and implant position.[4,6–8] Treatment of articular fractures with arthroscopy and a MIO technique has a significant learning curve. The technique should be practiced on cadavers if available. Novice surgeons can shorten the learning curve by assisting more experienced surgeons who are familiar with the MIO technique and by participating in minimally invasive plate osteosynthesis or MIO short courses that have lecture and laboratory components.

Shoulder

Supraglenoid fractures are uncommon and occur as a traumatic or pathologic articular fractures.[2,15] The bicep brachii tendon originates from the supraglenoid tuberosity. Fractures of the supragenoid tuberosity typically result in a weight-bearing forelimb lameness and shoulder pain. Swelling may be seen over the craniolateral aspect of the shoulder in some patients. Radiographic examination is usually diagnostic. The fracture line is usually clearly seen on the lateral shoulder view because of a distal displacement of the supraglenoid fragment caused by traction by the biceps brachii muscle. This articular fracture involves the cranial aspect of the glenoid cavity (**Fig. 1**). Supraglenoid fractures should be repaired because of the intra-articular nature and potential for chronic pain and future osteoarthritis. The fracture can be repaired using traditional open reduction and internal fixation (ORIF), but anatomic reduction is difficult without using an extensive surgical approach.[13,15,16] Supraglenoid fractures are amenable to a MIO technique.[2,11] Supraglenoid fractures are usually repaired by applying compression with pins or lag screws following anatomic reduction and percutaneous placement of implants (see **Fig. 1**; **Fig. 2**). The fracture can be

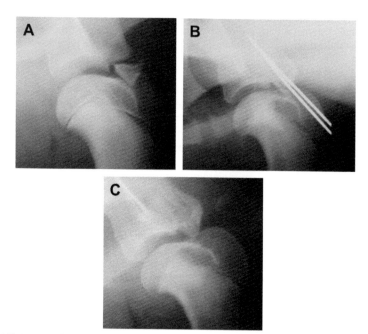

Fig. 1. (*A*) A supraglenoid fracture in a dog. (*B*) The fragment was deemed too small and fragile to place a lag screw. Stabilization was achieved using percutaneous divergent k-wires and a proximal biceps tendon release to remove the distractive force of the biceps. (*C*) Healed supraglenoid fracture following pin removal 8 weeks later.

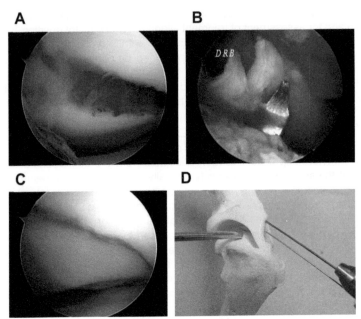

Fig. 2. (*A*) Arthroscopic view of a supraglenoid fracture in a dog seen in **Fig. 1**. (*B*) A percutaneous k-wire is placed in the supraglenoid fragment. The fragment is reduced by digital manipulation and use of the k-wire as a joystick. (*C*) The supraglenoid tuberosity is reduced under arthroscopic visualization using a lateral scope portal. Anatomic reduction is confirmed. (*D*) MIO technique for treatment of supraglenoid fractures is demonstrated on a bone model. A percutaneous k-wire is placed initially after anatomic reduction to provide temporary stabilization. A cannulated drill bit is used to drill a hole for placement of a cannulated lag screw.

initially reduced through percutaneous manipulation of the fragment using digital pressure with the surgeon's fingers or by application of a pointed reduction forceps. The ability to reduce the fracture should be confirmed arthroscopically, radiographically, or fluoroscopically. A traditional lateral scope portal or mini-arthrotomy is used when an arthroscope is used. Pointed-reduction forceps should be used to achieve fracture reduction when using imaging techniques to document temporary fracture reduction. It is often difficult to maintain fracture reduction while inserting implants used for stabilization. Final reduction is often performed after placement of a percutaneous k-wire. The k-wire is used to achieve temporary fracture stabilization. The size of k-wire varies depending on the size of patient but most commonly has a diameter of 0.045 or 0.062 inch. The wire is placed percutaneously from the distal cranial aspect of the supraglenoid fragment and it is directed in a proximal direction perpendicular to the fracture line. The pin should be strategically placed to allow room for an adjacent lag screw or a headless compression screw. The pin may also be used as the temporary guide pin when used with cannulated implant systems. The pin is placed to the level of the fracture line. Final fracture reduction is achieved and documented. The pin is driven across the fracture into the glenoid of the scapula. Anatomic reduction can be confirmed using the arthroscope or imaging. The fracture should be stabilized using an implant that will provide compression across the fracture line. Implants that are useful for supraglenoid fractures include lag screws, headless compression screws, and cannulated lag screws. An antirotational pin can also be used to provide adjunctive stabilization. Some surgeons perform a proximal biceps tenotomy to remove the distractive force on the fragment before reduction and stabilization of supraglenoid fractures. The reason for this is to ease reduction of the fragment and remove the risk of a potential distractive force postoperatively. The disadvantage of this practice is the potential for creating shoulder instability.[17] Arthroscopic biceps tendon release, however, has been found to result in clinical improvement in dogs with chronic tears of the tendon of origin of the biceps brachii muscle.[18,19]

Fractures of the glenoid cavity of the scapula involving other weight-bearing regions of the scapula occur uncommonly.[15] These fractures should be accurately reduced and stabilized with lag screws or compression pins when involving substantial regions of the glenoid and when fragments are of adequate size for fixation.[15] Reduction can be aided using fluoroscopy, arthroscopy, or arthroscopic-assisted arthrotomy. Surgical stabilization can also be accomplished using these MIO techniques by placing implants in a percutaneous fashion. Caudal glenoid fracture or fragmentation is typically treated with good outcome by arthroscopic excision of the small fragments.[2,20] Extensive or chronic fractures of the glenoid may necessitate shoulder arthrodesis.

Fractures of the humeral head are uncommon. Occasionally, proximal humeral physeal fractures can lead to displacement of the humeral head. MIO technique can be used to repair minimally displaced humeral head fractures. Fluoroscopy or arthroscope-assisted arthrotomy can be used to facilitate fracture reduction and placement of surgical implants. The fracture should be reduced anatomically and stabilized with a suitable implant, applying compression across the articular component of the fracture line. Compression should be avoided across the physeal component of the fracture if applicable. Lag screws or headless compression screws or pins are commonly used for this type of fracture. Typically, physeal fractures are repaired using k-wires or pins to decrease the chance of developing compression across the physis, leading to premature closure and disruption of growth.

Elbow

Fractures of the lateral or medial humeral condyle are very common, especially in growing dogs. Humeral condylar fractures require accurate anatomic reduction and rigid stabilization to achieve a favorable functional outcome. Complications are common if reduction is poor, if implant position is improper, or if surgical time is excessive.[4,21] Unicondylar humeral fractures can be repaired using a MIO technique, especially if minimal displacement is present. Lateral condyle fractures are much more common because of the forces acting though the relatively thin lateral epicondyle. Most lateral condyle fractures in immature dogs are Salter-Harris type III or IV physeal fractures. A MIO technique is easier to perform and recommended in fractures having mild or moderate swelling and a duration of less than 48 hours.[2,4] Traditional open reduction and internal fixation (ORIF) is recommended if substantial displacement has occurred because of the difficulty in achieving anatomic reduction. A MIO technique is not recommended for bicondylar fractures. These fractures are much more unstable and difficult to reduce without direct observation and open manipulation of the fragments. Closed reduction and stabilization of condylar fractures was found to result in minimal disruption of soft tissues and blood supply, decreased risk of infection, and earlier return to function.[4] Fluoroscopy was an effective method for evaluating the type of physeal fracture, assessing fracture reduction, and assisting in positioning implants used to stabilize the fracture.[4] Implants typically used to stabilize lateral or medial condyle fractures include traditional or cannulated lag screws, headless compression screws, or self-compression pins.[2,4–6,21] Reduction is performed using a combination of distraction, digital manipulation, and grasping with bone forceps placed in a percutaneous fashion. Vulsellum forceps, pointed reduction forceps, or a condyle clamp are often used to provide temporary stabilization. If reduction is accurate, both the condylar and epicondylar components should be anatomically aligned. Reduction is confirmed arthroscopically or fluoroscopically (**Fig. 3**). Stabilization is achieved in most patients with a transcondylar screw and a cross-pin placed across the epicondylar fracture line in percutaneous fashion. Some surgeons prefer to repair the epicondylar portion first, whereas others choose to place the transcondylar screw first (**Fig. 4**). The transcondylar lag or self-compressing screw is percutaneously placed to compress and stabilize the condylar component of the fracture. The most prominent aspect of the lateral and medial epicondyles can be palpated and used as a landmark to place the screw in a proper position. Ideally, the screw is placed parallel to the humeroradial joint near the center of the condyles. The physis should be avoided if possible, to reduce the chance of growth disturbances. The largest diameter screw that is appropriate for the patient should be used to decrease the chance of the screw breaking or loosening. Toy breed dogs and cats commonly require a 2.0- or 2.4-mm screw. Small, medium-size, large, and giant breed dogs typically require a 2.7-, 3.5-, 4.5-, or 6.5-mm screw, respectively.

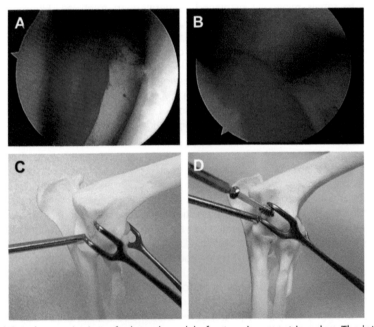

Fig. 3. (*A*) Arthroscopic view of a lateral condyle fracture is present in a dog. The intercondylar fracture gap is filled with the fracture hematoma. (*B*) The fracture is reduced with digital manipulation and compression with a vulsellum forceps. Reduction may be facilitated by slightly extending the elbow. Excellent reduction of the articular surface has been achieved and the fracture hematoma can be seen protruding from the compressed fracture gap. (*C*) MIO technique for treatment of humeral condyle fractures is demonstrated on a model. The arthroscope is placed through a medial portal to confirm anatomic reduction of the articular surface and compression of the fracture. The vulsellum forceps can be used to provide temporary stabilization. (*D*) A transcondylar lag screw is placed to apply compression and stabilization. A transcondylar pin can be placed first if desired to provide adjunctive stabilization and to help prevent rotation of the fracture during tightening of the lag screw.

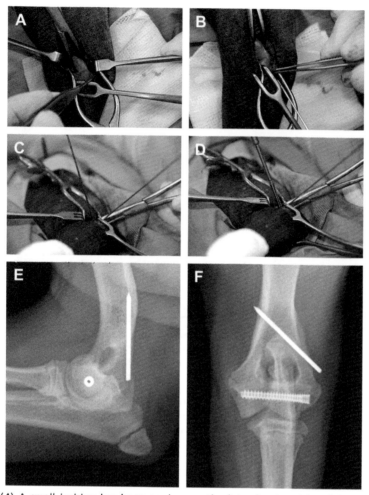

Fig. 4. (*A*) A small incision has been made over the lateral epicondyle of this dog with a lateral humeral condyle fracture. The epicondylar portion of the fracture is reduced. (*B*) A pin has been normograded across the epicondylar fracture and a vulsellum forceps has been applied to reduce the intercondylar portion of the fracture. Reduction was confirmed using a C-arm. (*C*) A transcondylar guide wire was placed across the humeral condyle under fluoroscopic guidance. (*D*) A cannulated self-compressing screw is inserted across the fracture over the guide wire, providing compression and stability. (*E*) Lateral postoperative radiograph. The lumen of the cannulated screw is evident. (*F*) Anteroposterior postoperative radiograph. Anatomic reduction and stabilization have been achieved with a headless, self-compressing screw in the humeral condyle and a pin in the lateral epicondyle.

A washer should be considered if the bone of the condyle is expected to be too soft to withstand the pressure of the screw head as it is tightened and compression is applied. Alternatively, intercondylar stability can be supplied using self-compressing screws or pins (**Fig. 5**).[5,6] An adjunctive antirotational k-wire can also be placed across the condyles to gain additional stability if room permits. It is essential to achieve accurate reduction to lessen the chance of future osteoarthritis. Rigid stabilization is required to prevent shifting of the fragments and proper healing. Early return to joint

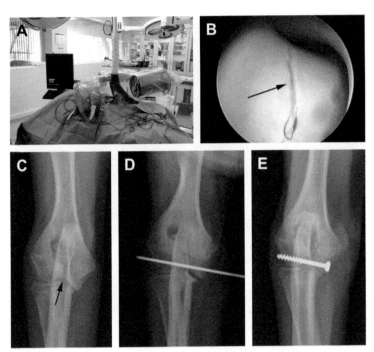

Fig. 5. (*A*) A dog is positioned and prepped for minimally invasive elbow surgery using fluoroscopy and arthroscopy. (*B*) Arthroscopic examination of the elbow confirmed incomplete ossification of the humeral condyle (*arrow*). (*C*) Incomplete ossification of the humeral condyle (*arrow*) is seen in the dog with forelimb lameness. (*D*) A guide pin has been normograded across the humeral condyle using fluoroscopic guidance. (*E*) A cannulated positional screw has been placed across the humeral condyle over the guide pin. The screw is used to buttress the gap in the condyle. Lameness resolved in this dog and potential condylar fracture did not occur 6 years after surgery.

mobility is critical to maintaining normal elbow range of motion and a successful outcome. A non–weight-bearing sling or carpal flexion bandage can be used postoperatively to protect the repair for the first 1 or 2 weeks after surgery but allow range of motion of the elbow. Physical rehabilitation exercises should be considered starting 2 weeks postoperatively by a trained physiotherapist if possible.

Incomplete ossification of the humeral condyle (IOHC) is a relatively common condition found in spaniel breeds (particularly the Brittney spaniel), but it has also been identified in other breeds including the Rottweiler and mixed-breed dogs.[6,22,23] IOHC predisposes the dog to condylar fracture with minimal trauma. The condition has also been associated with lameness without obvious fracture. IOHC is associated with a zone of incomplete ossification at the mid-portion of the humeral condyle. Fibrous tissue is found in this region. The adjacent bone of the condyle is more dense than normal. IOHC is diagnosed using radiographic examination, computed tomography, or arthroscopy.[2,6,22,23] IOHC is commonly bilateral and is often diagnosed in the opposite asymptomatic elbow in dogs that have sustained a Y-fracture of the distal humerus as a result of minimal trauma. A transcondylar positional screw can be placed in MIO fashion in asymptomatic or symptomatic dogs with IOHC in an attempt to prevent future fracture and resolve lameness if present (see **Fig. 5**).[2] The goal of the screw is simply to buttress the zone of incomplete ossification to prevent fracture. Compression should not be applied across this area as this may actually increase the chance of fracture because of tension placed on the thin lateral epicondyle. The screw should have maximal diameter to prevent breakage of the screw because of the effects of expected implant cycling and potential fatigue failure. Fitzpatrick and colleagues recently described a MIO technique to enhance healing in dogs with IOHC using an osteochondral autograft and a self-compressing screw.[6]

Other intra-articular elbow fractures and disorders that can be occasionally treated using a MIO technique include anconeal fractures, medial coronoid fractures (jumpdown syndrome), and radial head fractures.[2] The same principles of anatomic reduction and rigid stabilization apply to these fractures. Fractures with fragments that are too small to be reduced and stabilized, such as with the medial coronoid process, should be removed arthroscopically if possible.[2]

Ununited anconeal process (UAP) can also be stabilized using a MIO technique. This is best performed when the dog is immature and the fragment is minimally displaced and has viable hyaline cartilage and no evidence of radiographic remodeling. A distal dynamic ulnar osteotomy is initially performed through a small incision over the caudo-lateral aspect of the distal third of the ulna. The osteotomy gap is widened using a distraction forceps or by levering with an elevator. The interosseous ligament can be disrupted as needed to free the ulna from the radius to allow less restricted movement of the ulna. The elbow is evaluated arthroscopically through a standard medial portal.[2] Many patients having UAP also have a concurrent fragmented medial coronoid process.[2,24] Treatment of the fragmented medial coronoid process should be performed in routine fashion at the discretion of the surgeon. The UAP fragment is identified and evaluated. A decision should be made whether to remove or reduce and stabilize the UAP fragment. If needed, fibrous tissue can be removed and debrided at the interface between the fragment and the olecranon using an arthroscopic shaver.[2] If the articular surface of the fragment seems to be in good condition a small threaded k-wire is percutaneously placed from the olecranon to the gap adjacent to the fragment (**Fig. 6**). This wire will be used for as a guide wire for a cannulated lag screw or a headless compression screw. The fragment is reduced and partially immobilized by placing the elbow in full extension. Placing the elbow in this position aids reduction and stabilization of the fragment. A caudal instrument portal can be created proximal to the anconeal process if needed to insert a Freer elevator into the joint to lever the fragment against the olecranon.[2] This provides additional immobilization and resistance while the k-wire is driven into the fragment. Anatomic alignment is assessed using the arthroscope. The k-wire is driven into the fragment to provide initial stabilization. A small skin incision is made at the k-wire. An appropriate sized cannulated drill bit is used over the guide wire to drill a hole in the olecranon and the fragment. A cannulated lag screw or headless compression screw is applied over the guide wire, compressing the gap between the fragment and the olecranon.

Carpus

Distal radial articular and radiocarpal bone fractures are occasionally seen. Diagnosis is achieved using radiography, computed tomography evaluation, or arthroscopy. If displacement is minimal, these fractures can be reduced closed and temporarily stabilized with a percutaneous pointed bone reduction forceps. Arthroscopic or fluoroscopic assessment is needed to accurately reduce the fracture when using a MIO technique. The fractures are typically stabilized using a lag screw, headless compression screw, or self-compressing pin through a small incision.[8,25] A cannulated screw is often used to facilitate the repair. Screws should be placed in compression mode. Headless compression screws have been found to be an effective means of stabilizing

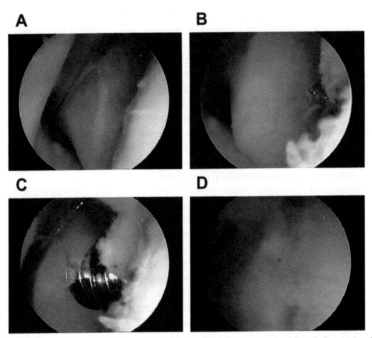

Fig. 6. (*A*) An ununited anconeal process is seen in this dog. A proximal dynamic ulnar osteotomy was performed initially. (*B*) A threaded guide pin is percutaneously placed in the olecranon under arthroscopic visualization. The pin exits at the gap between the olecranon and the ununited fragment. The elbow is then extended to partially close the gap and stabilize the fragment. The pin is inserted into the fragment. (*C*) A cannulated lag screw is inserted over the guide pin into the fragment. (*D*) The screw is tightened, compressing the gap and stabilizing the fragment.

radiocarpal bone fractures.[25] Small chip fractures or avulsion fractures associated with collateral ligaments are generally not of adequate size for fixation, but they can be removed minimally invasively using arthroscopy.[2,26]

Acetabular Fractures

Acetabular fractures are relatively common pelvic fractures in dogs and cats and are categorized by their location (cranial, middle, caudal). Caudal acetabular fractures and nondisplaced acetabular fractures in skeletally immature animals have been treated successfully with conservative management,[15,27,28] but all other acetabular fractures require surgical fixation to lessen the chance of osteoarthritis and a poor functional outcome.[29,30] These fractures are traditionally repaired via plating, screws and wire, or screws and polymethylmethacrylate.[29–31] Minimally invasive acetabular fracture repair has been reported in the human literature with assistance from computed tomography, fluoroscopy, arthroscopy, and, most commonly, a combination of fluoroscopy and arthroscopy.[10] Good candidates for percutaneous screw placement are articular fractures that are nondisplaced or minimally displaced. Use of a MIO technique for treatment of acetabular fractures in dogs and cats has not been reported to the authors' knowledge. The authors have used the arthroscope to assist in evaluation of the anatomic reduction of acetabular fractures in dogs. The arthroscope provides a magnified view of the articular fracture line along the dorsal acetabular rim so that optimal reduction can be achieved. Arthroscopy also gives a better view of the medial acetabulum to help ensure adequate reduction and ensure the absence of offending intra-articular fragments.

Capital Physeal Fractures

Capital physeal fractures are typically seen in dogs between the ages of 4 and 11 months of age.[15,31,32] However, spontaneous (atraumatic) capital physeal fractures have been described in cats as old as 16 months of age and are suspected to be to the result of delayed physeal closure.[33] Predisposed cats are male, neutered, and overweight. Spontaneous capital physeal fractures have also been reported in dogs, humans, and rabbits.[31–34] Capital physeal fractures in dogs and cats are most commonly repaired via divergent or parallel k-wires in an effort to preserve the physis.[15,31] Parallel K-wire fixation has been shown to be stronger than divergent k-wire fixation in an in vitro study in dogs.[35] In mature animals, lag screw fixation be used. In human children with capital physeal fractures, multiple k-wire fixation has been shown to have a higher complication rate than single cannulated screw fixation.[36] Prophylactic fixation of the contralateral hip, if unaffected, is recommended in children.[36] Feline capital physeal fractures are bilateral approximately 34% of the time according to one study; however, prophylactic fixation of the contralateral hip has not been reported in veterinary medicine.[33] The goals of capital physeal fracture fixation are anatomic reduction, restoration of stability, prevention of osteoarthritis, and avoidance of complications such as avascular necrosis and chondrolysis.[31–35] Femoral capital physeal closure should also be avoided in skeletally immature animals.[31,32,35] MIO repair can be used to treat minimally displaced femoral capital physeal fractures in dogs and cats (**Fig. 7**). Fracture reduction is usually accomplished by placing the hip in full extension while the patient is positioned in dorsal recumbency. Fluoroscopy or radiographic imaging is used to confirm adequate reduction. Fracture reduction can be adjusted slightly with manipulation of the proximal femur using percutaneous pointed reduction forceps attached to the greater trochanter. Minimally invasive placement of k-wires or screws can be accomplished in small animals with the help of fluoroscopic guidance and percutaneous placement. Implants should be well seated in the epiphysis of the femoral head but not disrupt the articular cartilage or the round ligament, which contains a portion of the blood supply to the femoral head.[31] Arthroscopy, fluoroscopy, or radiography of the hip can be used to verify adequate bone purchase and that pins do not penetrate the joint when using a MIO technique.

Femoral Head and Neck Fractures

Femoral neck fractures are most commonly seen in dogs less than 1 year of age and are typically associated with trauma.[16,37–39] Femoral neck fractures are also seen in kittens.[39] Simple fractures are typically repaired with a lag screw and an antirotational k-wire or divergent k-wires. Comminuted fractures in dogs are best treated with femoral head and neck ostectomy or total hip replacement. Fluoroscopic guidance can be used to place implants across the femoral neck in a similar manner as discussed for capital physeal fractures; however, compression is recommended for fixation of femoral neck fractures. A recent cadaveric study reported that the stability of femoral neck fracture repair achieved with Orthofix Magic Pins (Orthofix, Lewisville, TX, USA) has similar load to failure as traditional fixation methods.[37] Orthofix Magic Pins can be inserted under fluoroscopic guidance and can achieve compression without predrilling or pretapping. Cannulated screws or other self-compressing implants can be placed percutaneously in combination with fluoroscopy to evaluate reduction and proper implant placement.

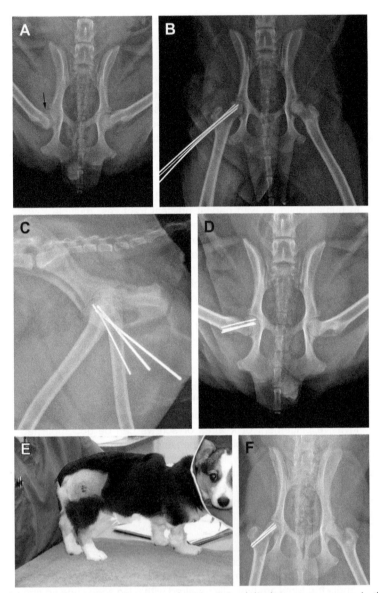

Fig. 7. (*A*) A capital physeal fracture (*arrow*) with minimal displacement was seen in this dog with a right hindlimb lameness. The frog-leg view was necessary to make the diagnosis because minimal displacement was seen on the ventrodorsal view. (*B*) The fracture was reduced by placing the hip in extension. Reduction was confirmed radiographically, and 3 divergent pins were placed across the fracture through a small incision over the lateral aspect of the proximal femur. (*C*) Adequate pin placement is checked on the lateral view of the hip. (*D*) The ventrodorsal postoperative radiograph confirms good reduction, stability, and positioning of the implants. (*E*) A small lateral incision was used to place the pins across the fracture of the capital physis in this corgi. (*F*) Follow-up radiographs at 6 weeks confirm healing of the fracture.

Femoral Condylar Fractures

Fractures of the femoral condyle are most commonly Salter-Harris type II fractures in immature dogs.[16,40] A variety of fixation methods have been described for these fractures including a single intramedullary pin, cross-pinning, and dynamic intramedullary pinning; however, the latter 2 methods have shown greater in vitro load to failure.[16,40] Slight overreduction of the distal segment during intramedullary pinning allows for greater pin purchase, especially in dogs. Femoral condylar fractures are typically good candidates for minimally invasive fluoroscope-guided repair if displacement is minimal because closed reduction is inherently stable as a result of the interdigitating pegs of the distal femoral physis. Cross-pinning and dynamic intramedullary pinning can both be performed percutaneously with fluoroscopic guidance; however, cross-pinning is less technically challenging. Cross-pins should be placed such that they cross proximal to the fracture site and do not penetrate the articular cartilage of the stifle.

Tibial Plateau Fractures

Tibial plateau fractures are also most commonly seen in immature animals and can be associated with femoral condylar fractures.[16] In human orthopedics, tibial plateau fractures are classified into 6 types with multiple subtypes according to the Schatzker system.[41] These fractures can be associated with cartilaginous depressions and ligamentous injuries, thereby indicating the use of arthroscopy in diagnosing concurrent pathology and assessing reduction. Salter-Harris fractures of the tibial condyle can be repaired using a minimally invasive cross-pinning technique similar to that discussed for the distal femur with use of fluoroscopic guidance. In immature dogs, care should be taken not to permanently close the physis. Compression of the physis should be avoided. Varus and valgus stress radiography may be helpful in the diagnosis of minimally displaced Salter-Harris fractures of the proximal tibia. Tibial physeal separations may also occur in combination with tibial tuberosity avulsions. Small terrier breeds may be overrepresented for this combination of injuries. This type of fracture can be managed with percutaneous cross-pins in the proximal tibial physis and 2 pins in the tibial tuberosity. The stifle should be immobilized in slight extension for 10 days. Pins may be removed when the fracture has healed in 3 to 4 weeks if desired. Some surgeons remove pins in an attempt to prevent compression of the physis caused by the cross-pins as the tibia grows. Successful management of proximal tibial physeal and tibial tuberosity fractures has been reported with pin and tension band fixation and crossed k-wires.[42] A side effect of using a stainless steel tension band across the physis of the tibial tuberosity is premature closure, leading to distal displacement of the tibial tuberosity and possibly patella baja. The authors typically use heavy nylon as a tension band rather than stainless steel, to reduce the chance of physeal closure in dogs that have substantial remaining growth. This provides adequate stability to prevent displacement of the tibial tuberosity when stabilized with pins only but may result in less compression of the physis. When using this technique, strict exercise restriction is needed, and ideally the stifle is bandaged in relative extension for approximately 2 weeks.

Distal Tibia and Fibular Fractures

Surgical stabilization of fractures of the medial malleolus (of the tibia) and the lateral malleolus (of the fibula) is recommended because of their intra-articular nature and because these are the sites of origin of the collateral ligaments of the tarsus. Conservative management leads to continued tarsal instability and eventual osteoarthritis in most patients. Malleolar fracture repair has been reported with lag screw fixation, pin and tension band fixation, and k-wire fixation. Malleolar fractures are often associated with shear injuries, and fracture fixation may be complicated by open wound management and delayed stabilization. Collateral ligament instability of the tarsus can be repaired using a transarticular external fixator for 6 to 8 weeks or by ligament reconstruction and/or malleolar fracture stabilization. If minimal displacement is present, closed reduction can be performed and percutaneous self-compressing pins, lag screws, or headless compression screws can be used. Lateral malleolus fractures are usually repaired with a pin and tension band. Arthroscopic or fluoroscopic evaluation can be used to assess anatomic reduction of the articular surface. Comminuted fractures of the distal tibia frequently require open reduction or arthrodesis, and these patients are not good candidates for minimally invasive repair. Postoperative coaptation is recommended for 2–8 weeks following malleolar fracture repair or collateral ligament repair in most patients.

Talar Fractures

Fractures of the trochlear ridges of the talus are generally associated with a traumatic episode, but are uncommonly reported. Talar ridge fractures must be differentiated from osteochondritis dissecans lesions. Diagnostic imaging in this location is challenging because of the superimposition of other tarsal structures. A flexed dorsoplantar (skyline) view or plantaromedial dorsolateral radiograph can be useful in diagnosis; however, computed tomography is more sensitive and very helpful in evaluating the severity and configuration of the fracture. Fracture fixation is commonly performed with k-wires or lag screws, with the latter being preferred if the fragments are large enough to permit screw fixation. Traditional implants should be countersunk so that they do not protrude on the articular surface, or headless compression screws should be used. There are limited case reports of minimally invasive repair of talar fractures in humans but none, to the authors' knowledge, in animals. However, tarsal arthroscopy may be useful to assess concurrent pathology in the joint before surgery and may be helpful in evaluating reduction. Postoperatively, exercise should be restricted to leash walks only until the fracture has healed. A soft padded bandage can be used for 2 weeks postoperatively if desired, but early range of motion exercise is recommended to improve patient outcome.

Central Tarsal Bone Fractures

Central tarsal bone fractures are most commonly fatigue fractures that are seen in the right hock of racing greyhounds, but they have also been reported in border collies and other breeds. Fractures of the plantar process of the central tarsal bone may look radiographically like luxations, with most of the central tarsal bone luxating in a dorsomedial direction. Repair of the central tarsal bone fractures typically involves lag screw fixation either within the central tarsal bone or to the fourth tarsal bone in the case of luxations. Minimally displaced central tarsal bone repair is amenable to percutaneous screw placement because of the paucity of soft tissue structures directly medial to the central tarsal bone, where the fixation would be placed. Fluoroscopic guidance can aid in the placement of screws and assess reduction of central tarsal bone fractures. Most central tarsal bone fractures have significant displacement and require traditional ORIF.

Calcaneal Fractures

Calcaneal fractures are another common injury in the racing greyhound, but are also seen less commonly in other dogs and cats. They are frequently associated with either a central tarsal bone fracture or plantar proximal intertarsal subluxation. These fractures are traditionally approached laterally and fixed either with a plate or pin and tension band. Calcaneal fractures that have articular involvement typically require ORIF or arthrodesis. No reports of minimally invasive repair of calcaneal fractures exist in the veterinary literature. The human orthopedic literature typically recommends ORIF of intra-articular calcaneal fractures; however, there is recent literature regarding a new implant similar to an interlocking nail that has been used with the aid of fluoroscopy. As with other tarsal injuries, significant comminution may require arthrodesis.

Implant Systems Used for Articular Fractures

Traditional implants used for repair of articular fractures can be applied in a minimally invasive manner. K-wires and screw fixation can be guided by the use of fluoroscopy. It may be useful to obtain radiographic images of the drill bit when it is positioned in the bone following drilling before proceeding with tapping and insertion of screws. Arthroscopy can be helpful to assess reduction and congruity of the articular surface after implant placement.

Cannulated systems are useful to achieve precision in implant placement before drilling. First, a guide wire is inserted, aided by the use of a drill sleeve, and placement is verified using fluoroscopy. The remainder of screw placement proceeds routinely, using a cannulated depth gauge, tap if needed, and a cannulated screw. If the screw head is placed on an articular surface, it should be countersunk.

Several headless compression screw systems are available that circumvent the need for countersinking of implants in articular surfaces. The headless compression screw by Synthes Vet (West Chester, PA, USA) is a partially threaded, cannulated screw. The threaded portion of the screw must be placed on the far side of the fracture segment to achieve compression. A compression sleeve is used to tighten the screw until the surgeon is satisfied with the reduction and compression, both of which can be verified with fluoroscopy and/or arthroscopy. Using the screwdriver while holding the compression sleeve stationary allows the surgeon to countersink the head of the screw, which is threaded to facilitate this purpose. Accutrak (Hillsboro, OR, USA) also produces a headless compression screw that is cannulated and fully threaded. Compression is achieved through a variable pitch throughout the length of the screw with a wider thread pitch at the tip of the screw and gradually finer threads.

Self-compressing pins are also available. Orthofix (Lewisville, TX, USA) produces a self-compressing pin (Orthofix Magic Pins) that is inserted in the same manner as a traditional k-wire. There is no need to predrill or tap, so length measurements must be accomplished beforehand on a radiograph or by overlaying the implant on the surgical site and estimating. The pins are all 120 mm in length and therefore need to be cut to size. These implants are partially threaded and achieve compression through a unique mechanism. When the chamfer, otherwise known as the thread–shaft interface, contacts the *cis*-cortex, advancement of the implant partially strips the threads cut in the bone in the *cis*-fragment. The threads maintain purchase in the *trans*-fragment, and compression is achieved. Orthofix Magic Pins are self-compressing pins that have been described for fixation of humeral condylar fractures in dogs and a variety of fractures in human orthopedic surgery including those of the hand, elbow, and femur.

POSTOPERATIVE CARE

The goal of fixation of articular fractures is to allow range of motion of the affected joint as soon as possible postoperatively to reduce joint stiffness and periarticular fibrosis.

Damage to articular cartilage, especially in situations where larger segments of articular cartilage are damaged, should be protected from heavy weight bearing in the early stages, to allow for healing. However, joint motion is required to maintain health and promotes healing of injured articular surfaces. Early joint motion while avoiding overloading can be accomplished via several mechanisms. Non–weight-bearing bandages, such as a carpal flexion bandage, can be used to allow joint motion without weight bearing. Passive range of motion exercises can also accomplish this goal. Passive range of motion is especially recommended in patients that are not bearing weight and can be accomplished by owners at home with proper instruction. Underwater exercises and sling walking can also allow for joint motion without excessive loading on implants.

Prolonged immobilization should be avoided to prevent bone atrophy, muscle atrophy, and articular cartilage damage. Movement is imperative for synovial fluid to nourish all cartilage within the joint. Articular cartilage changes resulting from immobilization may occur as soon as 2 weeks. In addition, immobilization can lead to periarticular adhesions between synovial folds and proliferation of fibrous connective tissue, all leading to decreased range of motion. Use of a canine rehabilitation specialist may be warranted for patients with a prolonged recovery or complications.

REFERENCES

1. Atesok K, Doral MN, Whipple T. Arthroscopy assisted fracture fixation. Knee Surg Sports Traumatol Arthrosc 2011;19:320–9.
2. Beale BS, Hulse DA, Schulz KA, et al. Small animal arthroscopy. Philadelphia: Saunders; 2003.
3. Miller J, Beale B. Tibiotarsal arthroscopy: applications and long-term outcome in dogs. Vet Comp Orthop Traumatol 2008;21:159–65.
4. Cook JL, Tomlinson JL, Reed A. Fluoroscopically guided closed reduction and internal fixation of fractures of the lateral portion of the humeral condyle: prospective study of the technique and results in 10 dogs. Vet Surg 1999;28:315–21.
5. Guille AE, Lewis DD, Anderson TP, et al. Evaluation of surgical repair of humeral condylar fractures using self-compress Orthofix pins in 23 dogs. Vet Surg 2004; 33:314–22.
6. Fitzpatrick N, Smith TJ, O'Riordan J. Treatment of incomplete ossification of the humeral condyle with autogenous bone grafting techniques. Vet Surg 2009; 38(2):173–84.
7. Hudson CC, Pozzi A. Minimally invasive repair of central tarsal bone luxation in a dog. Vet Comp Orthop Traumatol 2012;25(1):79–82.
8. Perry K, Fitzpatrick N, Johnson J. Headless self compressing cannulated screw fixation for treatment of radiocarpal bone fracture or fissure in dogs. Vet Comp Orthop Traumatol 2010;23:84–101.
9. Kregor PJ. Distal femur fractures with complex articular involvement. Orthop Clin North Am 2002;33(1):153–75.
10. Yang J, Chouhan DK, Oh K. Percutaneous screw fixation of acetabular fractures; applicability of hip arthroscopy. Arthroscopy 2010;26(11):1556–61.
11. Deneuche AJ, Viguier E. Reduction and stabilization of a supraglenoid tuberosity avulsion under arthroscopic guidance in a dog. J Small Anim Pract 2002;43(7): 308–11.
12. Salter RB, Harris WR. Injuries involving the epiphyseal plate. J Bone Joint Surg Am 1963;45:587–622.
13. Piermattei DL, Johnson KA. An atlas of surgical approaches to the bones and joints of the dog and cat. 4th edition. Philadelphia: Elsevier; 2004.

14. Beale BS, Hulse DA. Arthroscopy vs arthrotomy for surgical treatment. In: Muir P, editor. Advances in the canine cranial cruciate ligament. Ames (IO): Wiley-Blackwell; 2010.

15. Johnson A, Houlton J, Vannini R. AO principles of fracture management. Clavadelerstrasse (Switzerland): AO Publishing; 2005.

16. Piermattei DL, Flo G, DeCamp C. Handbook of small animal orthopedics and fracture repair. 4th edition. St. Louis (MO): Elsevier; 2006.

17. Sidaway BK, McLaughlin RM, Elder SH, et al. The role of the tendons of the biceps brachii and infraspinatus muscles and the medial glenohumeral ligaemtnin the maintenance of passive shoulder joint stability in dogs. Am J Vet Res 2004;65(9):1216–22.

18. Whitney WO, Beale BS, Hulse DA. Arthroscopic release of the biceps tendon for treatment of bicipital injury in the dog. Proceedings of the 28th annual conference of the Veterinary Orthopedic Society. February 24 - March 1, 2001. Lake Louise (Canada): Veterinary Orthopedic Society; 2001. p. 3.

19. Wall CR, Taylor R. Arthroscopic biceps brachii tenotomy as a treatment for canine bicipital tenosynovitis. J Am Anim Hosp Assoc 2002;38(2):169–75.

20. Morgan OD, Reetz JA, Brown DA. Complication rate, outcome, and risk factors associated with surgical repair of fractures of the lateral aspect of the humeral condyle in dogs. Vet Comp Orthop Traumatol 2008;21:400–5.

21. Olivieri M, Piras A, Marcellin-Little D, et al. Accessory caudal glenoid ossification centre as possible cause of lameness in nine dogs. Vet Comp Orthop Traumatol 2004;17(3):131–5.

22. Moores AP, Agthe P, Schaafsma IA. Prevalence of incomplete ossification of the humeral condyle and other abnormalities of the elbow in English springer spaniels. Vet Comp Orthop Traumatol 2012;15(3):211–6.

23. Marcellin-Little DJ, DeYoung DJ, Ferris KK, et al. Incomplete ossification of the humeral condyle in spaniels. Vet Surg 1994;23(6):475–87.

24. Meyer-Lindenberg A, Fehr M, Nolte I. Coexistence of ununited anconeal process and fragmented medial coronoid process of the ulna in the dog. J Small Anim Pract 2006;47:61–5.

25. Perry K, Fitzpatrick N, Yeadon R. Headless compression screw fixation for treatment of radial carpal bone fracture or fissure in dogs. Vet Comp Orthop Traumatol 2010;23(2):94–101.

26. Warnock JJ, Beale BS. Arthroscopy of the antebrachiocarpal joint in dogs. J Am Vet Med Assoc 2004;224(6):867–74.

27. Brinker WO, Braden TD. Pelvic fractures. In: Brinker WO, Hohn RB, Prieur WD, editors. Manual of internal fixation in small animals. New York: Springer-Verlag; 1984.

28. Denny HR. Pelvic fractures in the dog – a review of 123 cases. J Small Anim Pract 1978;19(3):151–66.

29. Boudrieau RJ, Kleine LJ. Nonsurgically managed caudal acetabular fractures in dogs: 15 cases (1979-1984). J Am Vet Med Assoc 1988;193(6):701–5.

30. Lewis DD, Stubbs WO, Neuwirth L, et al. Results of screw/wire/polymethylmethacrylate composite fixation for acetabular fractures in 14 dogs. Vet Surg 1997; 26(3):223–34.

31. Moores AP, Owen MR, Coe RJ, et al. Slipped capital femoral epiphysis in dogs. J Small Anim Pract 2004;45:602–8.

32. Simpson DJ, Lewis DD. Fractures of the femue. In: Slatter D, editor. Textbook of small animal surgery. 3rd edition. Philadelphia: Saunders; 2003. p. 2059–89.

33. McNicholas WT Jr, Wilkens BE, Blevins WE, et al. Spontaneous femoral capital physeal fractures in adult cats: 26 cases (1996-2001). J Am Vet Med Assoc 2002;221(12):1731–6.

34. Knudsen CS, Langley-Hobbs SJ. Spontaneous femoral capital physeal fractures in a Continental giant rabbit. Vet Rec 2010;166:462–3.

35. Tilson DM, Roush JK, McLaughlin RM. Biomechanical comparison of three repair methods of proximal femoral physeal fractures in shear and tension. Vet Comp Orthop Traumatol 1994;7:136–9.

36. Azzopardi T, Sharma S, Bennet GC. Slipped capital epiphysis in aged children less than 10 years. J Pediatr Orthop B 2010;19(1):13–8.

37. Fisher SC, McLaughlin RM, Elder SH. In vitro biomechanical comparison of 3 methods for internal fixation of femoral neck fractures in dogs. Vet Comp Orthop Traumatol 2012;26(1):36–41.

38. Daly WR. Femoral head and neck fractures in the dog and cat: a review of 115 cases. Vet Surg 1978;7:29–38.

39. Jeffrey ND. Internal fixation of femoral head and neck fractures in the cat. J Small Anim Pract 1989;30:674–7.

40. Beale B. Orthopedic clinical techniques femur fracture repair. Clin Tech Small Anim Pract 2004;19(3):134–50.

41. Markhardt BK, Gross JM, Monu JUV. Schatzker classification of tibial plateau fractures: use of CT and MR imaging improves assessment. Radiographics 2009;12(2):589–98.

42. Pratt JN. Avulsion of the tibial tuberosity with separation of the proximal tibial physis in seven dogs. Vet Rec 2001;149(12):352–6.

Minimally Invasive Repair of Sacroiliac Luxation in Small Animals

James Tomlinson, DVM, MVSc

KEYWORDS

• Sacroiliac • Luxation • Fracture • Fluoroscopy

KEY POINTS

- Sacroiliac fracture-luxation is a common injury that is associated with ilial and acetabular fractures of the opposite hemipelvis.
- A minimally invasive technique for repair of sacroiliac-fracture luxation is a viable option for repair.
- Closed reduction and screw fixation of sacroiliac fracture-luxation has been shown an effective method of treating this traumatic injury to the pelvis of dogs and cats.
- Reduction and fixation of a minimally invasive technique is comparable to an open technique without the associated morbidity of an open technique.
- A minimally invasive technique requires intraoperative fluoroscopy and associated possible radiation exposure.

INTRODUCTION

Sacroiliac fracture-luxation is a common injury that is associated with ilial and acetabular fractures of the opposite hemipelvis.[1] Sacroiliac fracture-luxation results in an unstable pelvis and potentially collapse of the pelvic canal. Bilateral sacroiliac fracture-luxations also occur without associate fractures of the ilium or acetabulum. Although conservative management of sacroiliac fracture-luxations is a treatment option, alignment and fixation is my preferred method of treatment. Surgery potentially allows a quick return to weight bearing and prevents obstipation from pelvic canal collapse.[1]

The approaches for open reduction and methods of stabilization have been described.[1] Difficulty in finding the exact place for screw insertion, especially on the lateral side of the ilium, is a drawback to the open approach for stabilization. Another difficulty with an open approach is directing the screw across the sacrum so that the spinal canal and the lumbosacral disk space is not penetrated yet allows the screw to

Department of Veterinary Medicine and Surgery, College of Veterinary Medicine, University of Missouri, 900 East Campus Drive, Columbia, MO 65211, USA
E-mail address: tomlinsonj@missouri.edu

Vet Clin Small Anim 42 (2012) 1069–1077
http://dx.doi.org/10.1016/j.cvsm.2012.06.005
0195-5616/12/$ – see front matter © 2012 Elsevier Inc. All rights reserved.

gain at least 60% purchase of the sacrum.[1,2] Angles for directing the screw across the sacrum have been described but may be difficult to execute during surgery.[3–5]

A minimally invasive approach to the reduction and insertion of a screw for fixation of sacroiliac fracture-luxation using fluoroscopic guidance has been described.[6] The advantages of using this technique is that a small incision can be made with minimal soft tissue disruption and the surgical time is short. Closed reduction and fixation of the sacroiliac fracture-luxation has been shown to produce results similar to an open repair technique.[2,6,7] Exact screw placement is facilitated by fluoroscopy to make sure that the disk space or vertebral canal is not penetrated yet allows an adequate length of screw purchase in the sacrum.[6,7] The big drawback to this procedure is that it requires the use of intraoperative fluoroscopy, which is expensive for the machine and exposes personnel to radiation.

SACROILIAC ANATOMY

The sacroiliac joint anatomy has been described.[8] Periarticular ligaments are located dorsal and ventral as the dorsal and ventral sacroiliac ligaments and also as cranial sacroiliac ligaments.[8,9] The dorsal sacroiliac ligament is the largest. The ligamentous portion and the synovial portion make up the 2 parts of the sacroiliac joint. The central and craniodorsal part of the joint is where the ligamentous portion of the joint is located.[8] The synovial part of the joint consists of the crescent-shaped articular surfaces of the ilium and sacrum lined with hyaline cartilage. A thin synovial membrane is present around the edge of the hyaline cartilage.[8,9]

Using a minimally invasive closed reduction repair technique using fluoroscopy, the 5 most important parts of the regional anatomy are the sacral body, the vertebral canal, the lumbosacral disk space, the ilial wings, and the transverse processes of the seventh lumbar vertebra. These structures can be easily seen by fluoroscopy (**Fig. 1**). The sacrum consists of the sacral body, sacral wings, vertebral canal, and dorsal spinous processes. The other anatomic structure that is important when performing a minimally invasive technique for repair of sacroiliac joint fracture-luxation is the lumbosacral joint space made up of the seventh lumbar vertebra and the first sacral vertebra.

The sacrum is comprised of 3 sacral vertebrae that are fused together. The correct part of the sacrum for screw placement is the body of the first sacral vertebra. The

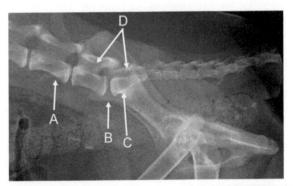

Fig. 1. Lateral view of the lumbar spine and pelvis in a true lateral position. (*Arrow A*) Superimposition of transverse processes of the seventh lumbar vertebra. (*Arrow B*) Lumbosacral disk space. (*Arrow C*) Points to the first sacral vertebra. (*Arrows D*) Points to the vertebral canal of the seventh lumbar and sacral vertebral canal.

surgeon needs to be aware of the vertebral canal and the lumbosacral disk space so that the screw is not inadvertently placed into these areas or out ventrally on the sacrum. The transverse processes of the seventh lumbar vertebra are also important landmarks for proper assessment of alignment of the sacrum in a true lateral position on the surgery table. From the lateral radiographic project of the caudal spine, the wings of the sacrum are not visible due to the overlap of the ilium. From the ventrodorsal projection, the wings of the sacrum are visible and can aid in determining if the sacroiliac joint is properly aligned (see **Fig. 1**).

PREOPERATIVE PATIENT ASSESSMENT AND DECISION MAKING

Preoperatively, standard orthogonal views of the pelvis are taken to assess the type and locations of the injuries that are present. Measurements of the length of screw needed to achieve at least 60% purchase of the sacrum are made. The total width of the sacrum is measured along with the thickness of the ilium at the sight of screw insertion from a ventrodorsal image of the pelvis. In most cases, it is easier to measure from the nonluxated side than from the luxated side of the pelvis.

In most instances, a fracture of the ilium or acetabulum is present on the opposite side of the pelvis from the sacroiliac fracture-luxation. Repair of the contralateral fracture decreases the displacement of the sacroiliac joint, making the final reduction of the sacroiliac joint easier. Placement of a bone plate on the ilium, however, potentially obscures the view of the sacrum, making it more difficult to correctly place that screw. Using the C-arm, placement of the bone plate on the ilium can be adjusted to prevent the bone plate from obscuring the sacrum in most cases. Repair of the sacroiliac luxation can be performed as the first procedure as an alternative. Exact reduction of the sacroiliac fracture-luxation is required, however, if this is done first or it makes acceptable repair of a contralateral ilial or acetabular fracture more difficult or impossible.

ORTHOPEDIC EQUIPMENT, IMPLANTS, AND ANCILLARY EQUIPMENT

Performance of minimally invasive surgery for repair of sacroiliac fracture-luxation requires the use of intraoperative fluoroscopy (C-arm) along with a radiolucent operating table. Proper radiation protection equipment (gowns and thyroid protectors) is also required to minimize radiation exposure.

Orthopedic equipment that is used for reduction of the sacroiliac luxation includes Kern bone holding forceps (or other similar bone holding forceps) and intramedullary (IM) pins. A Jacob's pin chuck can be used as a handle on the IM pin during reduction of the sacroiliac fracture-luxation.

The most common implants used for joint fracture fixation include Kirschner (K)-wires, screws, and washers. K-wires are used to locate the place for screw insertion and for temporary stabilization of the sacroiliac joint luxation after it is reduced. Tap sleeves, taps, screwdriver, and drill bits of the appropriate size for the screw that is inserted are also required. Cortical screws are the implant most commonly used to stabilize the sacroiliac fracture-luxation. The appropriate-sized washer can be used to increase the surface area of the implant to decrease the possibility of the screw head penetrating through cortex of the ilium.

PREOPERATIVE PREPARATION

A standard orthopedic aseptic preparation for surgery is performed. Just because a minimally invasive technique is used does not reduce the importance of performing aseptic surgery. The difference between draping procedure and performing an open repair is that a stockinette and/or adhesive drape is typically not used.

A patient is positioned in lateral recumbency so that the lower lumbar spine is in a perfect lateral position. It is important to position the patient in as a perfect lateral recumbent position as possible to facilitate correct screw placement. A beanbag that can be suctioned out to conform to the patient may be useful to maintain this position. A cantilevered table that allows rotation of the table side to side is also useful for perfect lateral positioning of the lumbar spine. Superimposition of the lateral spinous processes of the seventh lumbar vertebra is used to indicate that the vertebrae are in a true lateral position dorsal to ventral. The lumbosacral disk space is used to judge if the sacrum is positioned correctly cranial to caudal. It should be possible to look completely through the lumbosacral disk space without seeing an oblique view of the end of either vertebra.

SURGICAL TECHNIQUE

Reduction of the sacroiliac fracture-luxation is performed. Three basic methods of reduction are possible (or in combination). The first method involves manipulation of the hemipelvis by controlling the ischium with either an IM pin or a Kern bone holding forceps. This method requires that the hemipelvis is intact. If an ischial body fracture is present, this method does not work. A small approach to the ischium can be performed to facilitate placement of a Kern bone holding forceps. An IM pin can be driven directly through the tuber ischium and used as a traction device. The second method of manipulation of the hemipelvis involves pushing caudally on the wing of the ilium with one hand while using the femur to apply caudal and lateral force to the pelvis with the other hand. This method works best for small, thin, and lightly muscled dogs or cats. If ipsilateral ischial body fractures are present, this method of reduction can be tried. The third method (and my preferred method) of reduction involves pushing on the ilial wing using an IM pin. With this technique, the tip of the pin is inserted through the skin and driven into the cranial dorsal corner of the wing of the ilium. The pin is then used to push the ilium caudal and ventral as needed. The cranial aspect of the ilial wing can be pushed medially to move the caudal part of the hemipelvis laterally to widen the pelvic canal out to its normal position. Combining pushing and pulling is effective in reducing the sacroiliac joint in large dogs.

Assessment of reduction is estimated in the lateral view by superimposition of the 2 wings of the ilium and acetabuli. Comparison of the slope of the 2 sides of the pelvis gives an estimation of the angulation of the pelvis to the spine (normal, approximately 45°) (Fig. 2). The C-arm can be rotated 90° to assess reduction in the ventrodorsal projection. Once the sacroiliac joint appears reduced, a K-wire of appropriate size is driven across the sacroiliac joint caudal to the area that the lag screw will be placed to temporarily maintain reduction of the sacroiliac joint (see Fig. 2). A ventrodorsal view of the pelvis can also be taken, if desired, to assess appropriate reduction.

Two methods of screw application are available. For either technique, a K-wire is used to locate the proper place for insertion of the lag screw. Once the insertion site is found, a small incision is made through the skin and subcutaneous tissue. Instrumentation is tunneled through the fat and muscle to reach the bone.

Insertion of a cortical screw in lag fashion is performed in a routine manner except that the thread hole is drilled first because it generally is not possible to use the drill sleeve insert to center the glide hole and the thread hole. Once the correct position is found for insertion of the screw with the K-wire and viewing with the C-arm, a tap sleeve is slid over the K-wire and pushed down to contact the ilium. The tap sleeve

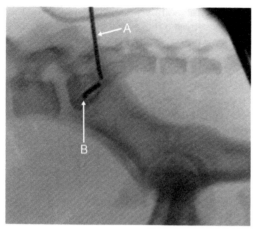

Fig. 2. Once the sacroiliac joint is reduced, a K-wire (*arrow A*) of appropriate size is driven across the sacroiliac joint caudal to the area that the lag screw will be placed to temporarily maintain reduction of the sacroiliac joint. (*Arrow B*) A K-wire that has been used to find the correct insertion position of the screw used to stabilize the sacroiliac joint.

is positioned such that one can see directly down the center of the tap sleeve (only seeing a round circle when viewing from the lateral position) (**Fig. 3**). Insertion of a tap sleeve allows all the drilling and tapping to be done without removal of the tap sleeve. If the sacrum is in a true lateral position and the tap sleeve is correctly positioned, the thread hole can be drilled completely across the sacrum without worry of penetrating the spinal canal or the disk space or coming out ventrally. The glide hole is next drilled by finding the entrance to the thread hole in the ilium with the tip of the glide hole drill bit and enlarging it just through the ilium. Usually the drill bit drop can be felt once it goes through the ilium. The length of the screw is determined by measuring the difference between a K-wire inserted to the bottom of the screw hole and a K-wire inserted to the lateral aspect of the ilium next to the screw hole. From preoperative measurements of the ilium and sacrum, the minimum length of screw

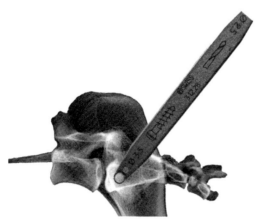

Fig. 3. The tap sleeve is positioned such that one can see directly down the center of the tap sleeve (only seeing a round circle when viewing from the lateral position).

that is acceptable (60% of sacral width) is determined. A screw that is slightly shorter than the measured distance is inserted to make sure that the screw does not bottom out on the hole. If the screw bottoms out, compression across the joint does not occur and there is a risk of stripping the screw threads. A washer can be added to the screw to decrease the chance of the head of the screw tearing through the ilial cortex (**Fig. 4**). A second screw can be added in some dogs. Typically, the K-wire is removed because it is difficult to cut it flush with the bone. A couple of sutures are placed to close the skin incision.

The second method uses a cannulated drill bit to correctly position the screw hole. In this technique, a K-wire that corresponds to the size of the cannulated drill bit used is positioned and driven across the ilium and sacrum. If the sacrum is in a perfect lateral position, the K-wire should be viewed perfectly on end (a dot) when viewing from the lateral aspect. Once the K-wire is in place, the cannulated drill bit is slipped over the K-wire and the screw hole drilled. This is the thread hole for the screw in the sacrum. The appropriate-sized drill bit for the glide hole is then inserted down to the ilium and a glide hole drilled just across the ilium. A cortical screw with an attached washer is then inserted through the tissue and tightened. A cannulated screw is not used because it is expensive and not as strong as a regular cortical screw.

Postoperative care of patients after closed reduction and lag screw fixation of sacroiliac fracture-luxation is the same as repair of any pelvic fracture/luxation case. Because most of these patients have contralateral pelvic injuries plus potentially other lower extremity fractures, restricted activity and weight support are required. Rechecking radiographic examination at 4 weeks and 8 weeks after repair is advised. In most cases, adequate healing is present at 4 weeks postoperatively such that the repair is unlikely to fail.

DISCUSSION

Closed reduction and screw fixation of sacroiliac fracture-luxation has been shown an effective method of treating this traumatic injury to the pelvis of dogs and cats.[6,7] Advantages of this procedure are minimal soft tissue disruption with less pain and chance for infection, good reduction of the luxation, precise screw placement, low percentage of screw loosening, and an early return to use of the leg on the luxation side. The minimally invasive technique for repair of sacroiliac fracture-luxations is fast, consistently more accurate, and less traumatic for patients than an open technique, in my experience.

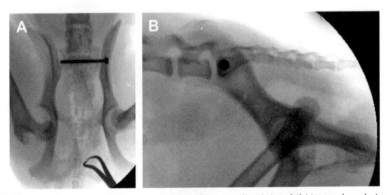

Fig. 4. Correct placement of the screw across the sacroiliac joint. (*A*) Ventrodorsal view; (*B*) lateral view. The sacroiliac joint has been anatomically reduced and the screw goes completely across the sacrum.

Accurate reduction of the sacroiliac joint is important for the success of the procedure. In a report about open reduction of sacroiliac fracture-luxation, screw loosening occurred in 22% of cases when greater than 90% reduction was achieved compared, with 41% when less than 90% reduction was achieved.[2] In the first report of closed reduction and screw fixation of sacroiliac joint fracture-luxation repair, no screw loosening occurred with a mean reduction of 92% (range 79.55%–100%).[6] In a subsequent report on closed reduction and screw fixation of sacroiliac joint fracture-luxation repair, the mean percent reduction of the sacroiliac fracture-luxation was 91% (range 51%–100%).[7] In this report, 3 cortical screws loosened and 2 of these sacroiliac joints had reduction of less than 90%. Five of the 24 sacroiliac joints had reduction less than 90%.[7] Reduction of greater than 90% should be easy to achieve with accurate fluoroscopic assessment.

Another method of assessing the adequacy of reduction is to measure the pelvic canal width. The mean pelvic canal diameter ratio has been reported greater than 1.1 (range 1.07–1.82).[10] In the first report of closed reduction and screw fixation of sacroiliac fracture luxation, the mean pelvic canal width ratio was 1.2 immediately postoperatively and 1.11 at the last examination.[6] In the second report of closed reduction and screw fixation of sacroiliac fracture luxation, the mean pelvic canal width ratio was 1.17 immediately postoperatively and 1.06 at the last examination.[7] This indicates that the pelvic canal had been returned to close to its normal width and that stenosis of the pelvic canal did not occur.

Cortical screws are the implant of choice for most cases. In the 2 reports of closed reduction and screw fixation of sacroiliac fracture-luxation, 1 cancellous screw broke and 1 cannulated screw bent.[6,7] The cannulated screw that bent was associated with catastrophic failure of the bone plate repair of an ilial fracture on the opposite hemipelvis.[6] A screw of the proper diameter compared with the size of the sacrum is probably more important in preventing screw breakage than screw type. Percutaneous fluoroscopically assisted placement of a transiliosacral rod to stabilize sacroiliac fracture-luxations after limited open reduction has also been described.[11]

Screw length has been shown an important factor in screw loosening after repair of sacroiliac fracture-luxation using an open repair technique.[2] In this study, a 7% screw loosening rate was found when the cumulative screw depth/sacral width was greater than 60%.[2] A 48% screw loosening rate was found when the cumulative screw depth/sacral width was less than 60%.[2] In the 35 sacroiliac fracture-reductions that were repaired with a closed reduction and screw fixation technique, 3 (8.5%) screws loosened.[6,7] The mean screw lengths/sacral widths were 79% and 64% postoperatively in these 2 reports of a closed reduction and screw fixation.[6,7] A significant difference between the open and closed techniques was that in the closed reduction technique only 1 screw was used, whereas in the open technique, 22% of the cases had more than 1 screw placed.[2,6,7] In the open repair technique, placement of multiple screws was not thought important in screw loosening.[2] In a study evaluating static strength of sacroiliac fracture-separation repairs, 2 screws were stronger than 1 screw of similar size, 2 small screws were stronger than a single larger screw, and a reduction pin added no significant strength to a single screw repair.[12] In this study, failure of the implant occurred by pullout of the screws and not breakage. Considering the low loosening rate of 1 proper length and properly placed screw (1/33 or 3%) for a closed reduction and screw fixation technique, a single screw of the correct diameter is recommended.[6,7]

Correct location of the screw is also important in repair of sacroiliac fracture-luxations. The screw needs to be placed in the first sacral vertebral body. The location of the screw can be easily visualized fluoroscopically. Use of a K-wire to find the spot on the first sacral vertebral body for screw insertion is easy accomplished. To allow the screw to be directed across the sacral body the proper depth (minimum of 60%), proper alignment of the sacrum in a true lateral position is required. A screw can be placed across the entire width of the sacrum. It is important to not place the screw into the vertebral canal, the lumbosacral disk space or intervertebral foramen, the body of the seventh lumbar vertebra, or pelvic sacral foramina.

The question arises as to the need to repair sacroiliac fracture-luxations. In the past, surgical wisdom has been that sacroiliac fracture-luxations can adequately heal on their own without repair. Some patients regain acceptable function without surgical repair. Some of the philosophy of not doing surgery probably comes from the difficulty that has been encountered in correct screw placement and reduction of sacroiliac fracture-luxations from an open technique. In my practice, just about all sacroiliac fracture-luxations are repaired because of the benefit to patients and the ease of performing the procedure. Most patients have significant injury to the opposite hemipelvis that requires surgical repair. Some patients also have injuries to the lower extremities, such as fractures of the tibia or femur. My philosophy about repair of sacroiliac fracture-luxations is that stability can be provided to this part of the hemipelvis, which translates into less pain and a quicker return to use and better function. In the first report of this technique, 9 of 13 dogs were willing to use the sacroiliac fracture-luxation side the day after surgery and 1 more dog was willing to walk on the leg 2 days after surgery. The only dogs (3) that did not walk on the leg soon after surgery had sciatic nerve injury due to the original trauma that caused the fracture-luxation.[6] In most cases, patients use the side with the sacroiliac repair before and better than the opposite side with an ilial or acetabular fracture repair. This all is in relationship to what other types of injuries that a patient has.

In summary, a minimally invasive technique for repair of sacroiliac-fracture luxations is a viable option for repair of this injury and has considerable benefits. Reduction and fixation of a minimally invasive technique is comparable to an open technique without the associated morbidity of an open technique. A minimally invasive technique, however, requires intraoperative fluoroscopy and associated possible radiation exposure.

REFERENCES

1. DeCamp CE. Principles of pelvic fracture management. Semin Vet Med Surg (Small Anim) 1992;7(1):63–70.
2. DeCamp CE, Braden TD. Sacroiliac fracture-separation in the dog a study of 92 cases. Vet Surg 1985;14(2):127–30.
3. Bowlt KL, Shales CJ. Canine sacroiliac luxation: anatomic study of the craniocaudal articular surface angulation of the sacrum to define a safe corridor in the dorsal plane for placement of screws used for fixation in lag fashion. Vet Surg 2011;40(1):22–6.
4. Shales CJ, Langley-Hobbs SJ. Canine sacroiliac luxation: anatomic study of dorsoventral articular surface angulation and safe corridor for placement of screws used for lag fixation. Vet Surg 2005;34(4):324–31.
5. Joseph R, Milgram J, Zhan K, et al. In vitro study of the ilial anatomic landmarks for safe implant insertion in the first sacral vertebra of the intact canine sacroiliac joint. Vet Surg 2006;35(6):510–7.
6. Tomlinson JL, Cook JL, Payne JT, et al. Closed reduction and lag screw fixation of sacroiliac luxations and fractures. Vet Surg 1999;28(3):188–93.
7. Tonks CA, Tomlinson JL, Cook JL. Evaluation of closed reduction and screw fixation in lag fashion of sacroiliac fracture-luxations. Vet Surg 2008;37(7):603–7.

8. Gregory CR, Cullen JM, Pool R, et al. The canine sacroiliac joint. Preliminary study of anatomy, histopathology, and biomechanics. Spine (Phila Pa 1976) 1986;11(10): 1044–8.

9. DeCamp CE, Braden TD. The surgical anatomy of the canine sacrum for lag screw fixation of the sacroiliac joint. Vet Surg 1985;14(2):131–4.

10. Averill SM, Johnson AL, Schaeffer DJ. Risk factors associated with development of pelvic canal stenosis secondary to sacroiliac separation: 84 cases (1985–1995). J Am Vet Med Assoc 1997;211(1):75–8.

11. Leasure CS, Lewis DD, Sereda CW, et al. Limited open reduction and stabilization of sacroiliac fracture-luxations using fluoroscopically assisted placement of a trans-iliosacral rod in five dogs. Vet Surg 2007;36(7):633–43.

12. Radasch RM, Merkley DF, Hoefle WD, et al. Static strength evaluation of sacroiliac fracture-separation repairs. Vet Surg 1990;19(2):155–61.

Percutaneous Plate Arthrodesis in Small Animals

Antonio Pozzi, DMV, MS*, Daniel D. Lewis, DVM,
Caleb C. Hudson, DVM, MS, Stanley E. Kim, BVSc, MS

KEYWORDS

- Minimally invasive • Arthrodesis • Percutaneous • Dogs • Cats • Small animals

KEY POINTS

- Arthrodesis is an elective salvage procedure designed to eliminate joint pain and/or dysfunction by deliberate osseous fusion.
- Open arthrodesis requires an extensive surgical approach that can cause vascular trauma leading to soft tissue complications.
- Percutaneous arthrodesis is performed using limited surgical approaches, which do not require joint disarticulation. The bone plate is inserted through small plate insertion incisions.
- Intraoperative imaging is used to guide cartilage debridement and implant fixation.
- Percutaneous arthrodesis has been successfully used for carpal and hock disorders.
- A traditional open arthrodesis may be preferable to a percutaneous approach in animals with chronic osseous malalignment.

INTRODUCTION

One of the most useful applications of percutaneous plating in small animals is percutaneous distal extremity arthrodesis. Carpal and hock arthrodeses can be associated with the development of substantial postoperative complications.[1] The risk of several specific postoperative complications can be decreased by performing these procedures with minimally invasive plate osteosynthesis (MIPO) techniques. Articular debridement performed through limited approaches and application of the plate through small insertion incisions minimizes the degree of periarticular iatrogenic soft tissue trauma. Preservation of the regional soft tissues facilitates tension-free closure, and mitigates disturbance of the extraosseous blood supply to the arthrodesis site. The MIPO technique for arthrodesis consequently may decrease the risk of infection, wound dehiscence, distal limb ischemia, and subsequent necrosis, as well as accelerate union of the arthrodesis sites.

Department of Small Animal Clinical Sciences, College of Veterinary Medicine, University of Florida, 2015 Southwest 16th Avenue, PO Box 100126, Gainesville, FL 32610-0126, USA
* Corresponding author.
E-mail address: pozzia@ufl.edu

Vet Clin Small Anim 42 (2012) 1079–1096
http://dx.doi.org/10.1016/j.cvsm.2012.07.001
0195-5616/12/$ – see front matter © 2012 Elsevier Inc. All rights reserved.

Arthrodesis is an elective surgical procedure that eliminates motion in a joint through deliberate osseous fusion.[2–24] Arthrodesis is considered a salvage procedure. The primary indication for any arthrodesis is unremitting joint pain or dysfunction that interferes with daily activities and that cannot be resolved by other treatment modalities (such as administration of analgesic and nonsteroidal antiinflammatory medications, weight loss, and physical rehabilitation). Arthrodesis is performed to relieve chronic joint pain, to resolve irreparable joint instability, to arrest progressively destructive arthropathies, and to resolve postural dysfunction resulting from neurologic deficits.[15,18] Arthrodesis must be distinguished from ankylosis. Ankylosis is joint immobility which develops secondary to a severe, progressive degenerative process. Although motion in the affected joint may become severely limited, the process does not progress to osseous fusion and ankylosis is often associated with chronic pain and dysfunction.

There are four surgical requirements for performing an arthrodesis[4,15,18]: (1) debridement of the articular cartilage, (2) placement of a bone graft,[25] (3) positioning the involved limb segment at a functional angle, and (4) application of stable fixation.[8,13] First, the articular cartilage needs to be debrided from the involved joint spaces to allow for eventual osseous fusion.[26] Debridement is typically performed using a high-speed pneumatic drill and a burr, but can be done manually with a curette.[15] After the cartilage has been removed to expose the subchondral bone, the debrided joint spaces are packed with autogenous cancellous bone graft (allogenic grafts or other graft substitutes can be used in place of an autogenous cancellous bone graft) to expedite osseous union of the arthrodesis.[15,18] The involved limb segment should be stabilized in a functional position and maintained in that position with appropriate, stable fixation. Most arthrodeses are rigidly stabilized with plates[2,5,6,11,17,26]; however, transarticular external fixators and, in some instances, transarticular pins or Kirschner wires can be used to provide stable, but not rigid, fixation.[10,16,27,28] Transarticular pins or Kirschner wires are more useful in younger dogs and cats, which usually obtain osseous union in a short period of time, typically between 8 and 12 weeks.[14]

Owners must be informed before surgery that an arthrodesis is an involved surgical procedure and there is considerable morbidity associated with the surgical approach, debridement of the involved joint, and implant application.[1] The extensive surgical approach typically used may cause vascular trauma leading to soft tissue complications. Plantar necrosis has been reported following tarsal arthrodeses, most likely caused by iatrogenic trauma to the dorsal pedal artery or the perforating metatarsal artery.[1] Bone plates are often applied on mechanically unfavorable bone surfaces. Plates are frequently placed on the compressive surface rather than the tensile surface of the secured bone segments because the compressive surface is more readily accessible. These mechanical inadequacies can predispose to both early and late implant failure. The involved limb segment is often placed in a cast or splint, or an adjunctive external fixator may be used to supplement plate stabilization in an effort to prevent early implant failure. Owners must also be warned that fusion of one joint may place abnormal stress on adjacent joints, and the lack of mobility in the arthrodesed limb segment may predispose the limb to future trauma. Owners need to be adequately forewarned of possible adverse sequelae and complications before surgery[1,29]; however, the benefits of arthrodesis generally outweigh potential risks and possible complications, and functional outcomes can be excellent.[17,30,31]

Percutaneous plating has evolved to allow plates to be applied through small insertion incisions made remote to the site being stabilized. Although this technique was developed to stabilize fractures, the technique can also be used when performing arthrodeses.[32] The MIPO technique conforms to the principles of biologic osteosynthesis because there is minimal disturbance of the adjacent soft tissues and vasculature supplying the bones undergoing stabilization.[33] Cadaveric studies have shown that periosteal vessels are preserved to a greater extent when using an MIPO technique compared with a conventional open plating application.[34,35] Conservation of the local circulation should accelerate osseous union with fewer postoperative complications.[35–37]

Minimally invasive arthrodesis techniques were first described for human patients to minimize soft tissue complications and decrease the risk of postoperative infection. Percutaneous interphalangeal,[38] metatarsal-phalangeal,[39] sacroiliac,[40] vertebral pedicle,[41] and ankle[42] arthrodeses have been reported in people. Cartilage debridement is not performed as extensively as in open approaches and the implants are applied through small plate insertion incisions. One of the unique aspects of some described percutaneous arthrodeses procedures is that cartilage debridement is performed via fluoroscopic guidance or arthroscopy.[39,40,42–44] Successful fusion following ankle arthrodesis without cartilage debridement has been reported in human patients with rheumatoid arthritis.[43] Arthrodesis without cartilage debridement has also been investigated in experimental animal models.[45,46] Patellofemoral arthrodesis was performed in rabbits using two lag screws without cartilage debridement.[45] Histologic evidence of osseous fusion was demonstrated in most animals, showing that compression and rigid fixation without cartilage debridement can result in successful joint fusion. The effect of synovial fluid depletion and immobilization of the articular surfaces was also evaluated in a rabbit patellofemoral model.[46] Synovial depletion in combination with drilling a hole through the cartilage and subchondral bone resulted in bone bridging across the joint, leading the investigators to recommend this technique for percutaneous arthrodeses without cartilage debridement.[46] A limited surgical approach that does not require joint disarticulation or complete articular cartilage debridement has been described to facilitate pastern arthrodesis in horses.[47] Pastern arthrodeses were performed in 12 limbs (11 horse) affected by chronic osteoarthritis. Limited cartilage debridement was performed by distracting the proximal interphalangeal joint and drilling holes through the articular surface. Good outcomes were obtained in 9 horses (10 limbs).[47] Although it is difficult translating experimental data[45,46] or clinical data in human patients[43] and horses[32,47,48] to dogs with naturally occurring joint disease, these studies suggest that a more conservative approach to cartilage debridement may be sufficient to promote successful joint fusion.

Although the high-motion joints such as the talocrural and antebrachiocarpal joints can be thoroughly debrided through an incision of 2 to 3 cm, a limited articular cartilage debridement may be performed of the other joints. Aggressive open debridement of articular cartilage and application of a bone plate and screws can result in vascular compromise following both pantarsal and tarsometatarsal arthrodeses.[1] In addition, swelling and edema may make closure of the soft tissues over implants difficult when using a traditional open approach. Tension induced by closure can produce a tourniquet effect that may further inhibit venous and lymphatic return from the paw. Preserving bridges of intact skin and soft tissue between the plate insertion incisions, as well as any additional incision required for articular debridement, are likely responsible for the nominal soft tissue swelling we have observed following percutaneous arthrodesis. In addition, avoiding disarticulation of the joint to facilitate cartilage debridement may further decrease the risk of vascular injuries. We have observed minimal postoperative soft tissue swelling and edema formation in hock arthrodeses performed using minimally invasive techniques compared with hock arthrodeses performed using an open surgical approach.

Obtaining and maintaining compression across the debrided joint space is of utmost importance when performing percutaneous arthrodesis with limited cartilage debridement. Cartilage surfaces that are sustained in direct contact become deprived of nutrients normally provided by synovial fluid and, in some instances, may fuse without cartilage debridement.[45] Compression of the joint space can be achieved using a plate, lag screws, pin and tension band fixation, or an external fixator. Maintaining articular surface congruency is important to obtain intimate contact of the articular surfaces and to achieve acceptable postoperative stability. When cartilage debridement is performed, it is important to preserve the underlying subchondral bone. Subchondral bone loss may increase the gap between the articular surfaces and delay osseous union.

Hock Arthrodesis

Indications

Hock arthrodesis is often necessary to restore hind limb function in dogs or cats with severe traumatic or degenerative conditions affecting the talocrural, intertarsal, and/or tarsometatarsal joints.[2,5,6,9,11,18,27,28,49] Indications for hock arthrodeses include shearing injuries, particularly injuries with substantial osseous trauma, marked degenerative joint disease, which is some dogs is secondary to osteochondritis dissecans, chronic ligamentous instability or intra-articular fractures, irreparable Achilles tendon injuries, and, in some instances, neurologic dysfunction associated with sciatic nerve damage.[18] Pantarsal arthrodesis is often performed to resolve pain and dysfunction affecting the talocrural joint irrespective of whether the disorder involves distal articulations of the hock. Partial tarsal arthrodeses that pertain to arthrodesis of the intertarsal and tarsometatarsal articulations are performed in animals with disorders involving the intertarsal or tarsometatarsal joints without evidence of talocrural disorder. Animals should be thoroughly evaluated before committing to a partial arthrodesis because a pantarsal arthrodesis may be preferable even if a minor talocrural disorder is present.

Percutaneous arthrodesis can be performed in most situations in which an open arthrodesis would be considered. The signalment of the animal does not limit consideration of percutaneous arthrodesis. Animals with marked preexisting conformational deformities may be better treated with an open arthrodesis, especially if a corrective ostectomy is indicated as a component of the procedure. In animals with chronic tarsal disorders, fibrous tissue may prevent proper alignment of stabilized bone segments. Percutaneous rather than open arthrodesis may be preferable in animals with acute distal extremity traumatic soft tissue injuries. The circulation to the hind paw may already be compromised as a result of the inciting traumatic incident, predisposing the paw to vascular complications following surgery. The amount of iatrogenic soft tissue trauma induced during a percutaneous arthrodesis is nominal compared with that of traditional arthrodeses using open approaches.

Surgical anatomy

The talocrural joint is a modified hinge joint consisting of the tibia, fibula, and talus.[50] The articular surface of the distal tibia is concave and conforms to the contour of the talus. The congruity of this joint should be maintained when performing a pantarsal arthrodesis to improve the postoperative stability. The proximal surface of the talocrural joint is bordered medially by the medial malleolus, which projects distal to the joint line and articulates with the medial surface of the talus. Performing a malleolar ostectomy allows ready access to the talocrural joint for cartilage debridement and obviates the need for extensive plate contouring when applying a medial plate to stabilize a pantarsal arthrodesis. The bones of the tarsus (**Fig. 1**A) articulate at several levels and are stabilized by a complex of ligaments on the plantar and dorsal surfaces. The medial and lateral collateral ligaments span the hock joint bilaterally. Numerous

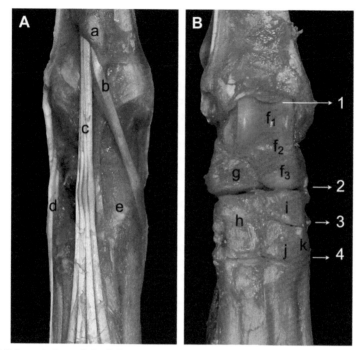

Fig. 1. (*A*) Dorsal view of the left tarsus after removal of skin, subcutaneous tissue, fascia, superficial veins and nerves: (a) proximal extensor retinaculum; (b) m. tibialis cranialis tendon; (c) m. extensor digitorum longus tendon; (d) m. extensor digitorum lateralis, m. peroneus longus, and m. peroneus brevis tendons; (e) short dorsal tarsal ligaments. (*B*) Dorsal view of the left tarsus after removal of ligaments and tendons: (f_1) talus, trochlea; (f_2) talus, neck; (f_3) talus, head; (g) calcaneus; (h) fourth tarsal bone; (i) central tarsal bone; (j) third tarsal bone; (k) second and first tarsal bones; (1) talocrural joint; (2) proximal intertarsal joint; (3) distal intertarsal joint; (4) tarsometatarsal joint.

short dorsal ligaments connect the individual tarsal bones (see **Fig. 1**A). A large ligament unites the talus with the third and fourth tarsal bones. Oblique ligaments connect the central and second tarsal bones, as well as the central with the third tarsal bone. The distal row of tarsal bones is joined to the proximal ends of the metatarsal bones by small ligaments. The ligaments on the plantar surfaces are thicker than those on the dorsal surface. A more distinct ligament extends from the body of the calcaneus to the fourth tarsal bone and distally inserts to the bases of metatarsals IV and V.[50]

Preoperative planning

Hock arthrodeses are major elective procedures and a complete evaluation of the animal is warranted before surgery. Obtaining a thorough history is essential because preexisting medical conditions such Cushing disease or diabetes may predispose the animal to delayed healing or increased risk of infection. A systematic orthopedic examination should be performed to identify conformational deformities and soft tissue injuries, and to define the location and extent of disorders. The animal should be evaluated for concurrent orthopedic abnormalities in the affected limb, as well as the other three limbs, to ensure that concurrent orthopedic problems will not impair function following arthrodesis. A neurologic evaluation should be performed to identify neurologic dysfunction that could impair function or predispose to hind paw ulceration.

Orthogonal radiographs of the distal tibia and fibula, tarsus, and hind paw should be obtained for preoperative planning. Stress radiography may be used to identify the level or levels of instability. The bone plate should be preselected and precontoured using the preoperative radiographs. The diameter of the metatarsal bones should be measured from a lateral view to determine the appropriate screw diameter. The diameter of screws to be placed in the metatarsal bones should not exceed 30% of the diameter of the metatarsal bones. Hybrid 2.0/2.7-mm or 2.7/3.5-mm plates (Veterinary Instrumentation, Sheffield, United Kingdom) can be used for proximal intertarsal and tarsometatarsal arthrodeses because these hybrid plates allow smaller diameter screws to be inserted distal in the metatarsal bones.[49] Precontoured angled plates of 2.0 to 2.7 mm or 2.7 to 3.5 mm are also available for medial plate application for performing pantarsal arthrodesis.[11] A medially applied plate for arthrodesis has the mechanical benefit of being loaded through the plate's widest dimension during weight bearing.[51] Locking implants can be used for hock arthrodeses. There are several advantages of using an angle stable plate to stabilize an arthrodesis.[52,53] The angular stability provided by the screw head–plate locking mechanism decreases the risk of implant failure caused by screw pullout. Another advantage of using a locking plate is that the implant does not need to be accurately contoured to the surface of the underlying bones if locking screws are used. The fixed angle of insertion of the locking screws can be problematic when placing screws in the metatarsal bones, and the plate must align so that screws properly engage the metatarsal bones.

Patient positioning

The animal is positioned in dorsal recumbency with the affected limb positioned at the end of the table. The ipsilateral proximal humerus should be prepared and draped for procurement of autogenous bone graft. Depending on which side of the limb the plate will be applied, the animal can be tilted laterally and the affected distal hind limb rested on a Mayo stand. Positioning should take into account the need for intraoperative image acquisition, with the ability to obtain both craniocaudal and lateral views.

Surgical technique: pantarsal arthrodesis using a medial plate

The procedure is usually performed through three incisions. The plate is used to mark the location of the incisions on the skin. The incision parallels the long axis of the tibia proximally and is centered over the anticipated location of the two most proximal holes of the plate. A centrally placed 3 cm incision is centered over the medial malleolus. The distal incision is marked at the anticipated location of the two most distal plate holes over the second metatarsal bone. After elevating the soft tissue from the medial malleolus and distal tibia, a malleolar ostectomy is performed (**Fig. 2**). The purpose of this ostectomy is to render the medial aspect of the distal tibia as flat as possible, which obviates the need for extensive contouring of the plate. Excision of the medial malleolus also allows exposure of the talocrural joint (see **Fig. 2**). The articular surfaces of the distal tibia and talus are denuded of cartilage without removing extensive amounts of subchondral bone, especially on the talus, so as not to compromise stability of the arthrodesis. Metzenbaum scissors are used to develop an epiperiosteal tunnel joining the three skin incisions. This tunnel should be developed adjacent to the cortical surface, deep to the overlying soft tissue structures, without damaging the periosteum.

The intertarsal articulations are debrided through the central incision (**Fig. 3A**), by retracting the commissure of the skin distally. The tarsometatarsal joints are debrided through two 3 to 5 mm long incisions positioned medially and laterally on the paw. Debridement performed through these bilateral incisions allows reasonable access

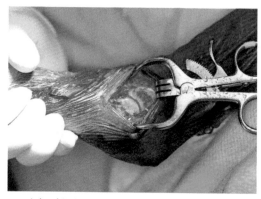

Fig. 2. A 2 cm linear straight skin incision was made over the talocrural joint. The incision is long enough to allow sufficient exposure to excise the medial malleolus. The ostectomy gives sufficient exposure of the talocrural joint to allow effective cartilage debridement.

to all 4 tarsometatarsal articulations. A hypodermic needle is used to identify the joint spaces. Small individual incisions are made over the joint spaces and a number 15 blade or tenotomy scissors are used to separate the soft tissues so that a burr can be inserted into the joint spaces. Fluoroscopy can be used, if available, to facilitate this process (see **Fig. 3**B). The intertarsal and the tarsometatarsal joints can be debrided with a modified fanning technique, as described for carpometacarpal arthrodesis in horses.[54,55]

Autogenous cancellous bone graft (or a suitable alternative) is packed into the debrided joint spaces, or bone marrow or platelet-enriched plasma can be injected in joints that have not been sufficiently exposed for the placement of a bone graft.[56] The plate is inserted through either the proximal, middle or distal insertion incision and maneuvered through the epiperiosteal tunnel until the end of the plate emerges in the other insertion incision (**Fig. 4**). The paw must be properly aligned with respect to the proximal tibia and stifle before inserting screws through the plate. Fluoroscopy

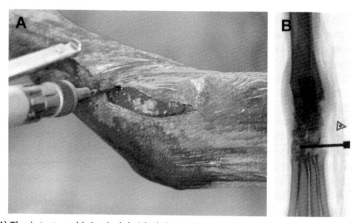

Fig. 3. (*A*) The intertarsal joint is debrided through the central skin incision by retracting the skin distally. Debridement of the tarsometatarsal joint is performed from the medial and lateral aspect through stab incisions. (*B*) Fluoroscopy is useful to evaluate the position and depth of the burr during debridement.

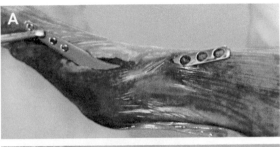

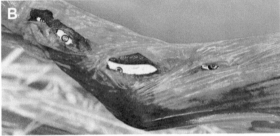

Fig. 4. (*A*) The plate is inserted through the middle incision toward the proximal skin incision, and then advanced distally (*B*).

can be used, if available, to assess the position of the plate and alignment of the limb before screw insertion (**Fig. 5**A). The first screw is inserted through the central hole of the plate into the talus. Two or more screws are inserted in the holes at each end of the plate, via the insertion incisions. The remaining screws are inserted in the holes in the plate through the insertion incisions or through stab incisions. All incisions should be closed routinely in two layers. Post-operative radiographs are obtained to assess the position of the implants and the alignment of the joint (**Fig. 6**C and D). Recheck radiographs are taken every 3 to 4 weeks until complete healing of the arthrodesis (**Fig. 6**E and F).

Surgical technique: partial tarsal arthrodesis

The procedure is usually performed through three small incisions and the plate is placed on the lateral aspect of the tarsus. The plate is used to mark the location of the incisions on the skin. The incision proximally parallels the calcaneus and is centered over the proximal aspect of the calcaneus. A centrally placed 2 cm incision is centered over the calcaneoquartal joint. The distal incision is marked at the anticipated location of the two most distal plate holes. After incising the skin and the subcutaneous tissue, the lateral intertarsal joints are exposed to allow cartilage debridement. The joints are debrided using a pneumatic drill and a burr through the central incision (**Fig. 7**A). The tarsometatarsal joint is debrided through separate medial and lateral stab incisions. Flattening the lateral aspect of the base of the fifth metatarsal bone decreases the amount of plate contouring required for plate application. Metzenbaum scissors are used to develop an epiperiosteal tunnel joining the three skin incisions (**Fig. 8**). Then the plate is inserted proximal to distal through the insertion incisions (**Fig. 7**B). The first screw is placed in proximally in the calcaneus. The second screw is placed in the most distal plate hole. It is important to place this screw in the center of the fifth metatarsal bone to decrease the risk of metatarsal fractures. The hole can be started using a Kirschner wire which is less likely to slip off the convex surface of the fifth metatarsal bone. At least three screws are placed in the

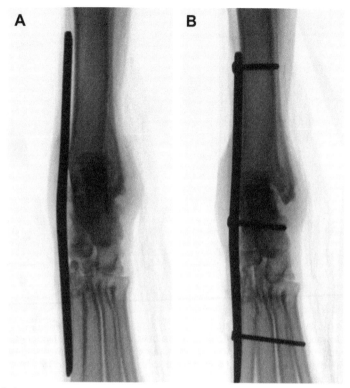

Fig. 5. (*A*) Fluoroscopy is used to assess limb alignment and the plate contouring. Performing an ostectomy of the medial malleolus, may obviate the need to contour the plate. (*B*) The first screw is inserted in the talus. Screws are then inserted in the metatarsus and in the tibia.

calcaneus, with the third screw engaging the head of the talus. One screw is placed into the fourth and central tarsal bone and at least three screws into the metatarsal bones. The skin incisions are closed routinely. Postoperative radiographs are obtained to assess the position of the implants and the alignment of the joint. Recheck radiographs are obtained every 3 to 4 weeks until complete healing of the arthrodesis (**Fig. 9**).

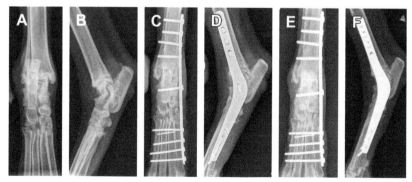

Fig. 6. (*A, B*) Preoperative radiographs (*C, D*), immediate postoperative radiographs (*E, F*) and 4 week postoperative recheck showing progressive healing.

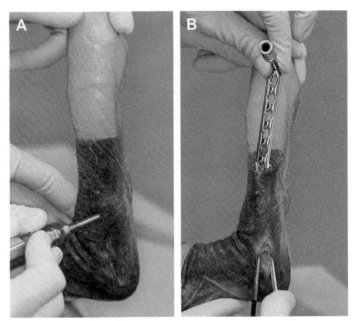

Fig. 7. (*A*) Articular cartilage debridement is performed with a high-speed pneumatic drill and a burr inserted through stab incisions made over the lateral and medial aspect of the intertarsal and tarsometatarsal joints. (*B*) The plate is inserted from distal to proximal through the epiperiosteal tunnel. Metzenbaum scissors can be used to facilitate the insertion of the plate.

Pancarpal Arthrodesis

Indications

Although pancarpal arthrodeses are associated with fewer postoperative complications than hock arthrodeses, percutaneous pancarpal arthrodeses afford many of the advantages previously alluded to for hock arthrodesis. Pancarpal arthrodesis is most commonly performed in dogs that sustain carpal hyperextension injuries or dogs with severe osteoarthritis.[4,7,10,14,15,19–22,57] Hyperextension injuries usually result in irreparable damage to the carpal palmar ligaments and palmar carpal fibrocartilage, which are the primary structures responsible for maintaining the carpus in a normal weight-bearing angle of 10° to 12° of extension. Medium and large breed dogs often sustain carpal hyperextension injuries as a result of falls or jumping. Acute traumatic carpal hyperextension or luxation injuries result in a painful, non weight bearing lameness; however, most animals attempt to bear weight on the affected limb within a few weeks of sustaining the injury. Chronic carpal hyperextension injuries typically do not seem to be overly painful and animals bear weight on the affected limb. Antebrachiocarpal arthrodesis is generally necessary to resolve the lameness and dysfunction associated with hyperextension injuries because conservative management typically fails to result in a functional outcome.[15] Other indications for pancarpal arthrodesis include erosive arthropathies and traumatic subluxation or luxation of the Antebrachiocarpal, intercarpal, and carpometacarpal joints. Most pancarpal arthrodeses can be performed using a percutaneous technique. A traditional open arthrodesis may be preferable to a percutaneous approach in animals with chronic osseous malalignment. For example, in an animal with chronic hyperextension injuries, an

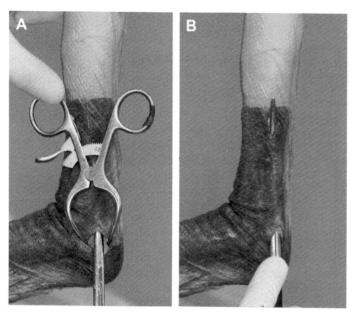

Fig. 8. (*A*) A linear incision of 5 to 10 mm is made lateral over the proximal aspect of the calcaneus. A longitudinal incision of 5 to 10 mm is made over the lateral aspect of the fifth metatarsal at the level where the plate will be positioned distally. A third middle stab incision is used to debride the intertarsal and tarsometatarsal joints. (*B*) The insertion tunnel is developed using straight Metzenbaum scissors that are advanced until a tunnel is created between the proximal and distal incisions.

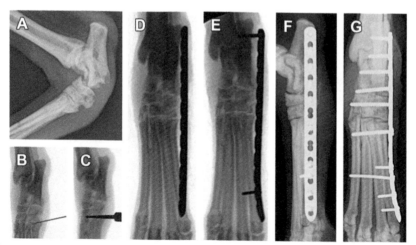

Fig. 9. (*A*) Preoperative medio lateral radiographic view of the tarsus showing a proximal intertarsal luxation, (*B*) intraoperative craniocaudal fluoroscopic view showing identification of the tarsometatarsal joints with a hypodermic needle (*C*) intraoperative craniocaudal fluoroscopic view showing cartilage debridement of the tarsometatarsal joints using a high-speed drill and burr; (*D*) intraoperative craniocaudal flouroscopic view demonstrating plate positioning to allow an estimation of the amount of plate controuring required; (*E*) intraoperative craniocaudal flouroscopic view demonstrating appropriate plate contouting and positioning after initial screw insertion; (*F, G*) postoperative mediolateral (*F*) and craniocaudal (*G*) radiographic views of a percutaneous partial arthrodesis performed with a 12-hole limited contact compression plate.

ostectomy may be necessary to realign the joint prior to plating. For this reason, dogs with overt deformity may be better suited for open arthrodesis.

Surgical anatomy

The carpus is composed of three joints: antebrachiocarpal, middle carpal, and carpometacarpal articulations (**Fig. 10B**). Several tendons and ligaments cross the joints (**Fig. 10A**). One of the unique anatomic features of the carpus is that the carpal collateral ligaments do not span all three joints. The ligaments of the carpus are generally short and most span only one joint level, connecting individual carpal bones together. Palmar stability of the carpus depends predominantly on the integrity of the palmar carpal fibrocartilage and ligaments.

Preoperative planning

Evaluation of a potential candidate for a pancarpal arthrodesis is similar to that described for hock arthrodesis. Obtaining a thorough history and performing a systematic orthopedic examination are necessary to exclude underlying systemic disease or orthopedic abnormalities that might prevent a full return to function. Orthogonal radiographs of the carpus including the distal third of the antebrachium and the reminder of the paw should be obtained to allow preoperative selection of the appropriate size implants. Selection of an adequate length plate and proper screw diameter can be problematic in some animals. The width of the third metacarpal bone is typically the limiting factor in implant selection because the diameter of the screw should not exceed 30% of the diameter of the bone. Hybrid plates are available, designed

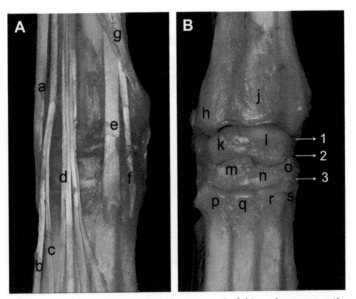

Fig. 10. (A) Dorsal view of the right carpus after removal of skin, subcutaneous tissue, fascia, superficial veins and nerves: (a) m. extensor carpi ulnaris tendon; (b, c) m. extensor digitorum lateralis tendons; (d) m. extensor digitorum communis tendon; (e, f) m. extensor carpi radialis tendons; (g) m. abductor pollicis longus tendon. (B) Dorsal view of the right carpus after removal of ligaments and tendons: (h) ulna; (j) radius; (k) ulnar carpal bone; (l) radial carpal bone; (m) fourth carpal bone; (n) third carpal bone; (o) second carpal bone; (p) fifth metacarpal bone; (q) fourth metacarpal bone; (r) third metacarpal bone; (s) second metacarpal bone; (1) antebrachiocarpal joint; (2) middle carpal joint; (3) carpometacarpal joint.

specifically for pancarpal arthrodesis.[20,21,23] The plate should extend at least half of the length of the third metacarpal bone to minimize the risk of postoperative fracture.[29]

Patient position
The animal is positioned in dorsal recumbency with the affected limb extended to allow the surgeon to access the dorsal aspect of the antebrachium and paw. The ipsilateral proximal humerus should be prepared and draped for the procurement of autogenous bone graft. For imaging with fluoroscopy, the limb is suspended vertically, which facilitates imaging. The animal's position on the table should allow the C arm of the fluoroscope to be rotated around the limb to obtain orthogonal view images of the carpus.

Surgical technique: pancarpal arthrodesis
Percutaneous arthrodesis is performed through three incisions. The central incision should be approximately 2 to 3 cm long and centered on the radiocarpal joint (**Fig. 11**). The plate is used to mark the location of the proximal and distal plate incisions on the skin. After the central incision is made, the articular cartilage of the antebrachiocarpal and intercarpal joints are debrided with a pneumatic high-speed drill and burr through that incision. The carpometacarpal joints can usually be accessed through a central incision by retracting the skin distally, or through separate stab incision positioned over the joint. Once the articular cartilage has been debrided, the carpus is flexed and cancellous bone graft is placed in the former joint spaces. Placing the graft prior to plate application facilitates effective packing the debrided joint

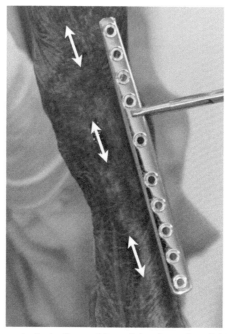

Fig. 11. The white arrows indicate the position of the three dorsal skin incisions to perform a percutaneous pancarpal arthrodesis. The middle incision is centered over the radiocarpal joint. The proximal and distal skin incisions are located at the level of the proximal and distal ends of the plate.

spaces with graft. The flare of the cranial surface of the distal radius can be flattened by partially debriding the protuberance with a high-speed drill and burr, which reduces the amount of plate contouring necessary for the plate to conform to the cranial aspect of the distal radius. The plate should be contoured to produce approximately 10° of carpal extension. The plate should extend as distal as possible on the third metacarpal bone.[15]

The plate insertion tunnel is developed using Metzembaum scissors and a periosteal elevator if necessary. Proximally, the plate is positioned under the extensor tendons. The tendons of the adductor pollicus longus muscle and extensor carpi radialis muscle on the second and third metacarpal bones can be elevated percutaneously using a periosteal elevator. The general principles of plate application for pancarpal apply to percutaneous plate arthrodesis. The first screw is placed in the radial carpal bone, but this screw is not tightened. The second screw is placed in the most distal plate hole. The screw hole should be in the center of the dorsal aspect of the third metacarpal bone. To ensure that the hole is drilled in the center of the bone, the plate is removed, two needles are inserted along the medial and lateral aspect of the third metacarpal bone, and a Kirschner wire is used to pre-drill a pilot hole for screw placement. The craniomedial proximal plate insertion incision allows placement of the screws in the proximal radius. A screw can be inserted in the distal radius through the central incision. The distal plate insertion incision is used to insert two or preferably three screws into the third metacarpal bone (**Fig. 12**). An additional screw may be placed in the base of the third metacarpal bone through a separate stab incision. Postoperative radiographs are obtained to assess implant position and joint alignment. Recheck radiographs are obtained every 3 to 4 weeks until there is radiographic evidence of bone bridging at the arthrodesis site (**Fig. 13**).

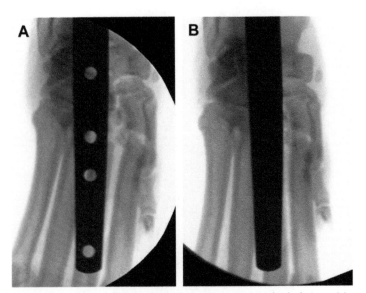

Fig. 12. (*A*) One of the distal screws is placed first to ensure that the hole is positioned in the middle of the third metacarpal bone. Note the valgus angulation of the paw caused by the metacarpal fracture. (*B*) Before placing a second screw in the third metacarpal bone, valgus is corrected by direct manipulation of the paw. After correcting the malalignment, the additional screws are inserted.

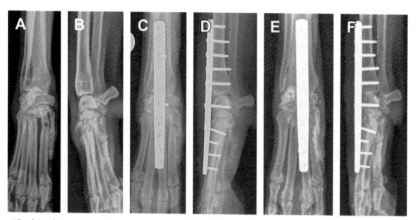

Fig. 13. (*A, B*) Preoperative radiographs, (*C, D*) immediate postoperative radiographs and (*E, F*) 4 week postoperative radiographs showing progressive healing.

Immediate postoperative care

Tarsal and carpal arthrodesis sites are protected by immobilizing the arthrodesed limb segment in an external coaptation splint for 2 to 3 months following surgery.[15,18] The duration of coaptation depends on the age of the animal and the radiographic progression toward union of the arthrodeses. A gradual return to normal activity is allowed over the subsequent 4 weeks following splint removal. Plate removal may become necessary in some animals following union because of screw loosening or extensor tendon inflammation. Motion between the metatarsal bones during weight bearing may cause loosening of the distal screws in animals that have undergone tarsal arthrodeses. Pancarpal arthrodeses are also predisposed to implant loosening as a consequence of the plate being applied to the compressive (dorsal) surface of the distal forelimb.[58]

SUMMARY

Most dogs and cats are able to resume normal activity following arthrodesis of the tarsus and carpus; however, major complications can develop following traditional open arthrodeses, especially following tarsal arthrodesis. The percutaneous arthrodesis technique described in this article may offer some advantages compared with open arthrodesis. When performing percutaneous arthrodesis, cartilage debridement is less extensive than when performed for open arthrodesis. The high-motion joints, such as the talocrural and antebrachiocarpal joints, can be thoroughly debrided through an incision of 2 to 3 cm, which allows the same exposure as with open approach. The other smaller, low-motion joints can be effectively debrided through separate stab incisions. Although cartilage debridement performed in this manner is conservative, we have noted a high rate of osseous union with a limited number of complications. Future comparative studies are needed to determine whether the percutaneous technique is superior to the traditional open arthrodesis technique and to define recommended guidelines for patient selection for percutaneous arthrodesis.

REFERENCES

1. Roch SP, Clements DN, Mitchell RA, et al. Complications following tarsal arthrodesis using bone plate fixation in dogs. J Small Anim Pract 2008;49:117–26.

2. Allen M, Dyce J, Houlton J. Calcaneoquartal arthrodesis in the dog. J Small Anim Pract 1993;34:205–10.

3. Benson JA, Boudrieau RJ. Severe carpal and tarsal shearing injuries treated with an immediate arthrodesis in seven dogs. J Am Anim Hosp Assoc 2002;38: 370–80.

4. Buote NJ, McDonald D, Radasch R. Pancarpal and partial carpal arthrodesis. Compend Contin Educ Vet 2009;31:180–92.

5. DeCamp CE, Martinez SA, Johnston SA. Pantarsal arthrodesis in dogs and a cat: 11 cases (1983-1991). J Am Vet Med Assoc 1993;203:1705–7.

6. Dyce J, Whitelock RG, Robinson KV, et al. Arthrodesis of the tarsometatarsal joint using a laterally applied plate in 10 dogs. J Small Anim Pract 1998;39:19–22.

7. Guerrero TG, Montavon PM. Medial plating for carpal panarthrodesis. Vet Surg 2005;34:153–8.

8. Johnson A, Houlton J. Arthrodesis of the carpus. In: Johnson AL, Houlton JE, Vannini R, editors. AO principles of fracture management in the dog and the cat. Stuttgart (Germany): Thieme; 2005. p. 446–57.

9. Klause S, Piermattei D, Schwartz P. Tarsocrural arthrodesis: complications and recommendations. Vet Comp Orthop Traumatol 1989;3:119–24.

10. Lotsikas PJ, Radasch RM. A clinical evaluation of pancarpal arthrodesis in nine dogs using circular external skeletal fixation. Vet Surg 2006;35:480–5.

11. McKee WM, May C, Macias C, et al. Pantarsal arthrodesis with a customised medial or lateral bone plate in 13 dogs. Vet Rec 2004;154:165–70.

12. Muir P, Norris JL. Tarsometatarsal subluxation in dogs: partial arthrodesis by plate fixation. J Am Anim Hosp Assoc 1999;35:155–62.

13. Vannini R, Bonath K. Arthrodesis of the tarsus. In: Johnson AL, Houlton JE, Vannini R, editors. AO principles of fracture management in the dog and the cat. Stuttgart (Germany): Thieme; 2005. p. 464–71.

14. Michal U, Fluckiger M, Schmokel H. Healing of dorsal pancarpal arthrodesis in the dog. J Small Anim Pract 2003;44:109–12.

15. Piermattei DL. Fracture and other orthopedic conditions of the carpus, meta-carpus, and phalanges. In: Piermattei DL, Flo GL, DeCamp CE, editors. Hand-book of small animal orthopedics and fracture repair. Philadelphia: Elsevier; 2006. p. 382–428.

16. Rahal SC, Volpi RS, Hette K, et al. Arthrodesis tarsocrural or tarsometatarsal in 2 dogs using circular external skeletal fixator. Can Vet J 2006;47:894–8.

17. Worth AJ, Bruce WJ. Long-term assessment of pancarpal arthrodesis performed on working dogs in New Zealand. N Z Vet J 2008;56:78–84.

18. Piermattei DL. Fracture and other orthopedic injuries of the tarsus, metatarsus, and phalanges. In: Piermattei DL, Flo GL, DeCamp CE, editors. Handbook of small animal orthopedics and fracture repair. Philadelphia: Elsevier; 2006. p. 661–713.

19. Denny H, Barr A. Partial carpal and pancarpal arthrodesis in the dog: a review of 50 cases. J Small Anim Pract 1991;32:329–34.

20. Diaz-Bertrana C, Darnaculleta F, Durall I, et al. The stepped hybrid plate for carpal panarthrodesis-part II: a multicentre study of 52 arthrodeses. Vet Comp Orthop Traumatol 2009;22:389–97.

21. Diaz-Bertrana C, Darnaculleta F, Durall I, et al. The stepped hybrid plate for carpal panarthrodesis-part I: relationship between plate and bone surfaces. Vet Comp Orthop Traumatol 2009;22:380–8.

22. Haburjak J, Lenehan T, Davidson C. Treatment of carpometacarpal and middle carpal joint hyperextension injuries with partial carpal arthrodesis using a cross pin technique: 21 cases. Vet Comp Orthop Traumatol 2003;16:105–11.

23. Li A, Gibson N, Bennett D, et al. Thirteen pancarpal arthrodeses using 2.7/3.5 mm hybrid dynamic compression plates. Vet Comp Orthop Traumatol 1999;12: 102–7.

24. Johnson KA, Bellenger CR. The effects of autologous bone grafting on bone healing after carpal arthrodesis in the dog. Vet Rec 1980;107:126–32.

25. Johnson K. A radiographic study of the effects of autologous cancellous bone grafts on bone healing after carpal arthrodesis in the dog. Vet Rad 1981;22: 177–83.

26. Clarke SP, Ferguson JF, Miller A. Clinical evaluation of pancarpal arthrodesis using a castless plate in 11 dogs. Vet Surg 2009;38:852–60.

27. Halling K, Lewis D, Jones R, et al. Use of circular external skeletal fixator constructs to stabilize tarsometatarsal arthrodeses in three dogs. Vet Comp Orthop Traumatol 2004;17:204.

28. Shanil J, Yeshurun Y, Shahar R. Arthrodesis of the tarsometatarsal joint, using type II ESF with acrylic connecting bars in four dogs. Vet Comp Orthop Traumatol 2006;19:61–3.

29. Whitelock RG, Dyce J, Houlton JE. Metacarpal fractures associated with pancarpal arthrodesis in dogs. Vet Surg 1999;28:25–30.

30. Andreoni AA, Rytz U, Vannini R, et al. Ground reaction force profiles after partial and pancarpal arthrodesis in dogs. Vet Comp Orthop Traumatol 2010;23:1–6.

31. Jerram RM, Walker AM, Worth AJ, et al. Prospective evaluation of pancarpal arthrodesis for carpal injuries in working dogs in New Zealand, using dorsal hybrid plating. N Z Vet J 2009;57:331–7.

32. James FM, Richardson DW. Minimally invasive plate fixation of lower limb injury in horses: 32 cases (1999-2003). Equine Vet J 2006;38:246–51.

33. Hudson CC, Pozzi A, Lewis DD. Minimally invasive plate osteosynthesis: applications and techniques in dogs and cats. Vet Comp Orthop Traumatol 2009;22: 172–85.

34. Garofolo S, Pozzi A. Effect of plating technique on periosteal vasculature of the radius in dogs: a cadaveric study. Vet Surg, in press.

35. Borrelli J Jr, Prickett W, Song E, et al. Extraosseous blood supply of the tibia and the effects of different plating techniques: a human cadaveric study. J Orthop Trauma 2002;16:691–5.

36. Field JR, Tornkvist H. Biological fracture fixation: a perspective. Vet Comp Orthop Traumatol 2001;14:169–78.

37. Perren SM. Evolution of the internal fixation of long bone fractures. The scientific basis of biological internal fixation: choosing a new balance between stability and biology. J Bone Joint Surg Br 2002;84:1093–110.

38. Ruchelsman DE, Hazel A, Mudgal CS. Treatment of symptomatic distal interphalangeal joint arthritis with percutaneous arthrodesis: a novel technique in select patients. Hand (N Y) 2010;5:434–9.

39. Bauer T, Lortat-Jacob A, Hardy P. First metatarsophalangeal joint percutaneous arthrodesis. Orthop Traumatol Surg Res 2010;96:567–73.

40. Al-Khayer A, Hegarty J, Hahn D, et al. Percutaneous sacroiliac joint arthrodesis: a novel technique. J Spinal Disord Tech 2008;21:359–63.

41. Anderson DG, Sayadipour A, Shelby K, et al. Anterior interbody arthrodesis with percutaneous posterior pedicle fixation for degenerative conditions of the lumbar spine. Eur Spine J 2011;20:1323–30.

42. Mader K, Verheyen CC, Gausepohl T, et al. Minimally invasive ankle arthrodesis with a retrograde locking nail after failed fusion. Strategies Trauma Limb Reconstr 2007;2:39–47.

43. Lauge-Pedersen H. Percutaneous arthrodesis. Acta Orthop Scand Suppl 2003; 74:1–30.

44. Lui TH. New technique of arthroscopic triple arthrodesis. Arthroscopy 2006;22: 461–5.

45. Lauge-Pedersen H, Aspenberg P. Arthrodesis by percutaneous fixation: patello-femoral arthrodesis in rabbits without debridement of the joint. Acta Orthop Scand 2002;73:186–9.

46. Lauge-Pedersen H, Aspenberg P. Synovial fluid depletion: successful arthrodesis without operative cartilage removal. J Orthop Sci 2003;8:591–5.

47. Jones P, Delco M, Beard W, et al. A limited surgical approach for pastern arthrodesis in horses with severe osteoarthritis. Vet Comp Orthop Traumatol 2009;22: 303–8.

48. Panizzi L, Barber SM, Lang HM, et al. Evaluation of a minimally invasive arthrodesis technique for the carpometacarpal joint in horses. Vet Surg 2011;40:464–72.

49. Fettig AA, McCarthy RJ, Kowaleski MP. Intertarsal and tarsometatarsal arthrodesis using 2.0/2.7-mm or 2.7/3.5-mm hybrid dynamic compression plates. J Am Anim Hosp Assoc 2002;38:364–9.

50. Evans HE. Arthrology. In: Miller's anatomy of the dog. Philadelphia: Saunders; 1993. p. 252–6.

51. Guillou RP, Frank JD, Sinnott MT, et al. In vitro mechanical evaluation of medial plating for pantarsal arthrodesis in dogs. Am J Vet Res 2008;69:1406–12.

52. Inauen R, Koch D, Bass M. Arthrodesis of the tarsometatarsal joints in a cat with a two hole advanced locking plate system. Vet Comp Orthop Traumatol 2009;22: 166–9.

53. Chodos MD, Parks BG, Schon LC, et al. Blade plate compared with locking plate for tibiotalocalcaneal arthrodesis: a cadaver study. Foot Ankle Int 2008;29: 219–24.

54. Lang HM, Panizzi L, Allen AL, et al. Comparison of three drilling techniques for carpometacarpal joint arthrodesis in horses. Vet Surg 2009;38:990–7.

55. Barber SM, Panizzi L, Lang HM. Treatment of carpometacarpal osteoarthritis by arthrodesis in 12 horses. Vet Surg 2009;38:1006–11.

56. Rao RD, Gourab K, Bagaria VB, et al. The effect of platelet-rich plasma and bone marrow on murine posterolateral lumbar spine arthrodesis with bone morphogenetic protein. J Bone Joint Surg Am 2009;91:1199–206.

57. Parker R, Brown S, Wind A. Pancarpal arthrodesis in the dog: a review of forty-five cases. Vet Surg 1981;10:35–43.

58. Guillou RP, Demianiuk RM, Sinnott MT, et al. In vitro mechanical evaluation of a limited contact dynamic compression plate and hybrid carpal arthrodesis plate for canine pancarpal arthrodesis. Vet Comp Orthop Traumatol 2012;25:83–8.

Index

A

Acetabular fractures
  MIO for, 1060–1061
Alignment
  in MIPO
    assessment of, 892–893
Antebrachium
  MIPO for
    alignment assessment, 893
    positioning for traction of, 876
Arthrodesis
  hock, 1082–1987
  pancarpal, 1088–1093
  percutaneous plate, **1079–1096**. *See also* Percutaneous plate arthrodesis
Articular fractures
  described, 1051
  MIO for, **1051–1068**
    goals of, 1052
    implants for, 1065
    indications for, 1052–1065. *See also specific indications, e.g.,* Shoulder fractures
    postoperative care, 1065–1066
    preoperative assessment, 1052

B

Bone healing
  after external fixation in MIO, 927–929
  in fracture fixation
    under conditions of absolute and relative stability, 861–863
Bone-holding forceps
  in MIPO, 887–888

C

Calcaneal fractures
  MIO for, 1063–1064
Capital physeal fractures
  MIO for, 1061
Carpus fracture
  MIO for, 1059–1060
Central tarsal bone fractures
  MIO for, 1064
Cerclage wires

Vet Clin Small Anim 42 (2012) 1097–1107
http://dx.doi.org/10.1016/S0195-5616(12)00136-2
0195-5616/12/$ – see front matter © 2012 Elsevier Inc. All rights reserved.

vetsmall.theclinics.com

Cerclage (*continued*)
    in MIO for femoral diaphyseal fractures, 1007
Circular external fixation
    in MIPO, 885–887
Coronal plane
    varus–valgus malalignment, 1019
Cortical step sign
    in axis and torsion assessment in MIO for femoral diaphyseal fractures, 1017

D

Deformation of materials
    in fracture fixation, 854–855
Diameter difference sign
    in axis and torsion assessment in MIO for femoral diaphyseal fractures, 1017
Direct reduction
    for MIO for femoral diaphyseal fractures, 1003
    for MIPO for humerus, 979
Distal fibula fractures
    MIO for, 1062–1063
Distal metaphyseal fractures
    MIO for, 1001–1021. *See also* Femoral diaphyseal fractures, MIO for
Distal tibia fractures
    MIO for, 1062–1063

E

Elastic plate osteosynthesis
    for femoral diaphyseal fractures, 1015
Elbow fractures
    MIO for, 1055–1059
ESF. *See* External skeletal fixation (ESF)
External fixation
    described, 913–914
External fixators
    in MIO, **913–934**
        articulations and diagonals and, 927
        biologic considerations in, 923–925
        bone healing due to, 927–929
        clinical application of, 927
        configurations of, 914–917
            clinical variations in frame, 916–917
        for femoral diaphyseal fractures, 1006
        frame configuration in, 927
        indications for, 914
        load sharing in, 925–926
        mechanical considerations in, 925–927
        minimally traumatic surgical approaches, 923–925
        pin number in, 926–927
        postoperative patient management, 929–931
        principles of, 917–923
            application technique principles, 919–921

decision-making/frame design principles, 921–923
general principles, 917–918
implant selection principles, 918–919
types of, 914
External skeletal fixation (ESF)
described, 913–914

F

Fatigue failure
in fracture fixation, 858–859
Femoral capital physeal fractures
MIO for, 999–1001
Femoral condylar fractures
MIO for, 1062
Femoral diaphyseal fractures
MIO for, 1001–1021
axis and torsion assessment, 1015–1018
coronal plane, 1019
implants and fixation, 1007–1015
bone plates with bridging function, 1011–1013
bone plates with compression or neutralization function, 1007–1011
elastic plate osteosynthesis, 1015
external skeletal fixation, 1013–1014
ILNs, 1013
screws placed in lag fashion, 1011
indirect reduction, 1003–1007
cerclage wires in, 1007
external fixators in, 1006
fractures distractors in, 1006
implants in, 1007
push-pull technique, 1006–1007
supports and pads in, 1006
traction in, 1006
limb-length discrepancy, 1020–1021
patient positioning, 1001–1002
prevention of femoral malrotation in, 1019
radiographs of intact opposite limb in, 1018
reduction methods, 1002–1003
sagittal plane, 1019–1020
surgical approach, 1001–1002
Femoral fractures. *See also specific types, e.g.,* Femoral diaphyseal fractures
ILNs for, 955
Femoral head and neck version sign
in axis and torsion assessment in MIO for femoral diaphyseal fractures, 1017–1018
Femoral head fractures
MIO for, 1061–1062
Femoral malrotation
prevention of
in MIO for femoral diaphyseal fractures, 1019
Femoral neck fractures
MIO for, 999–1001, 1061–1062

Femur
  anatomy of, 997–999
  IM pinning of, 883
  positioning for traction of, 878
Femur fractures. *See also specific types*
  MIO for, **997–1022**
    distal metaphyseal fractures, 1001–1021
    femoral capital physeal fractures, 999–1001
    femoral diaphyseal fractures, 1001–1021
    femoral neck fractures, 999–1001
    proximal metaphyseal fractures, 1001–1021
  MIPO for
    alignment assessment, 893
Fibula
  anatomy of, 1024–1027
Fibula fractures
  described, 1023–1024
  MIPO for, **1023–1044**
    acute *vs.* chronic, 1031
    assessment of repair and outcome, 1042–1043
    diaphyseal *vs.* metaphyseal fractures, 1029–1031
    immature *vs.* mature patient, 1028–1029
    indications for, 1027
    indirect reduction, 1037–1039
    locking *vs.* nonlocking plates in, 1031–1037
    patient positioning, 1037
    postoperative care, 1042
    preoperative evaluation, 1027–1037
    procedure, 1039–1042
    simple *vs.* comminuted fractures, 1027–1028
    surgical approach, 1039
Force of materials
  in fracture fixation, 854–855
Forceps
  bone-holding
    in MIPO, 887–888
Fracture(s). *See also specific types*
  repair of
    percutaneous pinning for, **963–974**. *See also* Percutaneous pinning, for fracture
      repair
Fracture distractors
  in MIO
    for femoral diaphyseal fractures, 1006
  in MIPO, 888–890
Fracture fixation
  biomechanical concepts in, **853–872**
    applied biomechanics, 859–866
      bone healing under conditions of absolute and relative stability, 861–863
      factors affecting stiffness of plate-bone construct, 863
      plate length, 865
      plate selection, 863–865

position of screws in plate, 865–866
mechanics of materials, 854–859
fatigue failure, 858–859
force, deformation, stress, and strain, 854–855
stiffness, 855–857
described, 853–854
Fracture healing
biomechanics of, 859–860
Functional reduction
described, 873

G

Greater trochanter position sign
in axis and torsion assessment in MIO for femoral diaphyseal fractures, 1017

H

Hip rotation test
in axis and torsion assessment in MIO for femoral diaphyseal fractures, 1015–1016
Hock arthrodesis, 1082–1987
anatomy related to, 1082–1083
indications for, 1082
patient positioning, 1084
preoperative planning, 1083–1084
techniques, 1084–1088
pantarsal arthrodesis using medial plate, 1084–1086
partial tarsal arthrodesis, 1086–1088
Humerus fractures
ILNs for, 955
IM pinning of, 882–883
MIPO for, **975–982**
alignment assessment, 893
anatomy related to, 975–976
biologic assessment, 976–977
case examples, 980–981
case selection, 976
direct reduction, 979
errors with, 981–982
implant selection, 978
indications for, 976
indirect reduction
alignment pin placement in, 979
mechanical factors in, 977–978
operating room setup, 978
preoperative planning, 976–978
surgical approach, 978–979
positioning for traction of, 876

I

ILNs. *See* Interlocking nails (ILNs)
IM pinning
for MIPO, 881–884

Indirect reduction. *See also specific indications and fracture types*
  described, 874
  for MIO
    for femoral diaphyseal fractures, 1003–1007
  for MIPO, 874
    for fibular and tibia fractures, 1037–1039
    for humerus fractures, 979
    for radius fractures, 987–988
    for ulna fractures, 987–988
Interlocking nails (ILNs)
  in MIO, **935–962**
    biomechanical properties of, 940–944
      general considerations, 940–941
      AS nail biomechanics, 943–944
      standard nail biomechanics, 941–943
    clinical use of, 950–959
      complications of, 955–959
      outcomes of, 955–959
    designs of, 937–940
      AS nail design and instrumentation, 938–940
      standard nail design and instrumentation, 937–938
    for femoral diaphyseal fractures, 1013
    general techniques, 952–954
    history of use, 936–937
    indications for, 944–950
      common indications, 945–946
      extended indications, 946–950
      general considerations, 944–945
    preoperative planning, 950–952
Intraoperative fluoroscopy unit
  for perioperative imaging in MIO, 902–904
Intraoperative skeletal traction (IST), 874
  with traction table, 875–876
IST. *See* Intraoperative skeletal traction (IST)

  K

Kirschner wires, 963

  L

Lesser trochanter shape sign
  in axis and torsion assessment in MIO for femoral diaphyseal fractures,
    1016–1017
Ligamentotaxis, 874
Limb hanging
  for MIPO, 880–881
Limb-length discrepancy
  in MIO for femoral diaphyseal fractures, 1020–1021
Linear external fixation
  in MIPO, 884–885

M

Meta-bone(s)
  anatomy related to, 1046
  described, 1045–1046
  minimally invasive repair of, **1045–1050**
    discussion, 1048–1049
    equipment for, 1046–1047
    implants for, 1046–1047
    preoperative assessment and decision making, 1046
    preoperative preparation, 1047
    technique, 1047–1048
Metacarpal fractures
  minimally invasive repair of, **1045–1050**. *See also* Meta-bone(s), minimally invasive
    repair of
Metatarsal fractures
  minimally invasive repair of, **1045–1050**. *See also* Meta-bone(s), minimally invasive
    repair of
Minimally invasive osteosynthesis (MIO). *See also specific indications and fracture types,*
  e.g., Femur fractures
  for articular fractures, **1051–1068**
  biologic considerations in, 923–925
  described, 897, 936
  external fixators in, **913–934**. *See also* External fixators, in MIO
  for femur fractures, **997–1022**
  ILNs in, **935–962**. *See also* Interlocking nails (ILNs), in MIO
  mechanical considerations in, 925–927
  minimally traumatic surgical approaches to, 923–925
  perioperative imaging in, **897–911**
    equipment for, 902–905
      intraoperative fluoroscopy unit, 902–904
      radiation safety equipment, 904
      surgery table, 904–905
    indications for, 901
    radioprotection in, 905–908
    technique, 908–909
  postoperative imaging in, 910
  preoperative imaging in, 898–901
Minimally invasive plate osteosynthesis (MIPO), **873–895**. *See also* Ulna fractures; *specific*
  indications and fracture types, e.g., Humerus fractures
  advantages of, 873
  alignment assessment in, 892–893
  bone-holding forceps in, 887–888
  circular external fixation in, 885–887
  for fibula fractures, **1023–1044**
  fracture distractor in, 888–890
  functional reduction by, 873
  goal of, 873–874
  for humerus fractures, **975–982**
  IM pinning for, 881–884
  indirect reduction by, 874, 1037–1039

Minimally (*continued*)
  intraoperative diagnostic imaging, 893–894
  limb hanging for, 880–881
  linear external fixation in, 884–885
  for radius fractures, **983–996**
  reduction through plate application in, 890–892
  skeletal traction table for, 873–880
  for tibia fractures, **1023–1044**
  for ulna fractures, **983–996**
MIO. *See* Minimally invasive osteosynthesis (MIO)
MIPO. *See* Minimally invasive plate osteosynthesis (MIPO)

O

Osteosynthesis
  elastic plate
    for femoral diaphyseal fractures, 1015
  minimally invasive. *See* Minimally invasive osteosynthesis (MIO)
  minimally invasive plate. *See* Minimally invasive plate osteosynthesis (MIPO)

P

Pancarpal arthrodesis, 1088–1093
  anatomy related to, 1090
  indications for, 1088–1090
  patient positioning, 1091
  postoperative care, 1093
  preoperative planning, 1090–1091
  technique, 1091–1092
Pantarsal arrthrodesis using medial plate, 1084–1086
Partial tarsal arthrodesis, 1086–1088
Percutaneous pinning
  for fracture repair, **963–974**
    case selection, 964
    clinical results, 972–973
    described, 963
    patient positioning for, 965
    postoperative care, 969–971
    preoperative planning and management, 964–965
    procedure, 967–968
    rehabilitation after, 969–971
    surgical approach, 965–965
Percutaneous plate arthrodesis, **1079–1096**. *See also specific types, e.g.,* Hock arthrodesis
  described, 1079–1082
  hock arthrodesis, 1082–1087
  pancarpal arthrodesis, 1088–1093
Pinning
  percutaneous
    for fracture repair, **963–974**. *See also* Percutaneous pinning, for fracture repair
Plate(s)
  in fracture fixation
    length of, 865

locking *vs.* nonlocking plates, 863–865
    position of screws in, 865–866
  in MIPO
    reduction through, 890–892
Procurvatum–recurvatum malalignment, 1019–1020
Proximal metaphyseal fractures
  MIO for, 1001–1021. *See also* Femoral diaphyseal fractures, MIO for

R

Radiation safety equipment
  for perioperative imaging in MIO, 904–905
Radioprotection
  in perioperative imaging in MIO, 905–908
    exposure time, 906
    OR personnel, 906–907
    shielding in, 907–908
Radioulnar fractures
  ILNs for, 955
Radius
  anatomy of, 984
  IM pinning of, 883–884
Radius fractures
  described, 983–984
  MIPO for, **983–996**
    acute *vs.* chronic fractures, 986
    assessment of repair and outcome, 995
    decision-making related to, 984–986
    for diaphyseal *vs.* metaphyseal fractures, 985
    implant placement, 993–994
    indications for, 984–986
    indirect reduction, 987–988
    locking *vs.* nonlocking plates for, 986
    patient positioning and preparation, 987
    postoperative care, 994
    preoperative planning, 986–987
    for simple vs.comminuted fractures, 984–985
    surgical approach, 989–993
Rehabilitation
  after percutaneous pinning for fracture repair, 969–971

S

Sacroiliac
  anatomy of, 1070–1071
Sacroiliac luxation
  described, 1069–1070
  minimally invasive repair of, **1069–1077**
    discussion, 1074–1076
    equipment for, 1071
    implants for, 1071

Sacroiliac (*continued*)
    preoperative assessment and decision making, 1071
    preoperative preparation, 1071–1072
    technique, 1072–1074
Sagittal plane
  procurvatum–recurvatum malalignment, 1019–1020
Shielding
  in radioprotection during perioperative imaging in MIO, 907–908
Shoulder fractures
  MIO for, 1053–1055
Skeletal traction table
  for fracture reduction, 874–880
    complications of, 879–880
    described, 874
    indications for, 874–875
    IST with, 875–876
    malalignment correction, 879
    patient positioning on, 876–878
    procedure technique, 878–879
Steinman pins, 963
Stiffness of materials
  in fracture fixation, 855–857
Stiffness of plate-bone construct
  factors affecting
    in fracture fixation, 863
Strain of materials
  in fracture fixation, 854–855
Stress of materials
  in fracture fixation, 854–855
Surgery table
  for perioperative imaging in MIO, 904–905

T

Talar fractures
  MIO for, 1063
Tibia
  anatomy of, 1024–1027
  IM pinning of, 883
  positioning for traction of, 877–878
Tibia fractures
  described, 1023–1024
  ILNs for, 955
  MIO for
    distal, 1062–1063
  MIPO for, **1023–1044**
    acute *vs.* chronic, 1031
    alignment assessment, 893
    assessment of repair and outcome, 1042–1043
    diaphyseal *vs.* metaphyseal fractures, 1029–1031
    immature *vs.* mature patient, 1028–1029

indications for, 1027
indirect reduction, 1037–1039
locking *vs.* nonlocking plates in, 1031–1037
patient positioning, 1037
postoperative care, 1042
preoperative evaluation, 1027–1037
procedure, 1039–1042
simple *vs.* comminuted fractures, 1027–1028
surgical approach, 1039
Tibial plateau fractures
MIO for, 1062

U

Ulna
anatomy of, 984
IM pinning of, 883–884
Ulna fractures
described, 983–984
MIPO for, **983–996**
acute *vs.* chronic fractures, 986
assessment of repair and outcome, 995
decision-making related to, 984–986
for diaphyseal *vs.* metaphyseal fractures, 985
implant placement, 993–994
indications for, 984–986
indirect reduction, 987–988
locking *vs.* nonlocking plates for, 986
patient positioning and preparation, 987
postoperative care, 994
preoperative planning, 986–987
for simple vs.comminuted fractures, 984–985
surgical approach, 989–993

V

Varus–valgus malalignment, 1019

Moving?

Make sure your subscription moves with you!

To notify us of your new address, find your **Clinics Account Number** (located on your mailing label above your name), and contact customer service at:

Email: journalscustomerservice-usa@elsevier.com

800-654-2452 (subscribers in the U.S. & Canada)
314-447-8871 (subscribers outside of the U.S. & Canada)

Fax number: 314-447-8029

Elsevier Health Sciences Division
Subscription Customer Service
3251 Riverport Lane
Maryland Heights, MO 63043

*To ensure uninterrupted delivery of your subscription, please notify us at least 4 weeks in advance of move.

ELSEVIER

Printed and bound by CPI Group (UK) Ltd, Croydon, CR0 4YY

03/10/2024

01040439-0009